Anatomy, Imaging and Surgery of the Intracranial Dural Venous Sinuses

Anatomy, Imaging and Surgery of the Intracranial Dural Venous Sinuses

Editor-in-Chief

R. SHANE TUBBS, MS, PA-C, PhD
Chief Scientific Officer
Vice President, Professor
Seattle Science Foundation
Seattle, WA, United States

List of Co-Editors

JOE IWANAGA, DDS, PhD
Senior Researcher
Seattle Science Foundation
Seattle, WA, United States

ROD OSKOUIAN, MD
Chief Executive Officer, President
Seattle Science Foundation
Seattle, WA, United States

MARIOS LOUKAS, MD, PhD
Chairman
Department of Anatomical Science
Dean of Basic Sciences
St. George's University, Grenada

MOHAMMADALI SHOJA
Chief Researcher
Department of Surgery
University of Texas Medical Branch
Galveston, TX, United States

STEPHEN MONTEITH, MD
Neurosurgeon
Swedish Neuroscience Institute
Seattle, WA, United States

ELSEVIER

ANATOMY, IMAGING AND SURGERY OF THE INTRACRANIAL DURAL VENOUS SINUSES
ISBN: 978-0-323-65377-0

Publisher: Cathleen Sether
Acquisition Editor: Belinda Kuhn
Editorial Project Manager: Megan Ashdown
Project Manager: Kiruthika Govindaraju
Cover Designer: Alan Studholme

ELSEVIER

3251 Riverport Lane
St. Louis, Missouri 63043

List of Contributors

Farzad Hami Adl, MD
California Institute of Neuroscience
National Skull Base Foundation
Thousand Oakes, CA, United States

Seleipiri Akobo, MD, MBA, MPH, RNC
Resident Physician
Hennepin Healthcare System
Minneapolis, MN, United States

Islam Aly, MD
Resident Physician
Obstetrics and Gynecology
St. Joseph's Regional Medical center
Paterson, NJ, United States
Research Fellow
St. George's University School of Medicine
St. George's, Grenada

Shenell Bernard, MD, MBA
Resident Physician
Department of Internal Medicine
Overlook Medical Center
Summit, NJ, United States

Amin Demerdash, MD
Resident Physician
Internal Medicine
Geisinger Medical Center
Danville, PA, United States

Graham Dupont, BS
Research Fellow
Seattle, Science Foundation
Seattle, WA, United States

Oded Goren, MD
Neurosurgeon
Gesinger Neuroscience Institute
Danville, PA, United States

Andre Granger, MD, MBA
Resident
Neurology
NYU Langone Hospital - Brooklyn
Brooklyn, NY, United States
Researcher
Department of Anatomical Sciences
St. George's University, Grenada

Galyna Ivashchuk, MSc, MBA, MD
Resident Physician
University of Texas Rio Grande Valley
Edinburg, TX, United States

Joe Iwanaga, DDS, PhD
Senior Researcher
Seattle Science Foundation
Seattle, WA, United States

Ghazaleh Ahmadi Jazi, MD
California Institute of Neuroscience
National Skull Base Foundation
Thousand Oakes, CA, United States

Shamfa C. Joseph, MD
Department of Anatomical Sciences
St. George's University
St. George's, Grenada

Lexian McBain, MD
Research Fellow
Department of Anatomical Science
St. George's University, Grenada

Martin M. Mortazavi, MD
Neurosurgeon/Chairman
California Institute of Neuroscience
Thousand Oakes, CA, United States

Kira Newell, BS
Research Fellow
Seattle, Science Foundation
Seattle, WA, United States

Rod Oskouian, MD
Chief Executive Officer, President
Seattle Science Foundation
Seattle, WA, United States

Chirag Patel, MD
The Pennsylvania State
University College of Medicine
Hershey, PA, United States

Matthew Protas, BS, MS, MD
Research Fellow
Department of Anatomical Sciences
St. George's University School of Medicine
St. George's, Grenada
Clinical Sciences
SUNY Upstate Medical University
Syracuse, NY, United States

Elias Rizk, MD, MSc
Associate Professor
Department of Neurosurgery
Penn State Medical Center
Hershey, PA, United States

Mohsen Sadati, MD
California Institute of Neuroscience
National Skull Base Foundation
Thousand Oakes, CA, United States

Diego San Millán, MD
Neuroradiologist
Department of Diagnostic and Interventional Radiology
Hospital of Sion
Sion, Switzerland

Maia Schumacher, BS
Research Fellow
Seattle, Science Foundation
Seattle, WA, United States

Alireza Shoakazemi, MD
Swedish Neuroscience Institute
Seattle, WA, United States

Amit Singla, MD
Swedish Neuroscience Institute
Seattle, WA, United States

Sajid S. Suriya, MD
California Institute of Neuroscience
National Skull Base Foundation
Thousand Oakes, CA, United States

Satoshi Tsutsumi, MD, PhD
Associate Professor
Neurological Surgery
Juntendo University Urayasu Hospital
Urayasu, Chiba, Japan

R. Shane Tubbs, MS, PA-C, PhD
Chief Scientific Officer
Vice President, Professor
Seattle Science Foundation
Seattle, WA, United States

Pamela Youssef, MD
Resident Physician
Neurology
Medical College of Wisconsin Affiliated Hospitals
Milwaukee, WI, United States

Contents

CHAPTER 1

The Embryology of the Dural Venous Sinus: An Overview

LEXIAN MCBAIN • ODED GOREN • R. SHANE TUBBS

INTRODUCTION

This review describes the embryologic development of the dural venous sinuses at different stages. It begins at the earliest stage with identification of the first venous structure and summarizes the development of the morphologic architecture of the dural sinuses. Data concerning the contribution of embryology were collected from authors such as Streeter and Padget, who comprehensively examined the Carnegie Institute's Mall Collection of a series of human embryos from 4 to 80 mm. Clinical correlations are made by examining malformations arising from developmental defects such as the vein of Galen aneurysm and arteriovenous malformation.

The main pattern of the dural sinuses is well established by the time the fetus reaches a length of 40 mm and is refined by the time it reaches 80 mm,[1] but the final arrangement even at birth does not necessarily fit the standard anatomical descriptions, partly because of the postnatal ossification of the skull.[2,3] A mesodermal mantle surrounds the developing nervous system and separates into three meningeal layers, each containing a distinct vascular pattern.[1] The dura mater will relate to the dural venous sinuses. There is extensive remodeling including the formation of new channels and resorption of old ones as the embryo develops.[1] Padget describes the evolution of cranial venous channels as an orderly sequence logically related to the changing environment like that of corresponding arteries.[1]

First Venous Vascular Structures

At 4 mm embryo (Fig. 1.1) length, the first vascular venous structure can be identified: the primordial vena capitis medialis. It is formed by the merging of the anterior cerebral vein, the maxillary vein, and the pituitary vein. It lies on the walls of the neural tube and runs medial to the trigeminal ganglion and the developing otic vesicle, whereas its caudal end proceeds laterally toward the surface of the embryo.[1]

The vena capitis medialis and the vena capitis lateralis are referred to together as the primary head vein,[4] and it constitutes the main channel of the developing embryo. Structurally, it first consists of a single layer of endothelial cells.[5] The most lateral part of the vena capitis medialis between the ganglia of cranial nerves V and VII is referred to as the posttrigeminal vein, and it joins the prootic vein before it continues caudally as the vena capitis lateralis.[1] At this stage, the primary head vein can be considered as having three portions: the vena capitis medialis, the posttrigeminal vein, and the vena capitis lateralis.[5]

The primary head vein receives many tributaries that aggregate into the three vascular plexuses of the meninges.[1] These drain mainly the dorsal and ventral portions.[4] The anterior group comes from the area of the diencephalon and mesencephalon.[4] Between the trigeminal and the acoustic facial complex is the middle or cerebellar portion, and in the neighborhood of the vagus nerve rootlets is the occipital or posterior group, as it bends sharply down into the neck region and drains into the duct of Cuvier.[4] This portion joins the cardinal vein to become the anterior cardinal vein and goes on to form the internal jugular vein. The cranial portion medial to the trigeminal ganglion will become the cavernous sinus. At this point, the only ventral contribution to the primary head vein is the primitive maxillary vein, which enters medial to the ganglion of the trigeminal nerve.[1]

Embryo at 10 mm

At around 10–14 mm, the mesenchyme around the sides and base of the brain has the developing dura mater and the chondrocranium.[1] There is also a separation between the superficial tributaries of the primary head vein and the deeper veins that drain the capillary sheets immediately surrounding the brain tube.[4] The ventral portion is completely separated from the deeper-lying plexuses of the neural tube.

Anatomy, Imaging and Surgery of the Intracranial Dural Venous Sinuses. https://doi.org/10.1016/B978-0-323-65377-0.00001-5

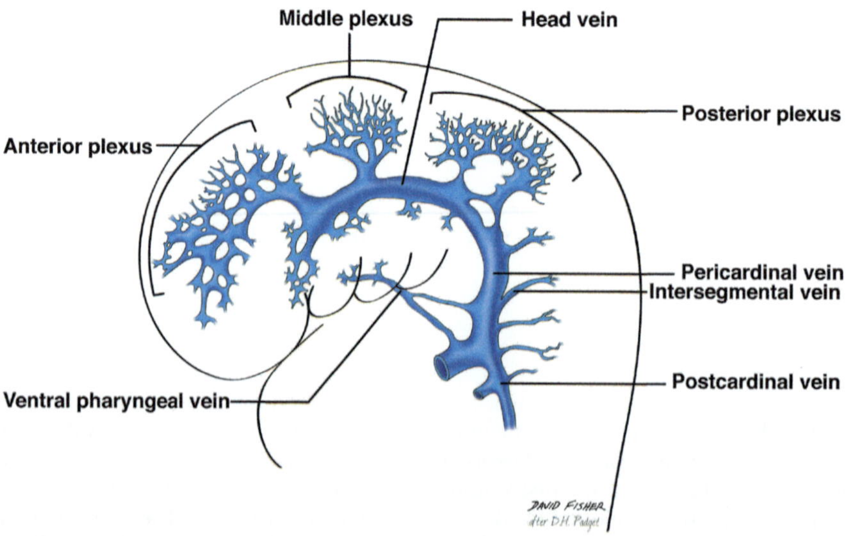

FIG. 1.1 Dural venous sinus development at stage 13, day 28, approximately 4–6 mm.

We can now see that the primary head vein is outside the dura mater and distinguish the veins of the dura mater from the cerebral veins, the former being the veins that form the dural venous sinuses.[4] At this point, the large channels do not cross the midline except at three points where the vessels appear to be bilaterally asymmetrical, anastomosing with the plexus on the opposite side. These points are (1) the caudal end of the roof of the fourth ventricle; (2) the junction of the midbrain and the hindbrain; and (3) over the diencephalon in the area along the caudal margin of the cerebral hemisphere.

Vein of Galen and the Straight Sinus

The choroid plexus, which develops much more rapidly than the cortical mantle, initially drains into the inferior choroidal vein. It is soon drained by the superior choroidal vein, which is the continuation of the primitive internal cerebral vein. At this early stage, there is only one very small thalamic extension. These bilateral internal cerebral veins fuse posteriorly into what will become the *vein of Galen* and *the straight sinus*.[1]

Embryo at 18 mm

The flow of the plexuses changes: the flow of the middle plexus travels into the posterior plexus owing to an anastomosis between the two plexuses that runs dorsal to the otic capsule and lateral to the endolymphatic sac[1] (Fig. 1.2). This then becomes the sigmoid sinus.[4] Drainage from the cerebellar region and the posterior part of the midbrain now travels directly into the channel to the posterior plexus.

The supraoptic vein, which will become the superior ophthalmic vein related to the ophthalmic division of the fifth cranial nerve, first extends backward to establish a temporary connection with the medial part of the primary head vein at the trigeminal ganglion.[1] It then migrates downward and laterally to merge with the maxillary veins, which become the inferior ophthalmic vein. They will enter the primary head vein at the line of the maxillary vein, the latter giving its facial and pharyngeal drainage to the developing jugular vein, maintaining its main drainage to the head vein and creating a potential collateral to the pharynx.[1]

The drainage of the cavernous sinus at this stage is upward through a channel that was originally the stalk of the middle dural plexus and what could be considered the superior petrosal sinus.[4] Dorsal to the otic capsule, there is enough free space for the development of a vascular channel, whereas growth of the cochlear and middle veins makes the region ventrolateral of the otic capsule crowded and most probably constitutes a change in the course of regional blood channels.[4,6]

The Embryo at 20 mm

By 20 mm the plexuses continue to change, the anterior plexus moving closer to the middle plexus and becoming attached to it. Its drainage now flows backward into the newly established channel dorsal to the otic capsule.[4,6] This channel drains all three plexuses and is considered the transverse sinus.[6] Streeter at this point refers to the conjoined anterior and middle plexuses as the tentorial plexus, which should not be confused with

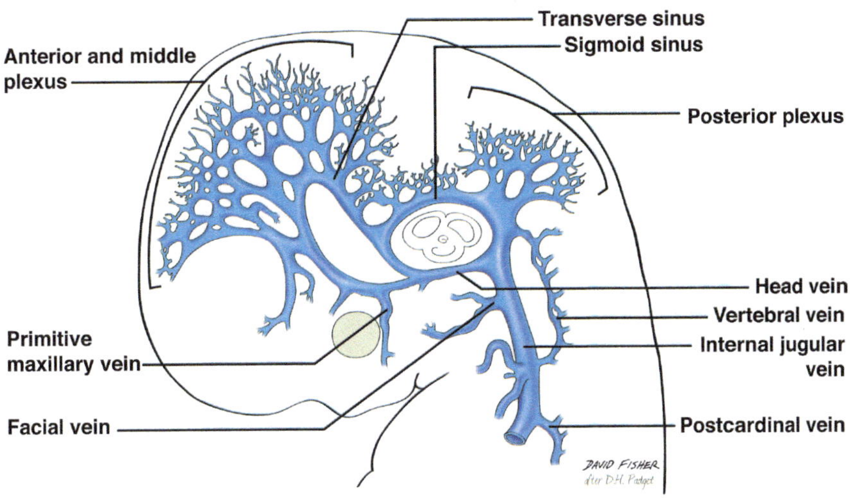

FIG. 1.2 Dural venous sinus development at stage 19, day 48, approximately 16–18 mm.

the adult venous tentorial plexus of the tentorium cerebelli. The posterior plexus changes less than the other two plexuses and later becomes the occipital plexus.[4,6]

The Superior Sagittal Plexus

At an embryo length of 21 mm, the superior sagittal plexus can be differentiated from the remaining anterior plexus from which it developed,[6] a process that began when the embryo was approximately 14 mm. The large tributaries of the anterior and middle plexuses merge into a longitudinal plexus that burrows into the developing hemisphere. At 14 mm it is not a single channel but a series of lakelets contributing to a narrow channel.[6] The choroidal body drains into it from below through a drainage channel that will become the straight sinus. By 20 mm it is a much simpler channel, still in the form of a plexus, asymmetrical with drainage mainly to the right side. There are also small anastomosing loops that connect the plexus usually to the left transverse sinus.

Owing to the growth of the cerebral hemispheres in 20 mm embryos, a well-marked cerebral longitudinal fissure is formed and is occupied by embryonic tissue. This rapidly takes the form of the adult falx cerebri. The meshes of the sagittal plexus are found in the dorsal part of this loose dural tissue.[6]

The Embryo at 50 mm

The superior sagittal plexus is established by the time the embryo is 50 mm. In its cephalic portion, there is a large characteristic channel, lacking only the dural connective-tissue investment to make it an adult type. In its more caudal portion, it still exhibits a plexiform character that indicates its transitional state.[6] Owing to the prolonged growth of the cerebrum and the readjustment of the tentorial plexus, several other sinuses take longer to establish their final positions.

By 50 mm the dura mater is separated by a layer of areolar tissue in which the large blood channels and their tributaries are found. The largest area of this kind is situated over the midbrain, extending from the caudal margin of the cerebral hemispheres to the cerebellum. There is also a lateral extension down to the base of the skull, narrowing as it travels. It constitutes what will later be known as the tentorium cerebelli, and the greater part of the dural venous system is included in it.[6]

A basal extension of the tentorium cerebelli widens in the region of the trigeminal ganglion, and the cavernous sinus is formed from this meshwork[6] (Fig. 1.3). A thinner area of the same tissue extends caudal from the cavernous sinus, median to the otic capsule, to join the jugular region. The slender plexus of veins extending through this constitutes the inferior petrosal sinus.[6]

The Embryo at 80 mm and Larger

The superior sagittal plexus grows caudally, corresponding to the growth of the cerebral hemisphere, resulting in shrinking of the tentorial plexus. The transverse and straight sinuses also follow and take a caudal course by a process described by Streeter as spontaneous migration. The channels form a caudal loop. The eventual torcular Herophili represents the point at which this caudal development reaches its

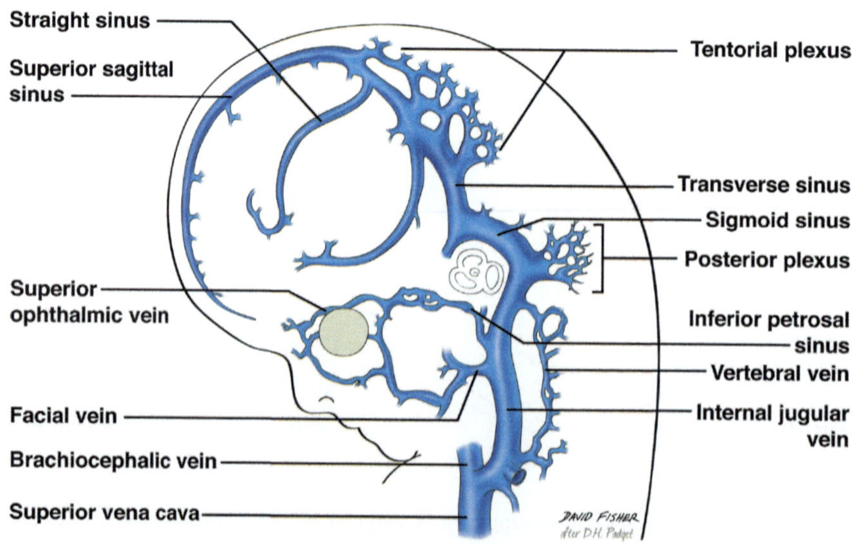

FIG. 1.3 Dural venous sinus development at early fetal period, ninth week, approximately 9 weeks.

completion—or, in other words, is a remnant of the embryonic tentorial plexus and usually retains a trace of the plexiform character that is found throughout the embryonic stage.[6]

The superior and inferior anastomotic veins (of Trolard and Labbé, respectively) are not primary venous structures and appear sometime after the third fetal month.[2] The great cerebral veins develop late and are a variable diverticulum of the straight sinus with negligible cerebral flow.[2] At this stage the tentorial sinus develops by receiving the middle cerebral veins and the ventral diencephalic veins; it drains into the transverse sinuses.[7] The diencephalon is drained by either the Galenic system or the lateral draining system. Between 80 and 120 mm the vein of Galen has not fully developed but shows an adult type of configuration at 170–210 mm with the development of the splenium of the corpus callosum. At this point the ventral diencephalic vein disappears with the development of the basal vein.[7] This embryonic tentorial sinus is elongated posteriorly and migrates medially in the middle cranial fossa base as the cerebral hemisphere enlarges, and anastomoses with the cavernous sinus during the late fetal or postnatal period.[8]

During the 17th to 18th weeks the transverse sinus begins to enlarge from its lateral border on each side. The enlargement is considered as ballooning and extends medially to the primitive torcular Herophili approximately 4–6 weeks later. The ballooning is more evident by the 20th week and can extend into the portion of the superior sagittal and superior petrosal sinuses.[9] At seven fetal months the transverse sinus stops enlarging and takes on its neonatal form (Fig. 1.4).

Extracranial drainage of the posterior cranial fossa dural sinuses, aside from the internal jugular vein, takes place via (1) the anterior condylar vein or the marginal sinus into the internal vertebral venous plexus, (2) the posterior condylar vein into the posterior external vertebral vein, (3) the mastoid emissary, or (4) the occipital emissary vein into the occipital vein.[9] The mastoid emissary veins and the anterior and posterior condylar emissary veins are easily identifiable around the third fetal month.

DISCUSSION

The primary head vein is the first identifiable venous structure in the developing embryo. It is seen as early as 4 mm embryo length, being preceded by the joining of the maxillary, pituitary, and anterior cerebral veins. Its course runs medial to the ganglia of cranial nerves V and VII. Its most lateral portion continues caudal-laterally of the acoustic-facial ganglion and is referred to as the vena capitis lateralis. This portion medial to the trigeminal ganglion goes on to form the cavernous sinus, whereas the caudal-lateral portion joins the cardinal vein to form the internal jugular vein.

Drainage into the primary head vein is via three plexuses: anterior, middle, and posterior. They drain the embryo dorsally, whereas the ventral drainage into the primary head is via the maxillary vein. Later, a channel running dorsal to the otic vesicle will develop and

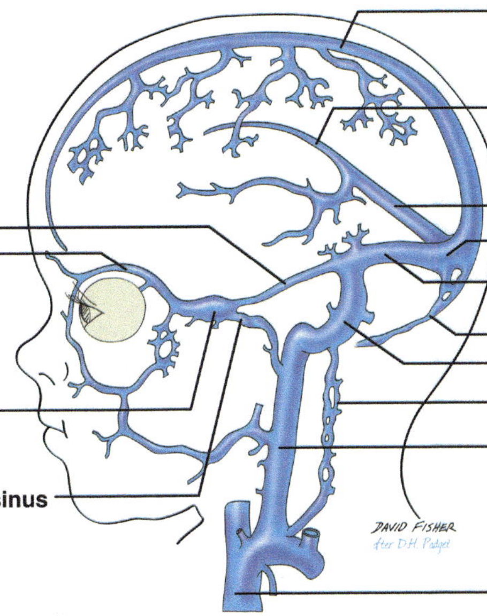

FIG. 1.4 Newborn dural venous sinuses.

will connect the middle and posterior plexuses; it will become the sigmoid portion of the transverse plexus. This anastomosis becomes the main drainage of what was formerly the middle dural plexus, causing the stalk of the middle plexus almost to disappear. The remaining stalk eventually becomes the superior petrosal sinus, which connects to the cavernous sinus.

At 18 mm the anterior plexus also forms a channel with the middle plexus, its drainage now flowing within the previous channel between the middle and posterior plexuses, producing a combined drainage of all three (Fig. 1.5). The middle and anterior plexuses change significantly, annexing each other to become the tentorial plexus. At this point the sagittal plexus is more noticeable; it was formed by the joining of the large branches of the middle and anterior plexuses. As the cerebral hemisphere develops, these branches form the longitudinal plexus, which merges in between the two hemispheres. The superior sagittal plexus is not yet a single channel and appears in the embryo at this stage as a network of plexuses. By 50 mm the superior sagittal plexus is well established. Its growth caudally along with the transverse and straight sinuses leads to the disappearance of the tentorial plexus.

While the dura mater develops, there is a clear demarcation between the cerebral and dural veins. By 21 mm the jugular portion of the dural sinus is identifiable. The rest of the developing structures progress slowly owing to the growth of the cerebrum, which causes readjustment of the tentorial plexus. Although the structure is established by 40 mm, it is not fully developed until birth.

Dural Sinus Fistula

The dural sinus fistula arises in areas of previous sinus occlusion. There can be many occluded areas, but not all become fistulae. A fistula will not produce serious symptoms unless veins entering the sinus become arterialized, whether in the orbit, the cranium, or both.[10]

It has been proposed that during thrombosis, there is also thrombosis of the venules within the wall and of the ends of the cortical veins entering the sinus. The fistula that develops drains into the sinus once the sinus lumen recanalizes, and this results in a standard sinus fistula. If the fistula volume is large or the sinus lumen is not completely open, back pressure will cause retrograde flow through the cortical or ophthalmic veins. Occasionally, the fistula will drain retrograde into one of the entering veins that has not regained continuity with the lumen.[10]

Vein of Galen Aneurysm

A vein of Galen aneurysm is the most common of the congenital sinus fistulae. Its development can be related to thrombosis during the period of venous remodeling.[1] It is characterized by the absence of the straight sinus in its normal position and the substitution of a falcine sinus higher up in the falx cerebri, entering

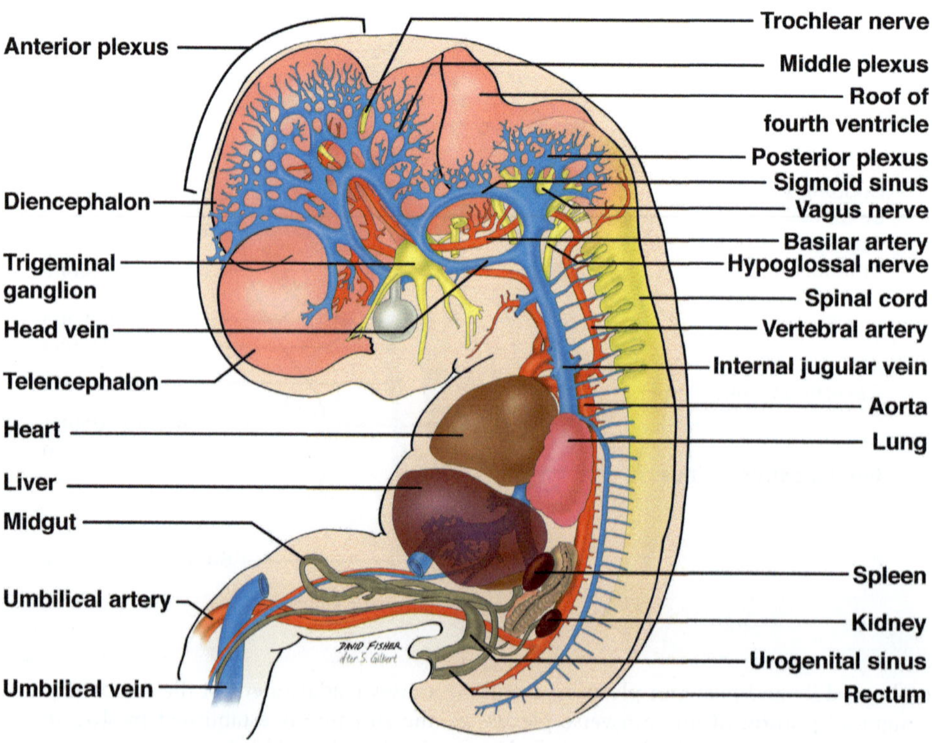

FIG. 1.5 Details of related neurovascular structures at stage 19, day 48, approximately 16–18mm. See Fig. 1.2 for reference.

the sagittal sinus or an enlarged torcular Herophili in an unusual manner.[10] Occasionally, the sinus is completely obstructed and the vein of Galen drains by an alternative route.[10] The most likely time for the vein of Galen aneurysm to form is approximately when the two primitive internal cerebral veins fuse, and no later than the point at which the fetus reaches 80 mm.[1]

Arteriovenous Malformation

Arteriovenous malformations (AVMs) can occur in the brain stem, which is well vascularized before the fetus reaches a length of 40mm (9–10weeks).[1] At 40mm the cortical mantle scarcely exists in the hemisphere, with the arterial and venous tubes being mainly indistinguishable. With the decrease in the number of pial-dural connections, areas that drain into veins that will disappear must find easy access by a pial anastomosis to adjoining veins that will persist. Venous malformation can occur if these connections are not developed or if the occlusive process spreads into the surface network served by the disappearing vessels.[1]

The fact that AVMs do not frequently drain into the tentorial sinus suggests that they originate after that channel has ceased to be a significant part of the hemispheric drainage, a period later than the 20mm and perhaps closer to the 80mm stage.[1] Their involvement with adult-stage vessels, such as the parasagittal veins or the vein of Labbé, suggests that they can occur after these have become established, which is before the fetus reaches 80mm.[1]

REFERENCES

1. Mullan S, MojtahediI S, Johnson DL, Macdonald RL. Embryological basis of some aspects of cerebral vascular fistulas and malformations. *J Neurosurg.* 1996;85:1–8.
2. Padget DH. The cranial venous system in man in reference to development, adult configuration, and relation to the arteries. *Am J Anat.* 1956;98:307–356.
3. Padget DH. The development of the cranial venous system in man from the viewpoint of comparative anatomy. *Contrib Embryol.* 1957;36:81–139.
4. Streeter GL. The development of the venous sinuses of the dura mater in the human embryo. *Am J Anat.* 1915;18:145–178.
5. Butler H. The development of mammalian dural venous sinuses with especial reference to the post-glenoid vein. *J Anat.* 1967;102:33–56.

6. Streeter GL. The developmental alterations in the vascular system of the brain of the human embryo. *Contrib Embryol.* 1918;8:5–38.
7. Yokota A, Oota T, Matsukado Y, Okudera T. Structures and development of the venous system in congenital malformations of the brain. *Neuroradiology.* 1978;16:26–30.
8. Mitsuhashi Y, Hayasaki K, Kawakami T, et al. Dural venous system in the cavernous sinus: a literature review and embryological, functional, and endovascular clinical considerations. *Neurol Med Chir.* 2016;56(6):326–339.
9. Okudera T, Huang YP, Ohta T, et al. Development of posterior fossa dural sinuses, emissary veins, and jugular bulb: morphological and radiologic study. *AJNR.* 1994;15(10):1871–1883.
10. Mullan S. Reflections upon the nature and management of intracranial and intraspinal vascular malformations and fistulae. *J Neurosurg.* 1994;80:606–616.

CHAPTER 2

The Superior Sagittal Sinus

SHENELL BERNARD • KIRA NEWELL • R. SHANE TUBBS

The superior sagittal sinus (SSS) (Figs. 2.1–2.6) is one of the major intradural venous sinuses, and because it is involved in various disease processes, it must be considered in intracranial neurosurgery. The SSS lies in a shallow midsagittal depression at the junction of the falx cerebri, with the dura lining the inner table of the calvaria. Enlarging as it passes from the foramen cecum toward the internal occipital protuberance, the SSS receives the superior convexity veins.[1] The SSS is triangular in shape, with its base positioned against the inner table.

EMBRYOLOGY

The embryology of the venous system is extremely complex, the development of which lags behind that of the arterial system in all embryonic stages and continues into the postnatal period.[2] As such, vascular malformations present at birth may result from failed regression of embryonic structures.[2]

The precursors of the venous system begin to take form in the third and fourth weeks of fetal life. The intracranial venous system begins with the capillary plexus, as well as the anterior, middle, and posterior dural plexuses that drain the neural tube into the lateral sinus, which at this stage is known as the head sinus, which then drains into the anterior cardinal vein, another element of the primitive venous system. By day 40 postgestation, the longitudinal sinus connects the anterior, middle, and posterior sinuses and drains them into the internal jugular vein. A section of the anterior venous plexus eventually will become the SSS.[2]

The SSS is formed from a plexiform channel of veins covering the telencephalon and diencephalon. Blood from these brain structures is collected by small vessels that unite to form three main stems: (1) the superior cerebral vein, which opens into the cranial end of the cavernous sinus; (2) the middle cerebral vein, which opens into the opposite end of the cavernous sinus, and (3) the inferior cerebral vein, which opens into the lateral vein of the head behind the ear vesicle.[3]

The branches of the superior cerebral veins extend over the cerebral hemispheres[3,4] (Fig. 2.6) and collect blood from the medial and convex surfaces.[4] The medial superficial cerebral veins (medial frontal, parietal, and occipital hemispheric veins[4]), together with the superior cerebral veins, unite with the corresponding veins on the opposite side to form the SSS.[3,4]

The SSS lies essentially in the midline (Figs. 2.7–2.9). The superior cerebral veins first drain it naturally, and as the cerebral hemispheres enlarge and extend farther toward the midbrain region, the superior cerebral veins are pushed back and join the middle cerebral vein; later, these veins are pushed even farther back and join the inferior cerebral vein.[3]

During these later changes, the connection between the SSS and the superior cerebral vein is lost. The middle cerebral vein becomes the superior petrosal sinus, which forms a communication between the cavernous and transverse sinuses.[3]

The transverse sinus represents the channel between the SSS and the cranial end of the cardinal vein; thus, the cranial portion of the transverse sinus represents the connection between the SSS and the inferior cerebral vein, whereas its caudal portion represents the inferior cerebral vein itself.[3] The caudal end of the SSS becomes dilated to form the confluence of sinuses[3] (Fig. 2.10).

The embryology of the venous sinuses has been documented extensively, from Streeter's account in 1915 and 1918 to Salzer's (1895)[5], who described dural venous sinus development in man, rabbit, pig, guinea pig, and cat, to Grosser's, who studied the development of the head veins in bats.[6] Butler demonstrated the embryologic development of the human venous system using human fetuses.[6] His observations were carried out with 24- to 48-day-old embryos with a crown-rump length (CRL) of 14.0 mm.

Streeter[7] observed and documented the development of the venous sinuses of the dura mater in human embryos and fetuses and studied in utero development in embryos with a CRL that ranged from 4 to 80 mm.[7]

Anatomy, Imaging and Surgery of the Intracranial Dural Venous Sinuses. https://doi.org/10.1016/B978-0-323-65377-0.00002-7

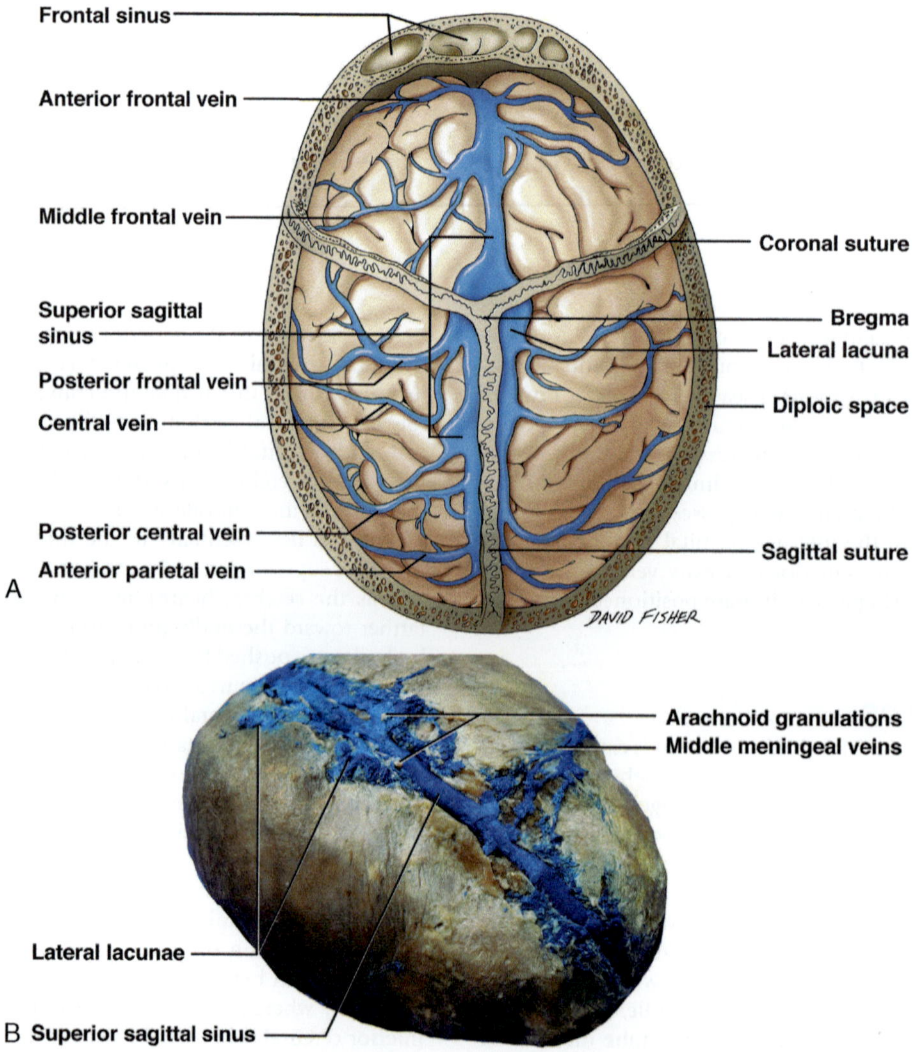

FIG. 2.1 **(A)** Superior view of the superior sagittal sinus and its tributaries. Note that the coronal and sagittal sutures are in place to show the relationship between the sinus and these sutures. **(B)** Anterolateral view of the superior sagittal sinus (latex injected) from a cadaveric specimen.

In 4-mm-CRL embryos, the primary head vein is present and receives the ventral and dorsal tributaries primarily. The ventral tributaries are more numerous near the optic stalk and around the nerve ganglions.[7] The branches of the superficial veins or dorsal dural plexuses entering the primary head vein comprise three groups: the anterior, middle, and posterior plexuses.[7,8] The anterior plexus drains venous blood from the diencephalon and mesencephalon into the primary head vein in front of the semilunar ganglion, whereas the middle or cerebellar plexus joins the primary head vein between the trigeminal nerve and the acoustic-facial complex. Finally, the posterior or occipital plexus drains venous blood from the medullary region and empties it into the primary head vein caudal to the otic capsule.[7,8]

The dura mater and arachnoid spaces begin to form as the embryo grows. Many of the anastomosing channels between the capillaries of the brain and the primary head vein close, and there is a general separation or cleavage of the more superficial head vein and its tributaries from the deeper veins that arise from and drain the deeper plexuses (capillary sheet) that envelop

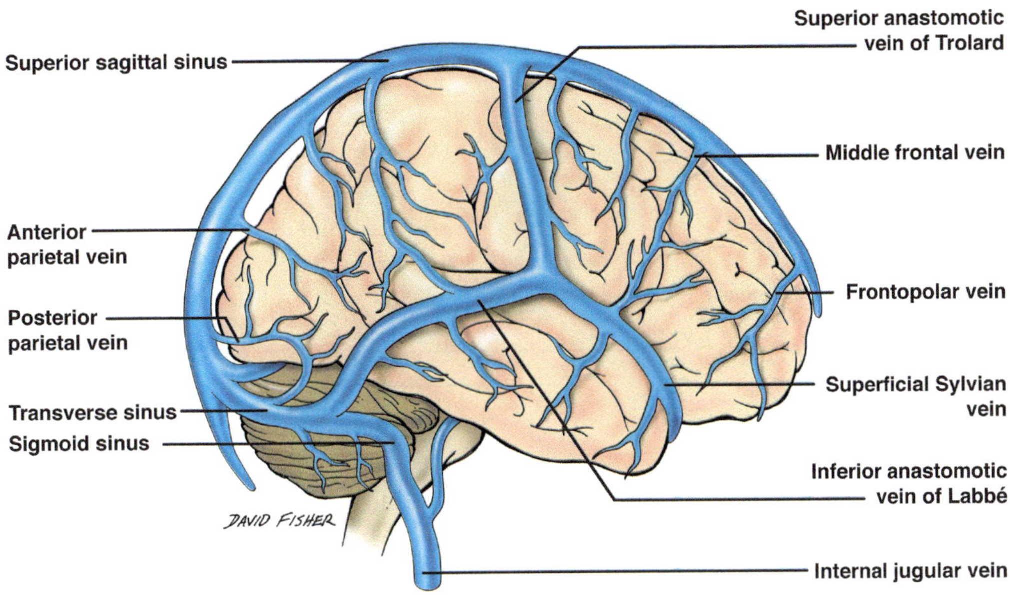

FIG. 2.2 Lateral view of the superior sagittal sinus and its tributaries.

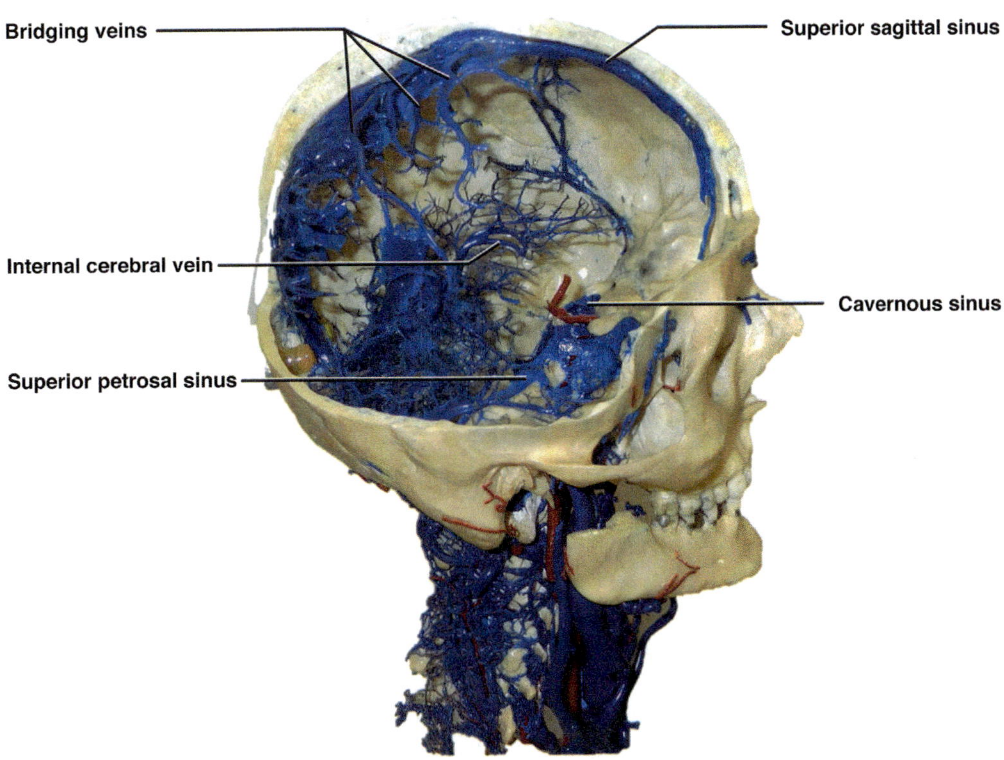

FIG. 2.3 Latex-injected specimen in situ noting the superior sagittal sinus and its tributaries.

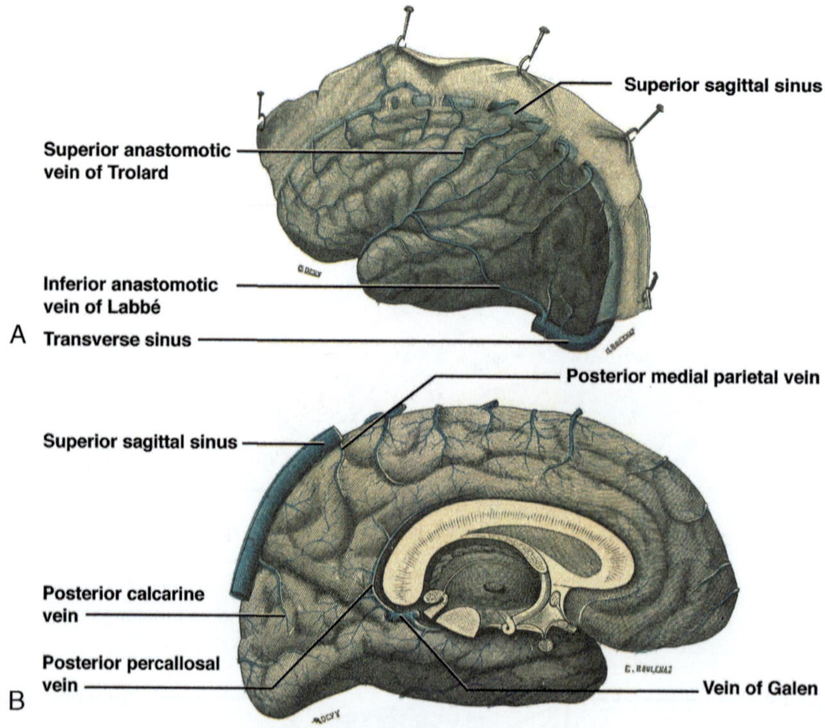

FIG. 2.4 **(A)** Lateral view of the superior sagittal sinus and its tributaries after Testut. **(B)** Medial view of the superior sagittal sinus and its tributaries after Testut.

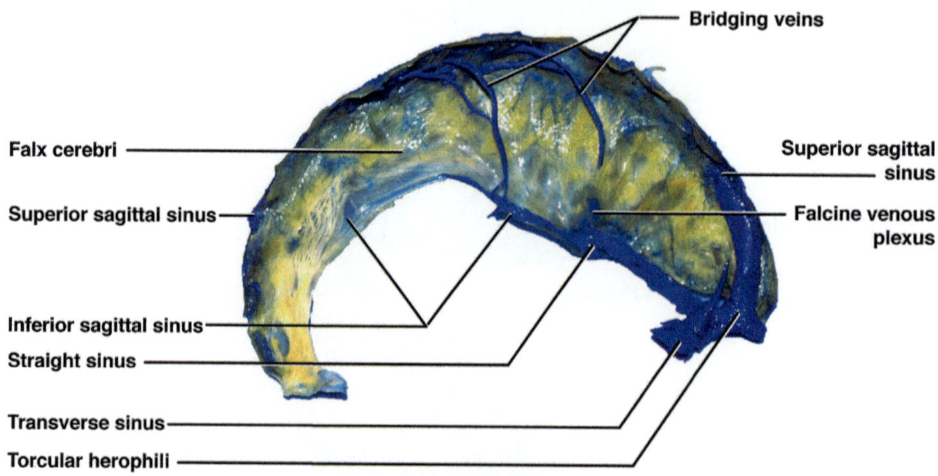

FIG. 2.5 Cadaveric falx cerebri removed and latex injected. Note the superior sagittal sinus and its tributaries.

the neural tube closely.[7,8] This can be seen in embryos with a 12 mm CRL.[8]

In tracing the anterior and middle dural plexuses dorsally toward the midline, there is an increasing frequency of communications between the deep and superficial veins. Near the midline, the veins are connected so intimately that it is impossible to distinguish between the two.[8]

In embryos with a CRL of 14 mm, the aforementioned anterior, middle, and posterior cerebral veins

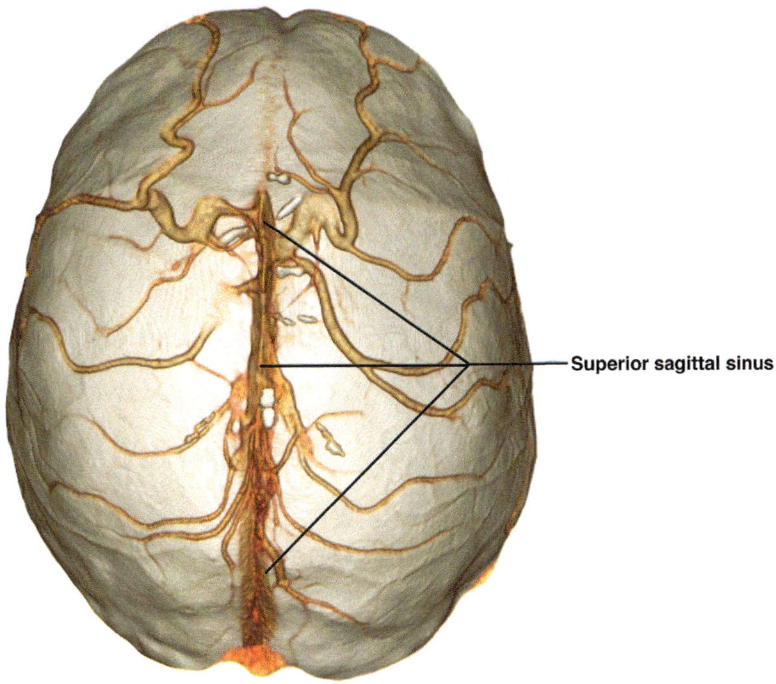

FIG. 2.6 CTA noting the superior sagittal sinus and its tributaries. Courtesy Dr. Joel Curé.

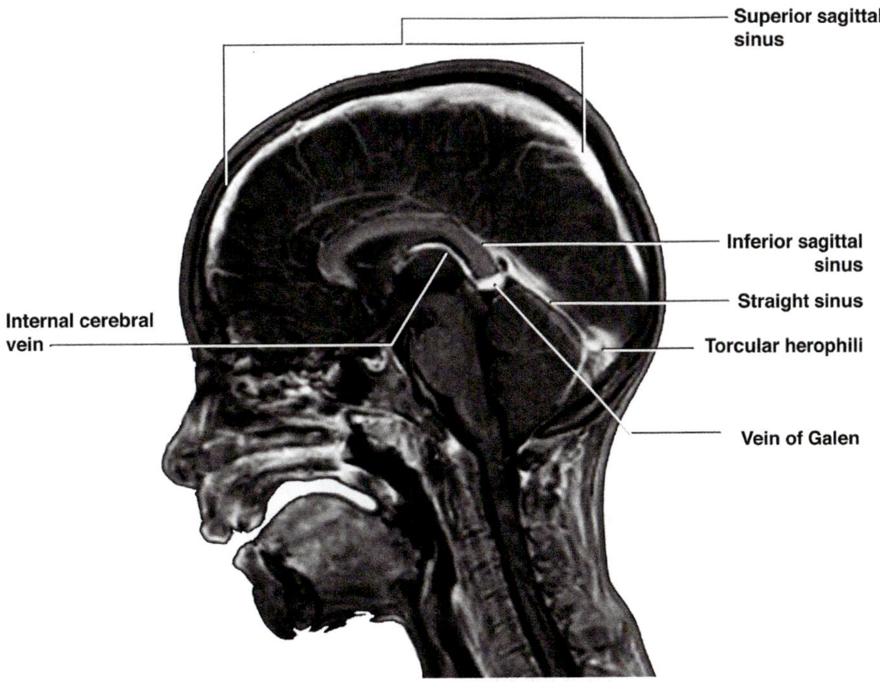

FIG. 2.7 Contrasted midsagittal T1-weighted MRI illustrating the superior sagittal sinus.

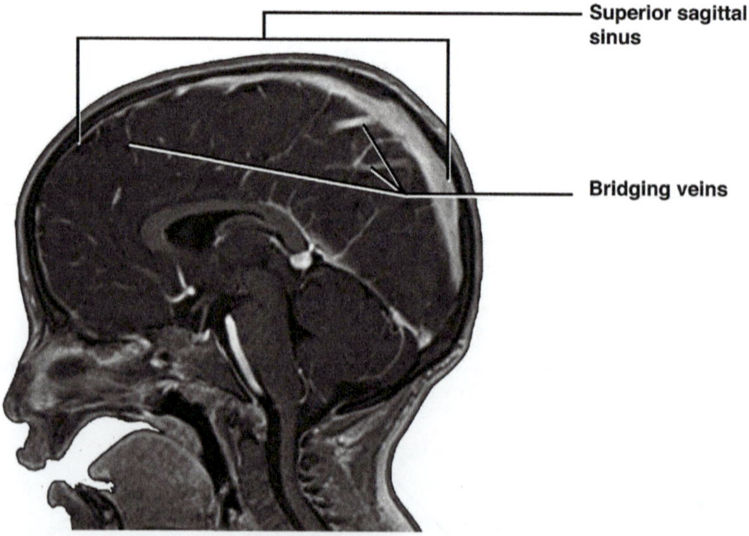

FIG. 2.8 Contrasted midsagittal T1-weighted MRI illustrating the superior sagittal sinus. Note that this sinus is less robust anteriorly compared with Fig. 2.7.

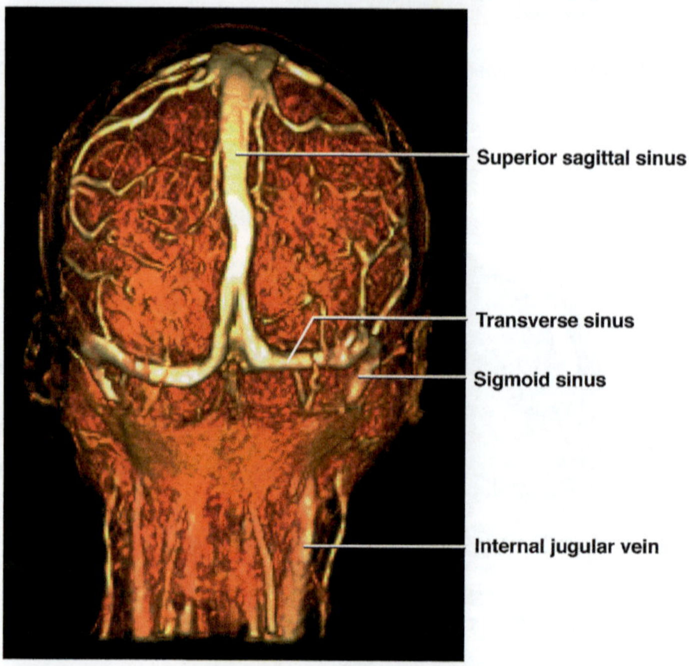

FIG. 2.9 CTA illustrating the superior sagittal sinus splitting more or less equally into the left and right transverse sinuses. (Courtesy Dr. Joel Curé.)

are seen, with the latter two both emptying into the main channel through a single trunk, whereas the anterior cerebral vein maintains the character of the original plexus and has multiple openings into the primary head vein.[7] The vascular mesh of the dorsal aspects of the anterior and middle dural plexuses advances toward the middorsal part of the telencephalon and form the sagittal plexus.[8]

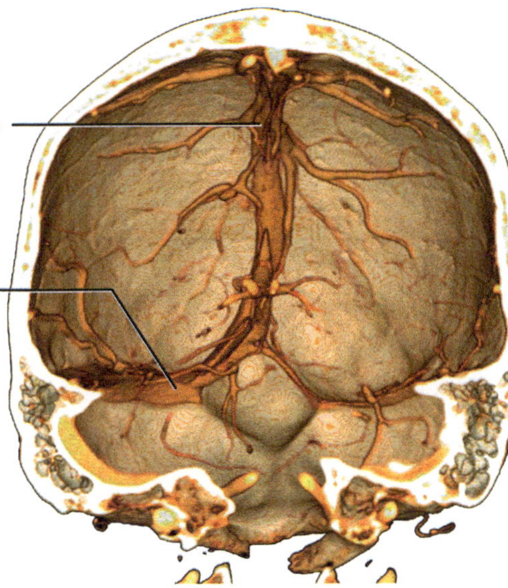

FIG. 2.10 Coronal CTA noting the superior sagittal sinus draining primarily into the right transverse sinus. (Courtesy Dr. Joel Curé.)

Rostrally, this venous network invaginates between the developing cerebral hemispheres, in which meshwork the superior and inferior sagittal sinuses originate.[8]

In the development of the SSS, large venous channels are connected first by a fine anastomosing network, which gives the appearance of small lakes connected by irregular coursing channels. Some of these lakes enlarge, whereas others dwindle, thus forming a sinus that grows asymmetrically with a tendency to drain more freely to one side than the other, usually to the right.[8]

According to Evan (1912)[9], the SSS is paired originally and fuses later into a single channel. The occasional finding of a duplicated segment of this sinus in adults supports this notion[8] (Figs. 2.11 and 2.12).

In 21-mm-CRL embryos, the veins of the head have an arrangement intermediate between the embryonic and adult types. The veins in the basal portion of the skull have features similar to those in the adult, whereas the dorsal veins retain many of the embryonic features.[7,8] With the alterations in the primary head vein, the anterior, middle, and posterior dural plexuses are drained by means of the new dorsal channel, which empties through the jugular foramen.[7] As the cerebrum and cerebellum grow, there are continual adjustments of the contained venous channels and repeated alterations in the pattern of the meshes.[7]

In the 21-mm fetus, the anterior dural plexus combines with the middle dural plexus to drain dorsally to the otic capsule. This forms a complete trunk that drains areas of the head dorsal to the primary head vein as far as the jugular foramen, where it is continuous with the internal jugular vein.[7] In embryos with a 50 mm CRL, the channels for venous drainage of the head correspond well to those found in the adult. The external, dural, and cerebral systems are now clearly separate entities,[8] and the SSS is established in part. In its cephalic or rostral portion, the dural connective tissue investments necessary for adults are lacking, and in its caudal region, the SSS still exhibits its plexiform character, which indicates a transitional state.[7]

In the early stages, the SSS consists of several collateral anastomosing veins. Eventually, a single channel forms in the anterior portions caused by the selection and enlargement of the most favorable vein and the disappearance of the others.[7] In the posterior position, some of the adjacent veins coalesce. The anterior aspect of the sinus completes its formation first,[7] whereas the caudal aspect remains plexiform, but with the growth of the cerebral hemispheres, the enlargement of one loop of the plexus, and the dwindling of the other plexuses, spontaneous migration of the sinuses occurs and the main channel of the SSS lengthens.[7,8]

ANATOMY

The cerebral venous system can be divided into the superficial and deep systems. The superficial system

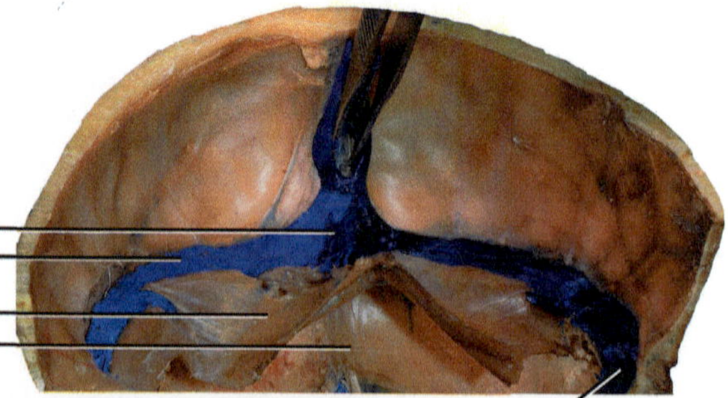

FIG. 2.11 Latex-injected cadaveric specimen noting a fenestrated superior sagittal sinus.

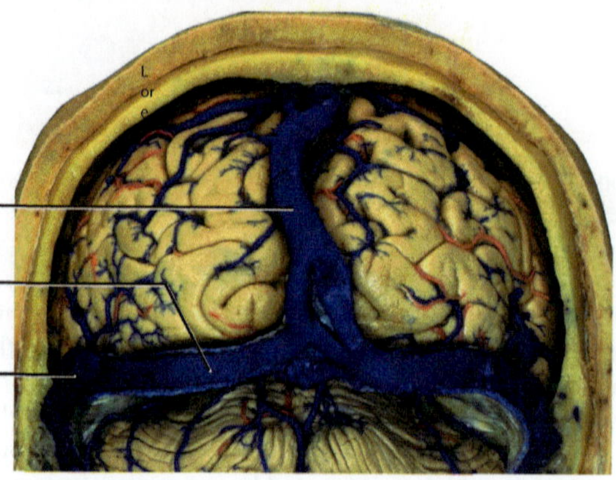

FIG. 2.12 Posterior view of latex-injected cadaveric specimen noting a fenestrated superior sagittal sinus. (Courtesy Dr. Albert Rhoton.)

comprises the sagittal sinuses and cortical veins, both of which drain the superficial surfaces of both cerebral hemispheres. The deep system consists of the lateral, straight, and sigmoid sinuses, together with the deeper draining cortical veins.[1,10] Both of these systems drain largely into the internal jugular veins.[10]

The superficial cerebral veins are interlinked with the anastomotic veins of Trolard and Labbé. The superolateral surface of the hemisphere drains into the SSS, whereas the posteroinferior aspect drains into the transverse sinus.[10]

The SSS runs in the attached, convex margin of the falx cerebri along the grooves of the internal surface of the frontal bone, the adjacent margins of the two parietal bones, and the squamous part of the occipital bone[11] (Fig. 2.13). It begins near the crista galli, a few millimeters posterior to the foramen cecum, and receives the primary tributaries from the cortical veins of the frontal lobes, the ascending frontal veins.[11] The cortical veins of the inferior surface of the frontal lobes may drain through the anterior cortical veins into the anterior third of the SSS, through the anterior cerebral veins into the basal vein of Rosenthal, or into the superficial middle cerebral vein.[12]

The vein of the foramen cecum (VFC) is mentioned frequently in the literature and often is described as an emissary vein. The VFC connects the nasal and paranasal mucosa to the SSS through the foramen cecum. However, various authors often have questioned the existence of this vein. Using digital subtraction angiography (DSA), Ruíz[12] demonstrated two cases of intracranial drainage of the nasal mucosa by a frontal cortical vein into the SSS, which could be analogous to a VFC. In rare cases, the nasal mucosa may drain intracranially through a vein traversing a foramen of the cribriform plate that joins the SSS ultimately. This connection may provide a pathway for the intracranial spread of sinunasal infectious or tumor, as well as provide an anatomic substratum for the genesis of dural arteriovenous fistulae of the anterior cranial fossa.[12]

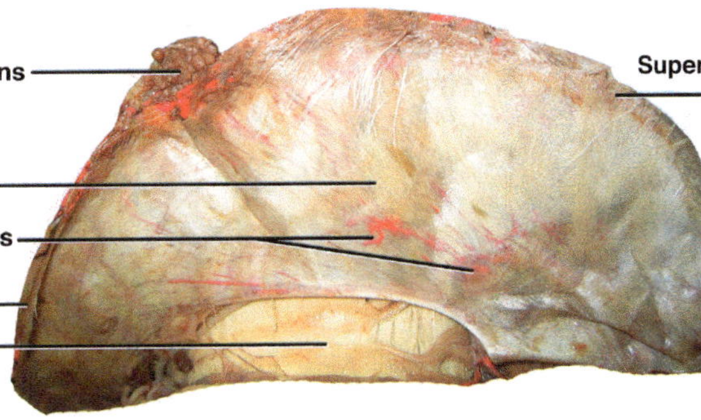

FIG. 2.13 Large arachnoid granulation within the superior sagittal sinus in a cadaveric specimen.

The SSS functions as a terminus of the superficial cortical venous system draining the anterior part of the inferior surface of the frontal lobe and the superior parts of the lateral and medial surfaces of the frontal, parietal, and occipital lobes.[13] The more anterior veins usually enter the sinus at more or less right angles. However, the more posterior, and usually larger, veins travel in an oblique fashion anteriorly to drain into the SSS in a direction opposite the blood flow within them.

Together with the straight and occipital sinuses, the SSS empties into the transverse sinus and causes a small excavation at the internal occipital protuberance (torcular Herophili)[13]: Although the SSS is narrow at its anterior end, the sinus runs backward and widens gradually to approximately 1 cm at its posterior end. Near the internal occipital protuberance, the SSS deviates, usually to the right (commonly three times), and continues as the transverse sinus[11] (Figs. 2.12 and 2.14).

In triangular cross section, the interior of the SSS includes the openings of the superior cerebral veins and arachnoid granulation projections. Many fibrous bands traverse the SSS (see Chordae Willisii section). It also communicates by small orifices with irregular venous lacunae situated in the dura mater near the sinus.[11]

There usually are two or three small frontal, large parietal, or intermediate-sized occipital lacunae on each side of the sinus.[11] In the elderly, the lacunae tend to become confluent, so there is one elongated lacuna on each side. Fine fibrous bands cross them, and numerous arachnoid granulations project into them.[11] The lacunae also drain the diploic veins and meningeal veins. Lateral lacunae frequently are so complex that they are nearly plexiform; they rarely are simple venous spaces. Plexiform arrays of small veins adjoin the sagittal, transverse, and straight sinuses, and ridges of such "spongy" venous tissue often project into the lumina of the superior sagittal and transverse sinuses.[11]

The mean length of the SSS was found to be 25.6 + 1.6 cm on computed tomography venographies (CTVs) and 19.2 + 1.4 cm in cadaveric dissections. The area of the SSS in cross section at the coronary suture measured 32.1 + 15.3 mm^2 and grows larger in the direction of flow.[13] The mean length of the SSS ranges from 23 to 28 cm measured from the foramen cecum to the torcular Herophili. The typical shape of the SSS in a coronal view in CTV appears not to be circular, but rather triangular or polygonal.[1,13,14] The transverse diameter of the SSS ranges from approximately 4 mm in the frontal region to 10 mm in the occipital region. In some cases, the SSS is atretic anterior to the level of the coronal suture.[1] In these cases, prominent superior frontal veins drain upward and posteriorly, converging near the coronal suture to form the SSS.[1] The posterior SSS may deviate more than 1 cm from the midline in up to 20% of patients.[1] Classically, the SSS converges with the straight sinus at the torcular Herophili, and their combined flow drains into the transverse sinuses.[1] However, a true sinus confluence (merger of the superior sagittal, straight, transverse, and occipital sinuses) exists in only a minority of individuals.[1]

Chordae Willisii

In 1664, Thomas Willis studied the venous sinuses of the dura mater and is credited with the original description of the inner walls of the dural sinuses (Browder et al., 1972).[25] Therefore, these structures are referred to as the chordae Willisii. The lumen of the SSS contains an average of 17 chordae Willisii (Fig. 2.15).[1,14]

The valvelike chordae Willisii are related intimately with the orifices of the SSS tributary veins. The terminal ends of the middle and posterior portions of the veins project forward and enter the SSS at an angle opposite to the direction of the flow, which creates an unfavorable physiologic angle at the vein orifice. Thus, most of the vein orifices in the sinus are half covered

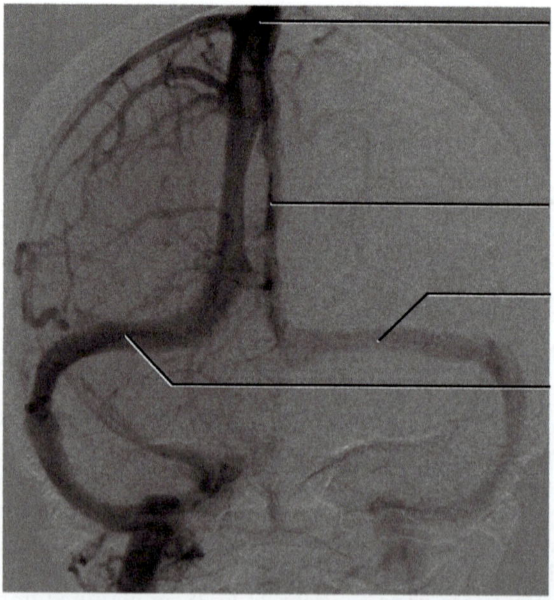

FIG. 2.14 Imaging of the superior sagittal sinus draining primarily into the right transverse sinus.

by valvelike chordae to prevent backflow of blood into the veins and to ensure drainage from the veins into the sinus. This is one of the characteristic physiologic functions of the chordae Willisii in the sinus and explains their shape and frequent location in the SSS.[14]

Browder et al. (1972) showed that the anterior 5–7 cm of the interior of the SSS has relatively few openings to join the cortical veins. However, there is a complex array of bands, bridges, cusps, and chords in the middle 12–14 cm of the sinus, which are the chordae Willisii. The authors recorded burrows that opened rostrally or caudally with cusp-shaped folds at their openings. They also recorded longitudinally oriented tunnels with cusp-shaped membranes at both ends. Bands of various shapes and lengths extend from one lateral leaflet of the sinus to the opposite side and are located most frequently in the parietal region of the SSS. Finer trabeculae also occasionally span from one lateral leaflet to another.

Several cadaveric studies have shown that no two specimens are similar in the placements of chordae Willisii. In a study of 10 sinuses, 172 intraluminal chordae Willisii were identified with an average of 17 chordae per sinus.[14] The minimum number of chordae in dissected SSSs was 12 and the maximum was 24. Sharifi et al.[15] published similar data. They recorded 432 total chordae in 25 sinuses with a mean of 17.2 chordae per sinus. The minimum and maximum numbers of chordae recorded were 11 and 25, respectively.

Shao et al.[14] identified three types of chordae: valvelike, trabecular, and laminar. Valvelike chordae were the most common and constituted 48.3% of the total recorded. Sharifi et al. found that 45.1% of chordae were valvelike, and Schmutz[16] found that 49% of all structures were valvelike lamellae. These authors noted that they generally are located at the lateral sinus wall, where they cover up to half of the openings of the superior cerebral veins. However, at the base, they are found only in the frontoparietal region. Shao et al.[14] indicated that the terminal parts of the middle and posterior portions of the veins are directed forward and enter the SSS at an angle opposite to the direction of flow, which, again, creates a physiologically unfavorable angle at the vein orifices. They concluded similarly that the valvelike chordae half cover most of the vein orifices in the sinus to preclude backflow of blood into the veins and ensure they drain to the sinus.

The second most common chordae were trabecular, 30.1% according to Sharifi et al.[15] Schmutz[16] recorded similar data that showed that 35% of all chordae were trabecular, whereas Shao et al.[14] found that 31.5% were trabecular. They determined that these chordae crossed the lumen at the sinus at different angles, were located in the lumen either centrally or peripherally, and varied in length and thickness. Schmutz[16] classified trabecular chordae as 19% isolated, 7.5% in small clusters, and 8.5% as a network. As Petroni and Marrone[17] detailed, most of the trabecular projections were unrelated to

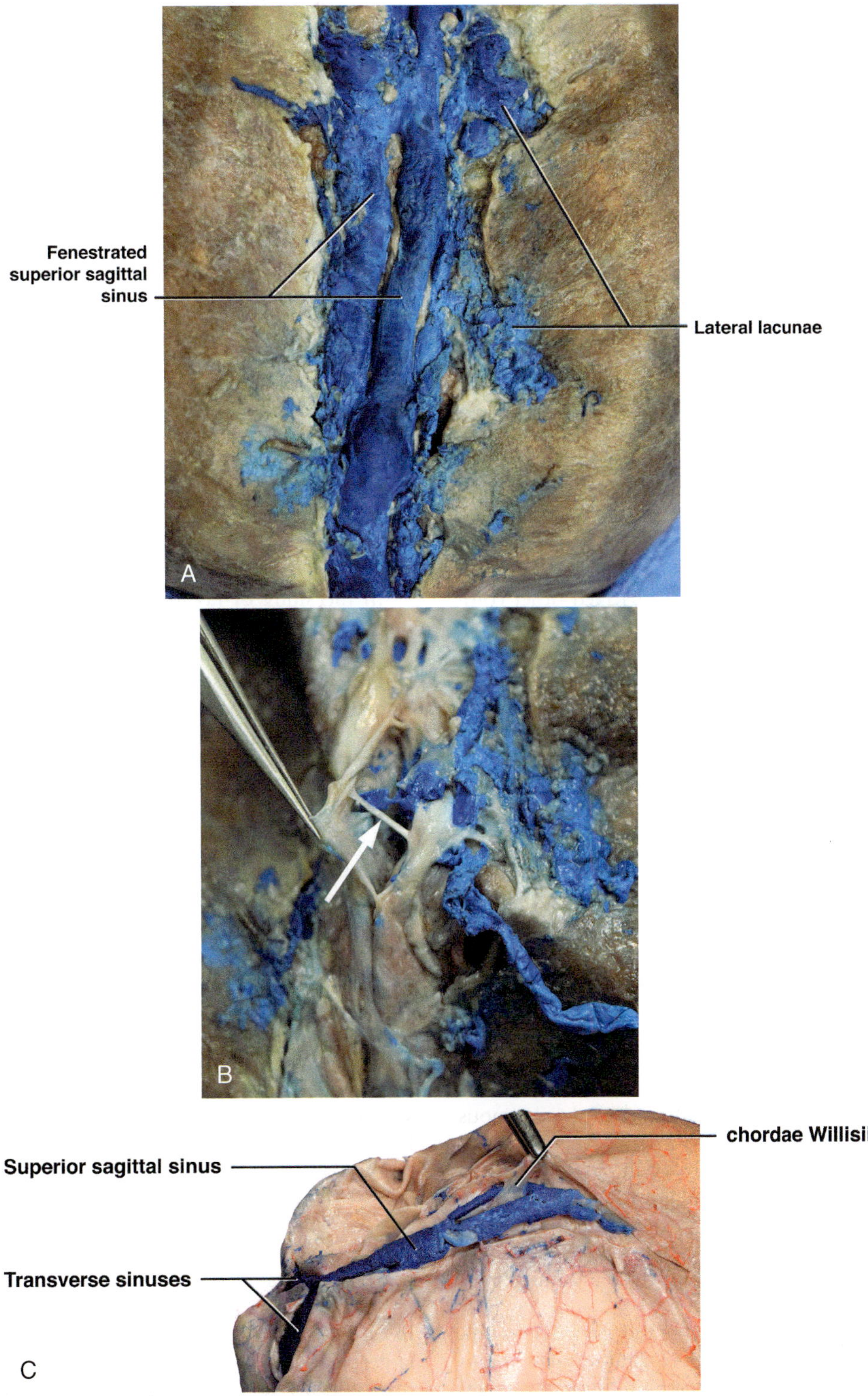

FIG. 2.15 **(A)** Superior view of latex-injected superior sagittal sinus noting lateral lacunae and partial sinus duplication. **(B)** Opened latex-injected superior sagittal sinus noting chordae Willisii. **(C)** Latex-injected superior sagittal sinus noting fenestration and chordae Willisii.

afferent veins. The numbers of trabecular projections related to veins were similar on both sides, whereas those unrelated to veins were more abundant on the left, which asymmetry would favor a more intense blood flow on the right.

The least common form of chordae was longitudinal lamellae.[16] Shao et al.[14] indicated that their form was laminar chordae and observed that they constituted 20.2% of all chordae, usually separating the lumen of the SSS into two or three single, independent channels. Sharifi et al.[15] found 23.1% of longitudinal chordae ranging from 2 to 35 mm in length. In contrast, Schmutz[16] found their length was 2–8 mm and that most lie in the median or parasagittal plane. He also observed that longitudinal lamellae generally are triangular or square with concave frontal and occipital borders. They support the lumen from within the sinus and prevent the build-up of pressure and resultant compression of the sinus walls.[14]

In addition to the three forms of chordae identified in most research, Sharifi et al.[15] observed other cordlike structures located in the lumina of cerebral vein ostia that were associated with valvelike chordae. They classified these as accessory cords and found that they constituted 1.6% of all structures in their study. These accessory cords formed networks that occupied the entrances to the venous lacunae.

Additional studies have elucidated the growth pattern of chordae Willisii. Kedzia and Kedzia[18] observed divisions in the SSS during the fetal period and an age-dependent increase in the chordae number and morphology. To provide a better platform for studies of the SSS and the functions of the chordae Willisii, Hoffmann et al.[19] studied bovine models and observed very similar chordae formations among all the animals examined.

VARIATIONS

Anatomic variations in the intracranial dural venous sinuses are found frequently.[20] These are associated with developmental anomalies of the brain and their corresponding anatomic variations having a strong potential to influence the interpretation of imaging and neurosurgical planning.[21] This represents a common diagnostic difficulty, particularly when a dural venous sinus thrombosis is suspected.[20]

Several anatomic variations of the SSS (such as unilateral hypoplasia, aplasia of the rostral segment, duplication, or fenestration) are typical findings in cerebral angiograms.[21] These abnormalities are common and include duplication of the rostral SSS, unilateral hypoplastic rostral SSS, complete hypoplastic rostral SSS, hypoplastic dorsal SSS, and atresia of the rostral SSS.[22]

Superior Sagittal Sinus Agenesis

Some anatomic variations of the SSS are uncommon, and agenesis is extremely rare.[22] Kocak et al.[22] reported an extremely rare variation, total agenesis of the SSS, and falx cerebri. Because of the shared anatomic and embryologic origin of both the falx cerebri and the SSS, cerebral falx abnormalities may be related to SSS abnormalities and the converse.[22]

In such imaging studies as computed tomography (CT), magnetic resonance imaging (MRI), and DSA, the absence or lack of contrast filling in all segments of the SSS primarily characterizes total agenesis of the SSS. Venous drainage is affected because of the absence of the SSS, but the lack thereof can be compensated by certain other enlarged venous structures situated around the region where the SSS usually lies.[22]

In the study of Kocak et al,[22] the tentorial sinus, frontal hemispheric veins, and parasagittal large venous channels compensated for the absence of an SSS. In clinical practice, these enlarged venous structures can lead to a misdiagnosis of an arteriovenous fistula or arteriovenous malformation.

Duplication of the Superior Sagittal Sinus

The SSS may be septated or duplicated in part, which occurs most frequently in its posterior portion.[1] The duplicated sinus can drain directly into one or both transverse sinuses.[23] Tubbs and Loukas[24] documented a case of duplication of the SSS in a cadaveric 81-year-old male. The left and right primordia of the SSS are seen during the 35th week of gestation, and these longitudinal channels usually fuse at approximately the 50th day of gestation. Hence, a duplication of the SSS represents persistence of this embryologic phenomenon.[23] Segmental or complete duplication of the SSS is associated sometimes with occipital or parietal meningoencephaloceles and an anomalous course of the straight sinus.[20]

Unilateral Hypoplasia

The most familiar variant of unilateral hypoplasia is that of the rostral third of the SSS. Overall, it constitutes the most frequent variation in SSS anatomy after preferential drainage to one of the transverse sinuses.[20] In cases of complete hypoplastic rostral SSS, a pair of large parasagittal superior frontal cortical veins that runs dorsally to join the origin of the SSS close to the coronal suture replaces the absent rostral portion of the SSS.[20]

In the most extensive form of rostral hypoplasia, the SSS originates in the vicinity of, or at, the coronal suture. In such instances, a rudimentary rostral segment has been documented occasionally by DSA, CTV, or MR venography, although no cortical or meningeal tributaries of this hypoplastic segment usually can be demonstrated by radiologic means.[20]

To distinguish clearly between a hypoplastic rostral SSS and thrombosis of the anterior third of the SSS, there should be a clear demonstration of prominent bilateral superior frontal veins that follow the parasagittal course extending from the pole of the frontal lobes to the origin of the SSS at the coronal suture.[20]

According to Kaplan and Browder,[25] hypoplasia of the rostral SSS is present in 1.8%–6% of cases, with the compensatory venous drainage occurring via an intradural venous channel that drains the cortical veins and runs parallel to the midsagittal plane toward the origin of the SSS.[25]

Kaplan and Browder reported one case of unilateral hypoplastic rostral SSS with a parasagittal dural venous sinus that collected the venous drainage of the adjacent frontal lobe, which likely was caused by a duplication of the rostral SSS.[25]

In a study Ruíz et al.[20] conducted, unilateral hypoplastic rostral SSS was present in 7% of cases. This is more than twice the incidence of complete hypoplastic rostral SSS. In one case, they were able to demonstrate compensatory drainage via the inferior sagittal sinus via an interhemispheric frontal vein.

Typically, in cases of SSS, outflow obstruction drainage via the inferior sagittal vein is prominent. In the case above, although there was no demonstrable outflow obstruction, the anomalous development of the rostral SSS may have resulted in rerouting part of its normal drainage territory to the inferior sagittal sinus.[20]

Manoj et al.[26] reported a case of a pediatric patient with an incidental persistent falcine sinus with a dominant straight sinus and hypoplastic SSS.

The SSS ends at the midline in only 50.9% of the population[1] and approximately half ends at the internal occipital protuberance as a true sinus confluence. In the remainder, the SSS bifurcates above the internal occipital protuberance and drains directly into the transverse sinuses. The SSS ending off the midline drains into the right transverse sinus approximately twice as often as into the left.[1]

IMAGING

CT

With the introduction of helical computed tomography (CT), the intracranial venous system can be assessed reliably using CT venography (CTV).[27] High-resolution CT has been reported to be comparable with magnetic resonance (MR) angiographic techniques that use either time-of-flight or motion-induced phase shifts to diagnose dural sinus thrombosis.[27]

Compared with MR techniques, CTV acquires images more rapidly and reduces the negative effect of patient motion-related artifacts. CTV also is subject to fewer contraindications and other artifacts that either may prevent or limit MR evaluation.[27] However, CTV requires the use of iodinated contrast material and exposure to ionizing radiation and includes complex postprocessing work. Hence, it plays a supportive role at most centers.[27]

A thrombosed SSS has a characteristic appearance on contrast-enhanced CT, where it presents as a triangular, low-density cast that occupies the full surface of the SSS, and is surrounded by a peripheral-high density area that appears as what some have referred to as an "empty triangle sign" or "delta sign." SSS thrombosis caused by tumor cells or damage secondary to trauma produces a similar appearance.[28]

MRI

The most sensitive technique to detect an SSS thrombosis is MRI with magnetic resonance venography (MRV).[28,29] Recent advances in MR angiography have made it possible to visualize the dural sinuses and cerebral veins without the use of invasive techniques or ionizing radiation.[27] In SSS thrombosis, T1- and T2-weighted MRIs demonstrate a hyperintense signal. The characteristics of the signal depend on the age of the thrombus, and T1-weighted images are isointense during the first 5 days and after 1 month.[29] The combination of an abnormal signal in the sinus and a corresponding absence of flow on MRV confirms the diagnosis of thrombosis, but expert radiologic judgment is required to avoid diagnostic and technical errors.[29]

If MRI is not available readily, CT imaging is a useful technique in the initial examination to rule out other acute cerebral disorders and to reveal venous infarcts or hemorrhages, but its results also can be entirely normal. High-resolution CT equipment may show the thrombus as a hyperintense signal of a cordlike density (the "cord sign") in a sinus or even in the cortical veins. CTV is a promising new technique to create images of the cerebral venous system.[29]

MRV and DSA demonstrate a good correlation, although some artifacts and potential diagnostic problems exist with individual MR techniques. Other advantages include the minimal risk of allergic or

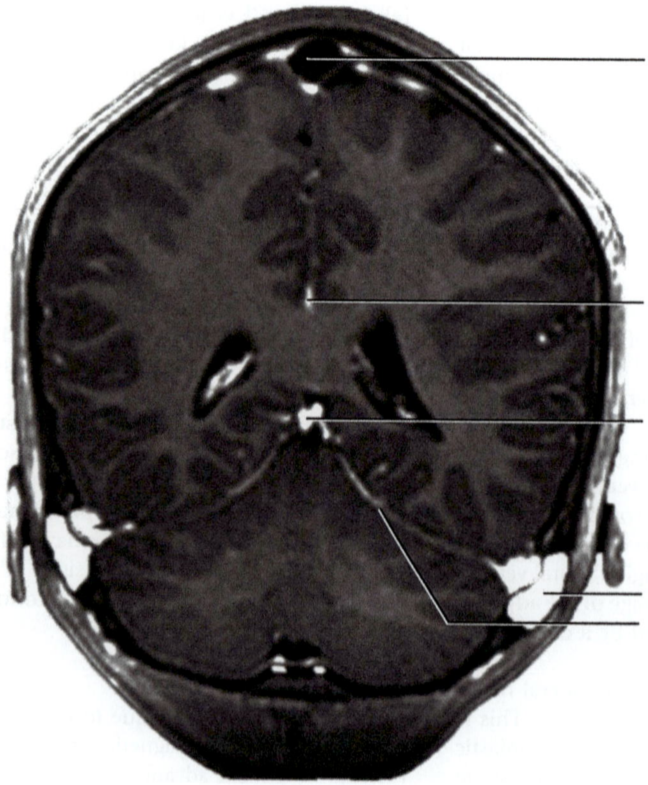

FIG. 2.16 Coronal MRI noting a large arachnoid granulation within the superior sagittal sinus. (Courtesy Dr. Joel Curé.)

nephrotoxic effects with intravenous administration of gadolinium. Disadvantages of MR angiography include poorer spatial resolution and slightly lower sensitivity and specificity for vascular patency relative to DSA.[29]

Magnetization-Prepared Rapid Acquisition Gradient Echo Imaging

Several entities can be encountered in the imaging evaluation of the dural sinuses to assess for thrombosis, including arachnoid granulations, intrasinus septa (fibrous bands), and hypoplasia or aplasia of the dural sinuses.[30] Arachnoid granulations are found in the SSS with frequencies ranging from 0.3% to 55% on imaging[30] (Figs. 2.13 and 2.16-2.19). These become more prominent with age and can indent the overlying calvaria.

High-resolution 3D contrast-enhanced magnetization-prepared rapid acquisition gradient echo (MPRAGE) imaging has been used to depict intracranial dural sinus thrombosis. It works via a pulse sequence that uses a 1.25-mm section thickness and 3D dataset. An intradural thrombosis generally is hypo- or isointense relative to the brain parenchyma and has a high contrast relative to the high signal intensity of flowing blood on 3D contrast-enhanced MPRAGE images.[30] Intradural sinus thromboses produce irregular margins, expand the sagittal sinus, and extend into other sinuses. This is in contrast to arachnoid granulations, which are isointense relative to the cerebral spinal fluid (CSF), do not widen the dural sinus or extend into other sinuses, and have sharp margins.[30]

The sensitivity in detecting dural sinus thrombosis was highest using 3D contrast-enhanced MPRAGE imaging (83%) compared with 2D time-of-flight MRV (51%) and T1-weighted MRI (33%). Specificity also was highest for 3D contrast-enhanced MPRAGE imaging (99%), compared with time-of-flight (92%) and T2-weighted MRI (84%).[30]

Angiography

Assessment of the intracranial venous system usually occurs during the venous phase of conventional

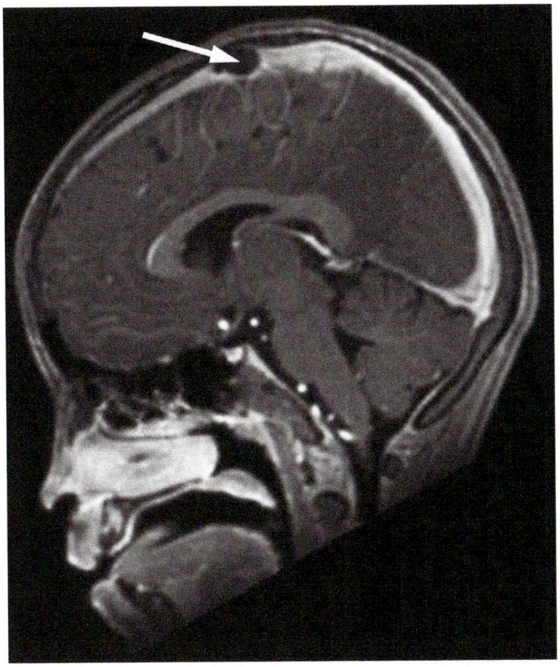

FIG. 2.17 Sagittal MRI noting a large arachnoid granulation within the superior sagittal sinus. (Courtesy Dr. Joel Curé.)

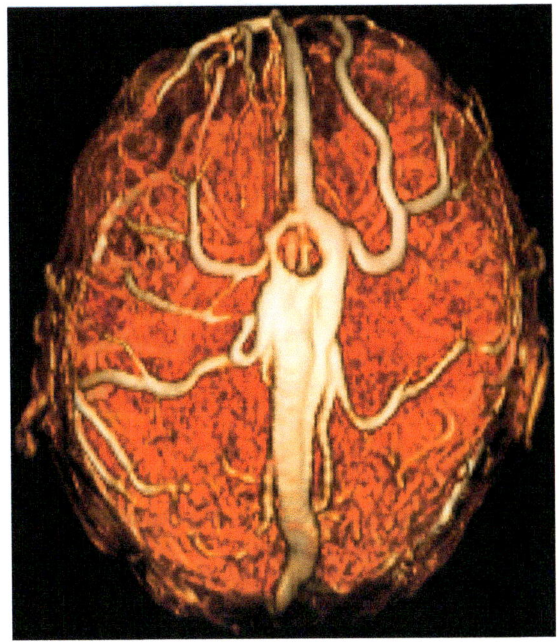

FIG. 2.18 CTA of patient seen in Figs. 2.16 and 2.17. (Courtesy Dr. Joel Curé.)

catheter digital subtraction angiography (DSA), which remains the most definitive diagnostic tool or reference standard in the investigation of intracranial venous disease.[27]

PATHOLOGY

Superior Sinus Thrombosis

Cerebral venous and sinus thrombosis are distinct cerebrovascular disorders[29] that account for <1% of all strokes[31] and affect young adults and children most often.[29,32] SSS thrombosis is an uncommon cause of stroke that has a highly variable symptomatology and clinical course.[29,31,33] The estimated annual incidence is three to four cases per 1 million,[29,31] and up to seven cases per 1 million among children[29]; approximately 75% of the adults are women.[31]

A prothrombotic risk factor or a direct cause is identified in approximately 85% of patients. SSS thrombosis is associated with a variety of hypercoagulable states, including diabetes insipidus, direct injury to the sinus, Crohn disease, iatrogenic causes, malignancy, nephrotic syndrome, pregnancy, oral contraceptives, paroxysmal nocturnal hemoglobinuria, polycythemia, puerperium, systemic lupus erythematosus, and ulcerative colitis.[31,33–35]

In a person who is at increased risk because of genetic factors, other precipitating factors, such as a head injury or obstetrical delivery, often can cause the formation of sinus thrombosis. For example, during the last trimester of pregnancy and after delivery, the risk of sinus thrombosis increases significantly, with a frequency of approximately 12 cases of peripartum and postpartum sinus thrombosis per 100,000 deliveries. This is slightly lower than the rate for peripartum and postpartum arterial stroke.[29]

Development of SSS thrombosis (SSST) results from multiple causes and includes three factors commonly: stasis of the bloodstream, abnormalities of the vessel wall, and hypercoagulability.[31,33] During the past decade, increased awareness of the diagnosis, improvements in neuroimaging, and effective treatment have improved the prognosis substantially, and more than 80% of all patients have a good neurologic outcome.[29]

The use of oral contraceptives, particularly third-generation derivatives that contain gestodene or desogestrel, has been studied, the results of which have shown an increased risk of sinus thrombosis in women who use these contraceptives. Additional evidence of this is found in computations of the sex ratio in cases of sinus thrombosis. Furthermore, laboratory findings have shown that oral contraceptives have a prothrombotic effect.[29]

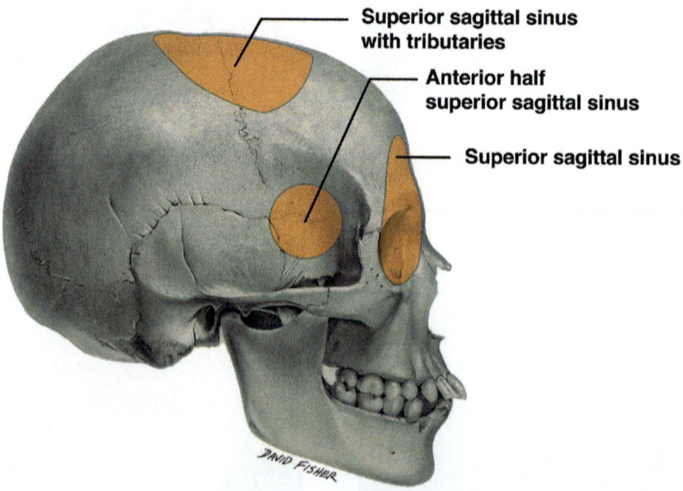

FIG. 2.19 Referred pain sites with stimulation of the superior sagittal sinus.

Mechanical causes of sagittal sinus thrombosis are head injuries and direct injury to the sinus or jugular veins via either catheterization or neurosurgical procedures.[29] Lumbar punctures also can lead to thrombosis because they decrease CSF pressure, which leads to the retention of intracranial blood, with particular stasis in areas of venous drainage (the cortical veins and sinuses). Diagnosis of sinus thrombosis after a lumbar puncture is difficult because the headache that follows often is attributed to the puncture itself.[29] Parenthetically, intraoperative stimulation of the superior sagittal sinus and its tributaries can in itself result in head pain as shown in Fig. 2.19.

Superior sagittal sinus occlusion can lead to the development of intracranial hypertension.[29,33,36] Normally, CSF is transported from the cerebral ventricles through the subarachnoid spaces at the base and surface of the brain to the arachnoid villi, where it is absorbed and drained into the SSS.[29] SSST leads to an increase in venous pressure, impaired absorption of the CSF, and consequently, an increase in intracranial pressure.[29] Approximately one-fifth of patients with SSST have intracranial hypertension only, without signs of cortical vein thrombosis.[29]

Approximately 15%–25% of cases of SSST are considered idiopathic.[31,33] Many authors have shown a link between SSST and hyperthyroidism, suggesting that hyperthyroidism is an independent risk factor for cerebral venous thrombosis.[31] Atrial fibrillation can be seen in patients with hyperthyroidism, which can lead to systemic and cerebral arterial infarctions, suggesting that an embolus might be the cause. In the study of Hwang et al., patients with hyperthyroidism and SSST had normal sinus rhythm on electrocardiography, and echocardiography results showed normal ventricular size and function with no evidence of intracardiac thrombus.

Many authors have concluded that SSST attributable to hyperthyroidism is caused by hypercoagulation through activation of the intrinsic clotting pathway, factor XI in particular. Normal activity of the clotting factor recovers after reaching the euthyroid state. Hence, antithyroid therapy constitutes an important element of treatment.[31,33]

Although the presentation of SSST is extremely variable, the diagnosis should be considered in any young and middle-aged patient with a recent unusual headache. They should be considered particularly in patients with (1) strokelike symptoms in the absence of the usual vascular risk factors; (2) intracranial hypertension, or (3) CT evidence of hemorrhagic infarcts, especially if there are multiple infarcts that are not confined to the arterial vascular territories.[29]

Superior Sagittal Sinus Arteriovenous Fistulas

Dural arteriovenous (AV) fistulas constitute 10%–15% of all intracranial arteriovenous malformations.[37] SSS fistulas are rare in the anterior and middle thirds of the SSS.[37,38] Quite frequently, they are limited and can be eliminated effectively by the endovascular route. The bridging veins entering the sinus can be the matrix of direct fistulas (types III and IV). These direct fistulas are managed best surgically with ligation of the draining vein.[38]

SSS AV fistulas are slightly more common in males, and the age range in patients is 23–78 years.[37] Sinus fistulas often are thought to be acquired, with etiologies attributable to cranial trauma, sinus thrombosis, venous hypertension, or idiopathy.[37,39,40] The majority of dural sinus fistulas are idiopathic, but trauma frequently has been reported as a possible etiology of SSS AV fistulas.[39] These fistulas can have severe neurologic consequences, including hemorrhage, intracranial hypertension, focal deficits, and seizures.[37,39] The incidence of bleeding caused by rupture of the draining veins or by venous hypertension is higher in SSS AV fistulas than in dural AV fistulas arising in other locations.[39]

INTERVENTIONAL RADIOLOGY

Superior Sagittal Sinus AV Fistula Embolization

SSS AV fistulas are difficult to treat because of their unique midline location, multiplicity of arterial feeders, and critical venous drainage.[37,39] Because the SSS drains the majority of the venous outflow of the cerebral hemispheres, surgical resection is tolerated only in the anterior third.[37] A variety of unusual and aggressive treatments, including endovascular embolization with particles or liquid adhesives, surgical techniques, and combined surgical and endovascular therapy, have been performed to close fistulas completely.[37,39]

Recent advancements in the treatment of SSS AV fistulas involve transarterial and transvenous embolization with particles and/or liquid adhesives. For cases in which total occlusion cannot be achieved or revascularization has occurred, combined endovascular techniques plus neurosurgical treatment is needed. Therapy should be chosen on an individual basis, considering the angiographic appearance of the lesions and the feasibility of safe endovascular access. If a fistulous channel is large enough to introduce a microcatheter into the draining vein, microcoils can be used as embolic material. If endovascular therapy fails to eliminate the fistula, simple surgical coagulation and division of the fistulous draining vein needs to be performed.[39]

SURGERY

Understanding anatomy and surgical landmarks is crucial for successful surgery and prevention of complications. In surgeries near the cranial venous sinuses, localization of the SSS, transverse sinus, and sigmoid sinus is critical to prevent sinus tearing and air embolism.[41] Neurosurgeons often assume that the sagittal suture is an external landmark of the SSS,[41] but Tubbs et al.[23] studied the relation of the SSS to sagittal suture and demonstrated that in the majority of cases, the SSS deviated to the right of the sagittal suture.

The SSS was deviated to the right side of the sagittal suture in 54% at the bregma and 64% at the midpoint of the sagittal suture and the lambda. The maximal deviation was approximately 10 mm to the right side. It was located approximately 3.5 mm at the bregma, 4.5 mm at the midpoint of the sagittal suture, and 5.7 mm at the lambda. Samadian et al.[41] noted that there were no sex-associated differences in the variations of SSS deviations.

Significant dural sinus injury occurs in 1.5%–5% of all head injuries, in which injury to the SSS accounts for 70%–80%. Injuries of the SSS are attributable to the direct impact of the fracture, extension of the fracture line over the sinus area, or coronal suture diastases. Injury to the anterior third of the sagittal sinus occurs in 80% of injuries, whereas injuries to the middle third occur in 20%.[42]

When parasagittal meningiomas invade the SSS, they can be extremely challenging lesions to remove completely without causing significant morbidity. This is especially true when the posterior two-thirds of the SSS are involved. Opening and resecting the sinus raises concerns of intraoperative and postoperative hemorrhage, sinus occlusion, and corticovenous thrombosis. Many neurosurgeons continue to consider sinus invasion a deterrent to radical surgery. However, subtotal resection is associated with a high rate of tumor recurrence. Some authors advocate aggressive resection of tumors followed by sinus reconstruction via a patch for meningiomas with partial sinus invasion and via a venous bypass for those with total sinus occlusion. Immediate mortality from surgery of parasagittal meningiomas is significant, ranging from 3.7% to 12.3% in different studies. Recent advances in neurosurgical evaluation, especially preoperative assessment of venous drainage pathways and the advent of microsurgical techniques, have played a major role in improving these patients' outcomes. Although meningiomas can arise along the anterior third of the SSS, their removal poses fewer anatomic challenges compared with tumors that arise along the middle and posterior thirds.[43] During surgery, the SSS can be ligated or resected safely anterior to the entry of the Rolandic veins. In contrast, ligation between the Rolandic veins and the torcular Herophili can cause hemiparesis and obtundation.[44]

REFERENCES

1. Curé JK, Tassel PV, Smith MT. Normal and variant anatomy of the dural venous sinuses. *Semin Ultrasound CT MR*. 1994;15:499–519.
2. Deshaies EM, Eddleman CS. *Handbook of Neuroendovascular Surgery*. New York, NY: Thieme; 2012.
3. Bailey FR, Miller AM. *Textbook of Embryology*. 2nd ed. York, PA: The MaplePress; 1989.
4. Jinkins JR. *Atlas of Neuroradiologic Embryology, Anatomy and Variants*. Philadelphia, PA: Lippincott Williams and Wilkins; 2000:369.
5. Salzer H. Über die Entwicklung der Kopfvenen des Meerschweinens. *Morph. Jahrb*. 1895:23–12. 232–255.
6. Butler H. The development of certain human dura; venous sinuses. *J Anat*. 1957;91:510.
7. Streeter GL. The development of the venous sinuses of the dura mater in human embryo. *Am J Anat*. 1915;18:2.
8. Browder J, Kaplan HA. *Cerebral Dural Sinuses and Their Tributaries*. Springfield, MA: Charles C Thomas; 1976:3–12. 45–56.
9. Evans HM. The development of the vascular system. In: Keibel F, Mall FP, eds. *Manual of Human Embryology*. Vol. 2. Philadelphia; 1912:676–680.
10. Kiliç T, Akakin A. Anatomy of cerebral veins and sinuses. *Front Neurol Neurosci*. 2008;23:4–15.
11. Mancall EL, Brock DG. *Gray's Clinical Neuroanatomy: The Anatomic Basis for Clinical Neuroscience*. Philadelphia, PA: Elsevier Saunders; 2011:71–74.
12. Ruíz SM. Systèmes veineux de la base du crâne et de la junction cranio-cervicale: anatomie macroscopique et radiologique et implications cliniques. *Thèse de doctorat: Univ. Genève, no. Méd*. 2006:10493.
13. Brockmann C, Kunze SC, Schmiedek P, Groden C, Scharf J. Variations of the superior sagittal sinus and bridging veins in human dissections and computed tomography venography. *Clin Imag*. 2012;36:85–89.
14. Shao Y, Sun JL, Yang Y, Qk C, Zhang QL. Endoscopic and microscopic anatomy of the superior sagittal sinus and torcular herophili. *J Clin Neurosci*. 2009;16:421–424.
15. Sharifi M, Kunicki J, Krajewski P, Ciszek B. Endoscopic anatomy of the chordae Willisii in the superior sagittal sinus. *J Neurosurg*. 2004;101:832–835.
16. Schmutz HK. The chordae Willisii in the superior sagittal sinus: morphology and classification. *Acta Anat*. 1980;108:94–97.
17. Petroni S, Marrone AC. Study of the trabecular projections (chordae Willisii) of the superior sagittal sinus. *Ital J Anat Embryol*. 1997;102:155–163.
18. Kedzia A, Kedzia W. Morphology of the Willis chords in the superior sagittal sinus during various periods of life. *Folia Morphol*. 2003;62:255–257.
19. Hoffmann A, Stoffel MH, Nitzsche B, et al. The bovine cerebral venous system: comparative anatomy, visualization, and implications for translational research. *PLoS One*. 2014;9:e92990.
20. Ruíz SM, Fasel JHD, Gailloud P. Unilateral hypoplasia of the rostral end of the superior sagittal sinus. *AJNR Am J Neuroradiol*. 2012;33:286–291.
21. Baltsavias G, Bhatti A, Valavanis S. Lateral convexial tributary sinus of superior sagittalsinus. A rare anatomic variation and the importance of its recognition. *Clin Neurol Neurosurg*. 2013;115:2268–2269.
22. Kocak B, Hasiloglu KO, Kocer N, Aydin S, Islak C. Total agenesis of superior sagittal sinus and falx cerebri in a patient who has a subacute subdural hematoma crossing midline: case report. *Neurosurgery*. 2013;5:863–867.
23. Tubbs RS, Salter G, Elton S, Grabb PA, Oakes WJ. Sagittal suture as an external landmark for the superior sagittal sinus. *J Neurosurg*. 2001;94:985–987.
24. Tubbs RS, Loukas M. Duplication of the superior sagittal sinus. *Clin Anat*. 2006;19:728.
25. Kaplan HA, Browder J. Atresia of the rostral superior sagittal sinus: substitute parasagittal venous channel. *J Neurosurg*. 1973;38:602–607.
26. Manoj KS, Krishnamoorthy T, Thomas B, Kapilamoorthy TR. An incidental persistent falcine sinus with dominant straight sinus and hypoplastic distal sagittal sinus. *Pediatr Radiol*. 2006;36:65–67.
27. Scott JN, Farb RI. Imaging and anatomy of the intracranial venous systems. Neuroimag. *Cin N Am*. 2003;13:1–12.
28. Brant WE, Helms CA. *Fundamentals of Diagnostic Radiology*. 3rd ed. Philadelphia, PA: Lippincott Williams and Wilkins; 2007:107–108.
29. Stam J. Thrombosis of the cerebral veins and sinuses. *N Engl J Med*. 2005;352:1791–1798.
30. Liang L, Korogi Y, Sugahara T, et al. Normal structures in the intracranial dural sinuses: delineation with 3D contrast- enhanced magnetization prepared rapid acquisition. *AJNR Am J Neuroradiol*. 2002;23:1739–1746.
31. Hwang J, Kwon K, Hur J, Lee J, Lee H. The role of hyperthyroidism as the predisposing factor for superior sagittal sinus thrombosis. *J Cerebrovasc Endovasc Neurosurg*. 2012;14:251–254.
32. Ferro JM, Canhao P, Stam J, Bousser MG, Barinagarrementeria F. Prognosis of cerebral vein and dural sinus thrombosis: results of the international study on cerebral vein and dural sinus thrombosis. *Stroke*. 2004;35:664–670.
33. Siegert CEH, Smelt AHM, de Bruin TWA. Superior sagittal sinus thrombosis and thyrotoxicosis: possible association between two cases. *Stroke*. 1995;26:496–497.
34. Ameri A, Bousser MG. Cerebral venous thrombosis. *Neurol Clin*. 1992;10:87–111.
35. Dai A, Wasay M, Dubey N, Giglio P, Bakshi X. Superior sagittal sinus thrombosis secondary to hyperthyroidism. *J Stroke Cerebrovasc Dis*. 2000;9:89–90.
36. Forbes J, Reig A, Tomycz L, Tulipan N. Intracranial hypertension caused by a depressed skull fracture resulting in superior sagittal sinus thrombosis in a pediatric patient: treatment with ventriculoperitoneal shunt insertion. *J Neurosurg Pediatr*. 2010;6:23–28.

37. Kurl S, Saari T, Vanninen R, Hernesniemi J. Dural arteriovenous fistulas of superior sagittal sinus: case report and review of literature. *Surg Neurol*. 1996;45:250–255.
38. Schmid-Elsaesser R, Muacevic A, Bruckmann H, Wowra. *Neurosurgery of Arteriovenous Malformations and Fistulas: A Multimodal Approach*. New York, NY: Springer-Verlag Wien; 2012:132.
39. Fukai J, Terada T, Kuwata T, et al. Transarterial intravenous coil embolization of dural arteriovenous fistula involving the superior sagittal sinus. *Surg Neurol*. 2001;55:353–358.
40. Acton QA. *Arteriovenous Malformations: Advances in Research and Treatment*. Atlanta, GA: Scholarly Editions; 2012.
41. Samadian M, Nazparvar B, Haddadian K, Rezaer O, Khormaee F. The anatomical relationship between the superior sagittal sinus and the sagittal suture with surgical considerations. *Clin Neurol Neurosurg*. 2011;113:89–91.
42. Behera SK, Senapati SB, Mishra SS, Das S. Management of superior sagittal sinus injury encountered in traumatic head injury patients: analysis of 15 cases. *Asian J Neurosurg*. 2015;10:17–20.
43. DiMeco F, Li KW, Casali C, et al. Meningiomas invading the superior sagittal sinus: surgical experience in 108 cases. *Neurosurgery*. 2004;55:1263–1274.
44. Andrews BT, Dujovny M, Mirchandani HG, Ausman JI. Microsurgical anatomy of the venous drainage into the superior sagittal sinus. *Neurosurgery*. 1989;24:514–520.

FURTHER READING

1. Caso V, Agnelli G, Paciaroni M. In: *Handbook on Cerebral Venous Thrombosis*. Karger; 2008.
2. Curé JK, Van Tassel P. Congenital and acquired abnormalities of the dural venous sinuses. *Semin Ultrasound CT MR*. 1994;15:520–539.
3. Lasjaunias P, Kwok R, Goh P, Yeong KY, Lim W, Chang SM. A developmental theory of the superior sagittal sinus(es) in craniopagus twins. *Childs Nerv Syst*. 2004;20:526–537.
4. Steiger HJ, Reulen HJ, Huber P, Boll J. Radical resection of superior sagittal sinus meningioma with venous interposition graft and reimplantation of the rolandic veins. *Acta Neuroschi (Wien)*. 1989;100:108–111.
5. Yaşargil MG, Teddy PJ, Duverno HM. *AVM of the Brain, History, Embryology, Pathological Considerations, Hemodynamics, Diagnostic Studies, Microsurgical Anatomy*. New York, NY: Thieme; 1987.

CHAPTER 3

Inferior Sagittal Sinus

GALYNA IVASHCHUK • R. SHANE TUBBS

ANATOMY

The inferior sagittal sinus (ISS) (Figs. 3.1–3.3) is a part of the superior group of dural venous sinuses,[1] and as a member of the superficial cerebral venous system, it drains the superficial surfaces of both cerebral hemispheres. The ISS is established by drainage of veins from the medial aspect of the frontal lobes of the brain, collecting veins coursing for the most part in the rostral sulci of the cingulate gyri.[2,2a] The ISS begins above the level of the anterior body of the corpus callosum from the crista galli and receives blood from the medial cerebral hemispheres, falx cerebri, corpus callosum, and cingulate gyri before draining into the straight sinus together with the vein of Galen[1]. Veins typically enter the ISS just above the anterior portion of the corpus callosum, where the entrance forms an acute bend in the lateral projection, with the apex of the bend being the actual origin of the sinus itself.[3] Small veins from the inferior part of the cingulate gyrus join it in its course caudally, where it is joined frequently by branches of veins from the dorsal surface of the corpus callosum. It receives tributaries from the falx cerebri, some of which establish substantial connections between the superior sagittal sinus (SSS) and the ISS[2a]. The ISS runs caudally in the free border of the falx cerebri to join the rostral aspect of the straight sinus and increases in size, while remaining very narrow and flat, unlike the other dural venous sinuses that tend to be triangular in shape.[2] It may lay up to 3 mm from the midline in normal patients.[1]

The ISS is cylindrical in form and usually increases in diameter as it passes posteriorly. In 15% of specimens, there is a bulbous termination, which continues caudally to form the rostral aspect of the straight sinus.[2a] The inner aspect of the ISS is smooth except for an occasional slitlike orifice that joins venous channels from the falx cerebri. The ISS is absent in approximately 1% of cadavers and is often more pronounced in young children and infants than in adults.[2a] It may communicate with the SSS via veins that lie within the falx cerebri.[1]

EMBRYOLOGY

A chain of angioblasts forms along the border of the hindbrain and produces a capillary meshwork to cover the structure. Then, a capillary plexus forms from the aortic arch and creates a vascular network that spreads upward to invest the fore and midbrains. These plexuses unite to cover the entire brain and are referred to as the primary head plexus, the precursor of blood vessels in the brain.[2a] As the meninges develop dorsally, intermediate venous connections from the deep to superficial venous plexus are cut off, except those that unite major dural sinuses. In the early phase of formation of the superficial dural venous plexus, channels at the ventral midline coalesce to form larger venous lakes.[2a] Large lakes lying between the diencephalon and optic bulb represent forerunners of the rostral part of the primary head vein, which ultimately becomes the cavernous sinus. Tributaries that drain into the primary head vein join it primarily along the dorsal margin. Ventral tributaries are numerous around the optic stalk and trigeminal ganglion. Branches of the superficial dural plexus of the primary head vein comprise three groups—anterior, middle, and posterior.[2a] In 14 mm CR embryos, the vascular mesh of the dorsal aspects of the anterior and middle dural plexuses advances toward the mid-dorsal aspect of the telencephalon to form the sagittal plexus. Rostrally, this network dips between the developing cerebral hemispheres, and the superior and inferior sagittal sinuses originate in this mesh.

VARIATIONS

The entrance of the veins into the ISS can be variable and has a double hook effect, with small veins draining the upper portion of the corpus callosum. In addition, it can form a gradual hook, with large veins draining the medial hemisphere more anteriorly than usual. Least commonly, most of the veins enter the anterior portion of the sinus from above.[3] Tributaries that drain the posterior aspect of the ISS usually are seen as collaterals in patients with SSS obstruction.[3] Furthermore, embryogenic drainage of the ISS can persist. In these

Anatomy, Imaging and Surgery of the Intracranial Dural Venous Sinuses. https://doi.org/10.1016/B978-0-323-65377-0.00003-9

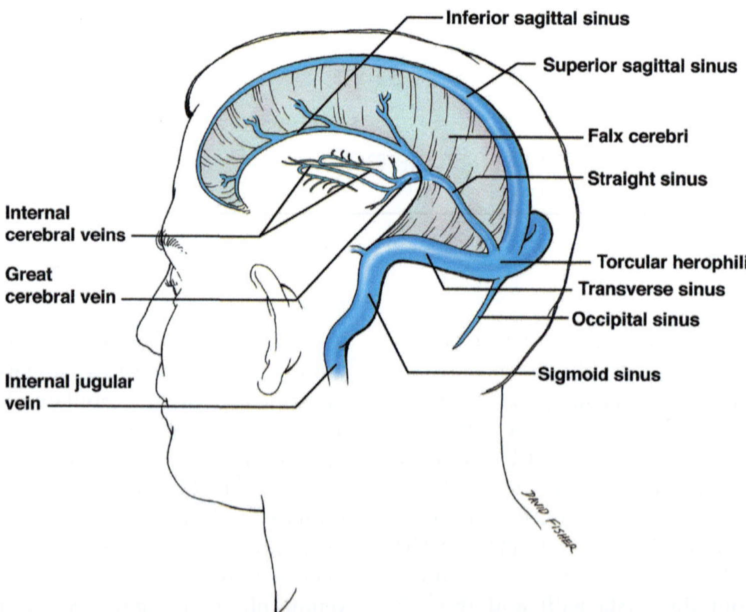

FIG. 3.1 Schematic drawing of the major intradural venous sinuses noting the inferior sagittal sinus.

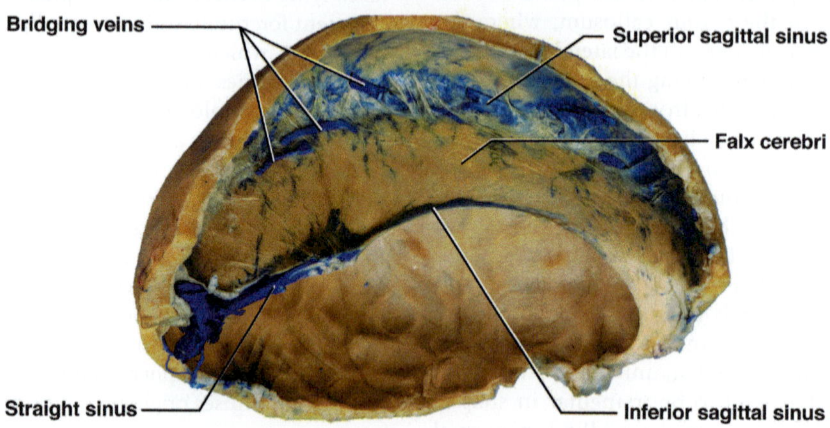

FIG. 3.2 Internal view of the calvaria with intact falx cerebri and inferior sagittal sinus. Note the drainage of the inferior sagittal sinus posteriorly into the straight sinus.

cases, the ISS runs upward and backward between the dural layers of the falx cerebri and drains into the SSS approximately 4 cm above the internal occipital protuberance.[4] The ISS also may drain directly into the SSS, above the torcular Herophili.[1]

A hypoplastic rostral SSS has been found to be associated with additional compensatory drainage through a large ISS by way of the interhemispheric frontal vein.[5]

The SSS may communicate with the ISS in the falx cerebri through a venous channel, and the connection can be sufficiently significant that the SSS will drain primarily into the ISS and straight sinuses.[6] Falcine plexus veins ranging in size from 0.5 to 1.1 cm all have been found to communicate with the ISS and can be divided into subtypes according to their communication with the SSS. Type I have no communication, type II have

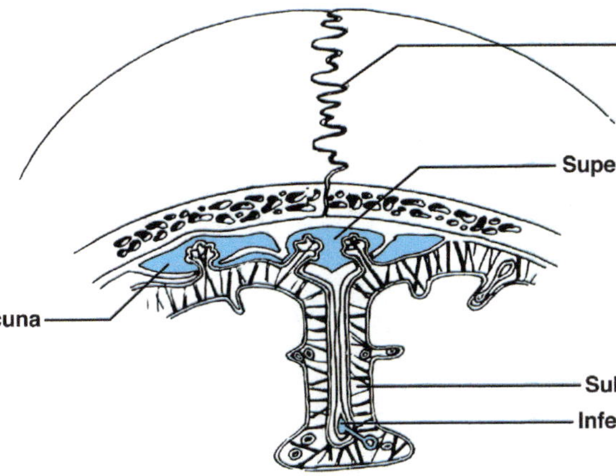

FIG. 3.3 Schematic drawing of a coronal slice through the skull and brain noting the relationship of the inferior sagittal sinus.

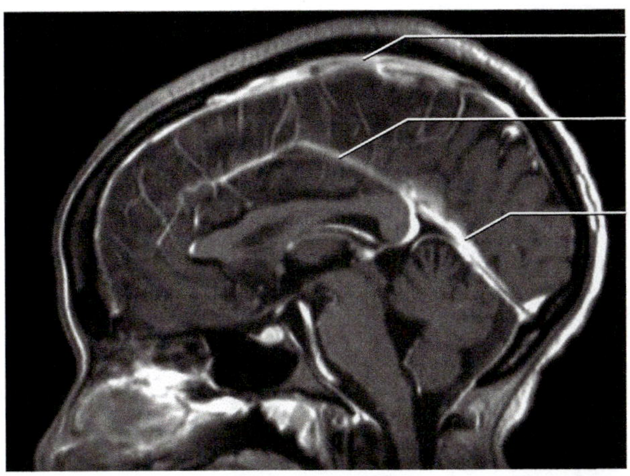

FIG. 3.4 Midsagittal T1-weighted MRI postcontrast illustrating the inferior sagittal sinus.

limited, and type III have significant communication with the SSS, such that the majority of falcine vessels communicate with it.[6] Most of these vessels exist in the posterior inferior one-third of the falx cerebri.

IMAGING

The ISS and its tributaries may be useful in identifying other structures in the brain during imaging (Figs. 3.3–3.6). It can help localize the anterior midline of the brain during the venous phase of a cerebral angiogram, as well as the position of the anterior portion of the callosal cistern and inferior margin of the falx cerebri.[3]

Options for imaging dural venous sinuses (DVSs) include conventional (intraarterial digital subtraction) angiography, intravenous digital subtraction angiography, computed tomography (CT), magnetic resonance imaging (MRI), and magnetic resonance angiogram (MRA).[1] The traditional "gold standard" for radiologic diagnosis of DVS disease has been conventional angiography; however, MRI and magnetic resonance venography (MRV) essentially have replaced conventional angiography. MRV is a useful, rapid, and noninvasive tool that allows visualization of thrombus within a dural sinus (Erabs et al., 2006), and angiographic methods enable 3D visualization of blood vessels.[7] Conventional angiography is performed through

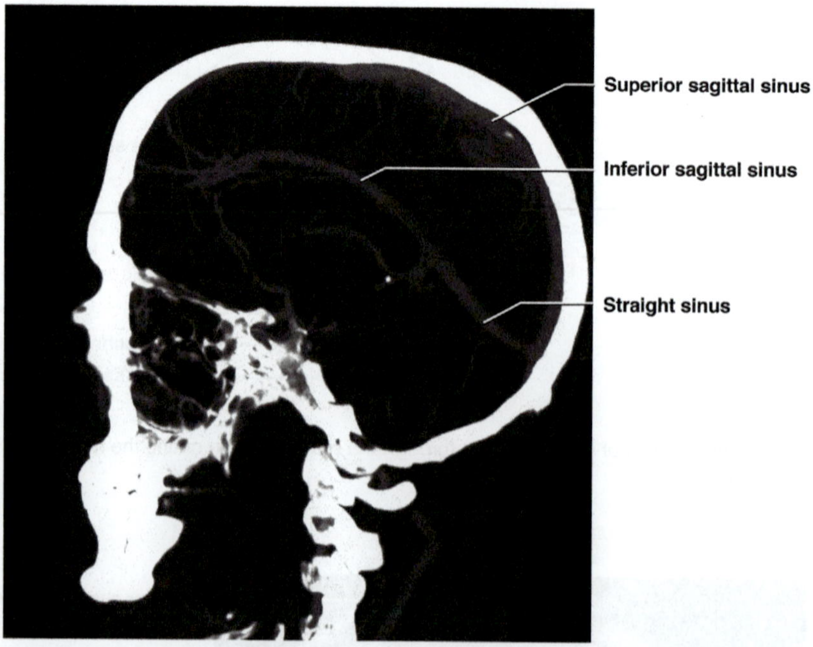

FIG. 3.5 CT image illustrating an enlarged inferior sagittal sinus.

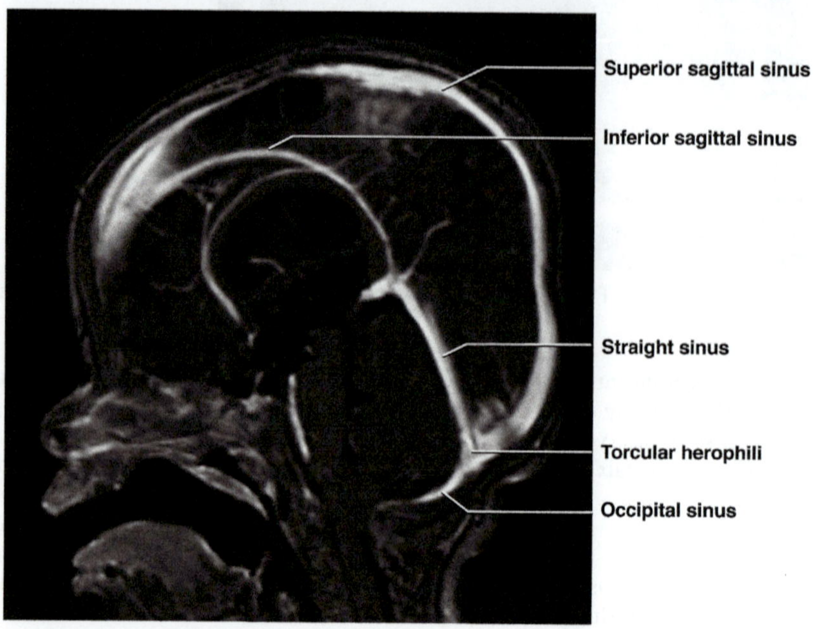

FIG. 3.6 Midsagittal T1-weighted MRI postcontrast illustrating the inferior sagittal sinus. Also note this pediatric patient has ventriculomegaly and Chiari I malformation.

internal carotid artery catherization, although it may fail to demonstrate the ISS.[8] Bilateral simultaneous common carotid artery injections achieve consistently good venous opacification without streaming artifacts and without the high volumes of contrast media required for the intravenous method.[8] Visualization of DVS is optimized with photographic or digital subtraction techniques. Ten degree anterior-posterior (AP) oblique and lateral projections are ideal for showing the DVS pathway. On MRI, patent DVS shows signal voids.[1] Flow-related enhancement may be seen on entry slices of short repetition time imaging series, but this artifactual high signal is not seen in all imaging planes within patent sinuses. The presence of phase shift–induced flow artifacts propagated for the vein with a bright luminal signal confirms the presence of at least some flow. Sinus thrombosis may be overlooked in long TR images when the luminal clot consists largely of constituents that produce T2-weighted shortening (deoxyhemoglobin, intracellular methemoglobin). However, the luminal signal in these thrombosed sinuses is abnormal in short TR images, such that they are either isointense (deoxyhemoglobin) or hyperintense (methemoglobin) to gray matter.[1] When there is some doubt, large flip angle 2D gradient-echo sequences oriented perpendicular to the long axis of the vessel can show occlusion or flow in the vein in question. If there is further doubt thereafter, phase contrast MRA techniques can be implemented. It is more practical to perform MRV using the 2D time-of-flight (TOF) technique, although some report only 52% visualization of the ISS with the technique.[9] The ISS is seen best on axial acquisitions with 75%, using thinner slices, which visualized the ISS in the majority of patients imaged coronally.[1]

The ISS has been shown to be visualized better with VIBE (steady-state contrast-enhanced 3D) than TR (time-resolved, contrast-enhanced 3D MR angio), with the worse visualization using MRV.[7] Conventional CT and MR are unable to diagnose cerebral venous disease correctly, although CT venography is available widely and is a rapid method to diagnose dural sinus thrombosis.[7] There are some challenges in delineating between patent sinus, chronic sinus obliteration, and occlusion by intravenous thrombus with a steady-state, contrast-enhanced MRV (VIBE MRV). Magnetic resonance is superior to CT in evaluating parenchymal abnormalities that are associated with cerebral venous disease.

DVS thrombosis in non–contrast-enhanced cranial CT can be seen as a cord sign (hyperdense bridging vein) or empty delta sign.

Ultrasound has been used to visualize DVS in neonates. Blood flow in the ISS can be visualized in almost all newborns but can be resolved as a distinct vessel in only 50% of neonates because of its course along the inferior margin of the falx cerebri.[10] The ISS can be visualized distinctly from the vein of Galen in a fraction of cases.

PATHOLOGY

Dural Venous Sinus Thrombosis

DVS thrombosis is a rare form of stroke that is responsible for 10% of cerebral ischemic lesions, and 1%–2% of strokes in young adults, in which a third of cases involve more than one sinus,[8,11] and it presents more commonly in young patients.[11] Cerebral venous thrombosis (CVT) is similar to Virchow's triad and presents as stasis of blood, changes in vessel walls, and changes in the composition of blood.[11] DVS thrombosis is associated with severe dehydration, hypercoagulable states (antithrombin III, protein C and protein S deficiency, antiphospholipid and anticardiolipin antibodies, resistance to activated protein C and factor V Leiden, mutation G202101 of factor II, hyperhomocysteinemia), infection, tumor invasion, dural sinus compression, CNS lymphoma, Behcet disease, inflammatory bowel disease, and oral contraceptive use.[9,11] Some of the hypercoagulable states can be attributable to low protein S levels.[8]

ISS thrombosis can present as unsteady gait, foot drop, focal seizures, headache, vomiting, papilledema, and loss of consciousness[8]. Acute occlusion of cerebral venous outflow is tolerated poorly, and venous HTN leads to stasis of blood in the capillaries and transudation of fluid, causing hypoxia and venous infarctions. Hemodynamic and parenchymal effects of dural sinus thrombosis depend on many factors, such as site extent, rapidity of occlusion, and anatomy of collateral pathways.

A unique case has been presented of ISS thrombosis associated with lipoprotein(a) increase and iron deficiency anemia (IDA).[11] A case of a 21-year-old female who presented with headache, abnormal movement, weakness of the right arm and leg, and blurred vision and was found to have bilateral papilledema, right hemiparesis, negative myoclonus of the right upper extremity, bilateral Babinski sign, and brisk deep tendon reflexes of the right side has been described in the literature.[11] MRI and MRV were performed, and T2-weighted and FLAIR-weighted sequences showed an increased signal in the splenium of the corpus callosum, and frontal and parietal subcortical regions bilaterally. T1-weighted MR showed thickening and diffuse enhancement of the dura mater over the falx cerebri. MRV showed patent SSS, straight, transverse, and sigmoid sinuses, with irregular appearance and poor detection of the ISS. The CBC was remarkable for iron deficiency anemia and increased Lp(a). Several reasons have been postulated why iron deficiency can lead to thrombosis. Thrombocytosis secondary to IDA causes thrombosis, as iron is a regulator of thrombopoiesis. Normal iron levels are needed to prevent thrombocytosis by inhibiting thrombopoiesis. IDA leads to a hypercoagulable state, because microcytosis causes RBCs to deform and increases viscosity. Anemic hypoxia causes ischemic damage in the brain supplied by terminal arteries.[11]

A third of all cases of dural sinus thrombosis present with thrombi in more than one sinus. One case was that of a patient who had both ISS and SSS thrombosis.[12] A 27-year-old female who had headache and right facial nerve paresis for 25 days, and left hemiparesis for 2 days, which had been improving, developed horizontal and vertical diplopia suddenly, as well as vomiting and generalized seizures the same day. On neurologic examination, she was found to be somnolent, disoriented with GCS of 9, had neck stiffness, right fourth, sixth, and mild seventh cranial nerve palsies, papilledema, right orbital venous congestion, and mild left hemiparesis. Lumbar puncture was significant for increased intracranial pressure and xanthochromia. On the day of admission, MR showed sagittal sinus thrombosis, whereas carotid angiography and MRV showed complete SSS and ISS thrombosis and prominent collateral venous circulation. The patient was treated with medical therapy, and at follow-up, neurologic symptoms had resolved.[12]

Aneurysms and Arteriovenous Malformations

The ISS also can develop aneurysms. One case of autopsy of a 23-year-old demonstrated that the diameter of the straight sinus was twice the normal size, the lumen was like a cylindrical tube, and was 8 mm in diameter, the cavity in the falx cerebri measured 28 × 16 × 11 mm, and the rostral segment of the ISS was not dilated. There was a plicalike fold over the superior half of the opening at the junction with the anterior-inferior aspect of the cavity in the falx cerebri. Caudally, the walls of the sac were funnel-shaped, tapering to the enlarged straight sinus. In addition to aneurysm of the ISS, the vein of Galen, two veins from the left cerebral hemisphere, and a third more caudal in the upper falx cerebri were involved.[2a]

Intracranial tumors can efface the ISS. Parasagittal astrocytoma has been reported to displace the ISS and its tributaries across the midline and displace the lateral colossal vein inferiorly.[3] Corpus callosum gliomas have been reported to displace the ISS from the midline and also are associated with displacement of the lower edge of the falx cerebri, and elevation of veins above the corpus callosum.[3] A left frontal pole glioma can shift the anterior cerebral artery and the anterior colossal vein that drains into the ISS. A left frontal pole meningioma has been reported to be associated with tributaries entering the sinus at a prominent bend and the ISS shifting from left to right associated with displacement of its tributaries. Intracranial tumors also can lead to pathologic circulation, with AV shunting to a tributary of the ISS and to the septal vein in a patient with a deep frontal malignant glioma.[3]

Congenital venous aneurysms can form when arterial blood is shunted under high pressure through a maldeveloped capillary system, and high-pressured blood under arterial pressure enters thin-walled veins, which dilate and become aneurysmal in appearance.[13] The ISS also can develop aneurysms that lead to fistulae. Typical symptoms of arteriovenous fistula with intracranial venous hypertension include entry into thin-walled veins, which dilate and become aneurysmal in appearance.[13]

REFERENCES

1. Cure JL, Van Tassel P, Smith MT. Normal and variant anatomy of the dural venous sinuses. *Semin Ultrasound CT MRI*. 1994;15(6):499–519.
2. Swedenborg E, Tafel RL. The brain considered anatomically, physiologically and philosophically. *James Speirs*. 1887;2:275–276.

2a. Browder J, Kaplan HA. *Cerebral Dural Sinuses and Their Tributaries*. Springfield, MA: Charles C Thomas; 1976:3–13. 89–97.

3. McCord GM, Goree JA, Jimenez JP. Venous drainage to the inferior sagittal sinus. *Radiology*. 1972;105:583–589.
4. Lang J. *Clinical Anatomy of the Head*. Berlin: Springer-Verlag; 1983:1–489.
5. Ruiz DSM, Fasel JHD, Gaillloud P. Unilateral hypoplasia of the rostral end of the superior sagittal sinus. *AJNR*. 2012;33:286–291.
6. Tubbs RS, Loukas M, Louis RG, et al. Anatomy of the falcine venous plexus. *J Neurosurg*. 2007;107:155–157.
7. Meckel S, Glucker TM, Kretzschmar M, Scheffler K, Radu E-W, Wetzel SG. Display of dural sinuses with time-resolved, contrast-enhanced three-dimensional MR venography. *Cerebrovasc Dis*. 2008;25:217–224.
8. Elsherbiny SM, Grunewald RA, Powell T. Isolated inferior sagittal sinus thrombosis: a case report. *Neuroradiology*. 1997;39:411–413.

9. Ayanzen RH, Bird CR, Keller PJ, McCully FJ, Theobald MR, Heiserman JE. Cerebral MR Venography: normal anatomy and potential diagnostic pitfalls. *AJNR*. 2000;21:74–78.
10. Taylor GA. Intracranial venous system in the newborn: evaluation of normal anatomy and flow characteristics with color Doppler US. *Radiology*. 1992;183(2):449–452.
11. Karakurum-Goksel B, Karaca S, Alkan O, Yildirim T. Isolated inferior sagittal sinus thrombosis caused by a rare combination of elevated lipoprotein (a) and iron deficiency anemia. *Neurosciences*. 2012;17(4):374–377.
12. Topsakal C, Cihangiroglu M, Kaplan M, Akdemir I, Tiftikci M. Complete superior and inferior sagittal sinus thromboses with multiple cranial nerve pareses and transient ischemic attack. *Neurol Med -Chir*. 2002;42:383–386.
13. Seljeskog EL, Rogers HM, French LA. Arteriovenous malformation involving the inferior sagittal sinus in an infant. *J Neurosurg*. 1968;29:623–628.

FURTHER READING

1. Cure JK, Van Tassel P. Congenital and acquired abnormalities of the dural venous sinuses. *Semin Ultrasound CT MRI*. 1994;15(6):520–539.
2. Morgan MK, Sundt Jr TM, Houser OW. Arterio-inferior sagittal sinus fistulae: case report. *Neurosurgery*. 1989;25(6): 971–975.

CHAPTER 4

The Transverse Sinus

JOE IWANAGA

EMBRYOLOGY

In 18-mm embryos, the transverse sinus forms first when the middle dural plexus drains over the otic capsule.[1] In 21-mm-long embryos, the transverse sinus, which begins at the torcular Herophili and empties into the lateral cerebral vein, forms from the anterior cerebral vein. The transverse sinus runs across the cavum epiptericum between the two layers of the tentorium cerebelli, and as the cavum epiptericum reduces in size, it comes to lie in the attached margin of the tentorium cerebelli. The transverse sinus and the tentorium cerebelli then will rotate backward 180° as the cerebral hemisphere expands caudally.[2] In the 23-mm embryo, the transverse sinus divides into two equal channels as it approaches the anterosuperior aspect of the otic capsule.[2] During the period of growth between the 50-mm embryo and the adult, the transverse sinus bends backward until it reaches a 90° angle with the internal jugular vein.[1]

Many studies of fetal venous circulation of the transverse sinus have been reported using ultrasound.[3] The transverse sinus exhibits a triphasic and pulsatile forward-flow velocity pattern similar to that of the other fetal venous vessels.[4]

ANATOMY

The paired transverse sinuses (Figs. 4.1 and 4.2) begin at the torcular Herophili most often located at the internal occipital protuberance,[5–7] and the majority of the external occipital protuberances are located inferior to the internal occipital protuberance.[6] Typically, the superior sagittal sinus continues into the right transverse sinus, and the straight sinus is more likely to drain into the left transverse sinus. Thus, in such cases, the right transverse sinus drains blood from the more superficial parts of the brain and the left transverse sinus drains deeper parts of the brain[8] and is located inferior to the left in roughly 50% of cases.[6] Anatomic asymmetry of the transverse sinuses is common and is considered normal variation because unilateral hypoplasia or aplasia has been observed in 20%–39% of cases.[8–10] On each side, the transverse sinus passes along the posterolateral attached margins of the tentorium cerebelli, anterolaterally along the transverse sinus sulcus, reaching the posterolateral part of the petrous part of the temporal bone, and then turns into the sigmoid sinus. The transverse sinus receives blood draining from the superior petrosal sinus, bridging veins from the occipital lobe and cerebellum (Fig. 4.3), diploic veins, and the labyrinthine vein if it does not drain into the superior petrosal sinus.

Strydom et al.[11] found that 53% of transverse sinuses contained arachnoid granulations and trabeculae/septa, both of which could result in potential venous filling defects, and were more commonly on the right side. These authors mentioned that these fibrous bands or septa may act as wall reinforcements to prevent the sinus walls from overdilating or collapsing.[11]

VARIATIONS

Although the transverse sinuses can be symmetrical (Figs. 4.4 and 4.5), left and right sides are asymmetrical. According to Hollinshead,[12] the most clinically significant variation in the region of the torcular Herophili is the hypoplasia or absence of a transverse or sigmoid sinus. It is important to identify such variations because they may yield false-positive results for venous thrombosis, for example, Tobey-Ayer-Queckenstedt tests. These are used in the diagnosis of unilateral and bilateral sinus thrombophlebitis. In cases where the sinus is obstructed on one side, compression of the internal jugular vein on the intact side causes a rise in CSF pressure, whereas compression of the obstructed side does not raise CSF pressure.

Lower (1881) was the first to report that the right transverse sinus is slightly moderately larger than the left, especially in men[13] (Fig. 4.6). This is thought to be due to the natural continuation of the sagittal sinus to the right side.[14,15] In almost all related studies, the right transverse sinus was dominant four times more frequently than was the left.[16] However, the left transverse sinus also has been reported to be larger and

Anatomy, Imaging and Surgery of the Intracranial Dural Venous Sinuses. https://doi.org/10.1016/B978-0-323-65377-0.00004-0

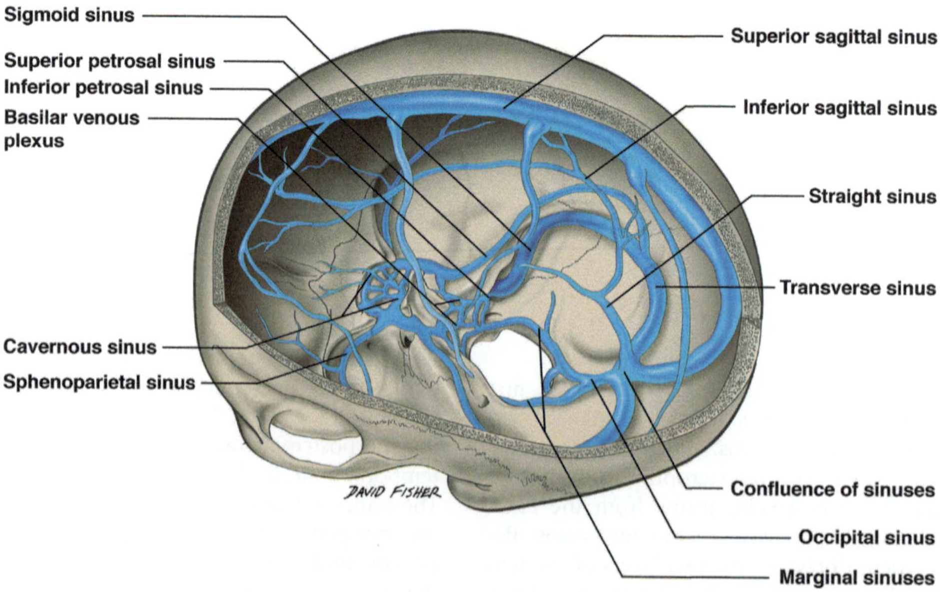

FIG. 4.1 Schematic drawing of the intracranial venous sinuses.

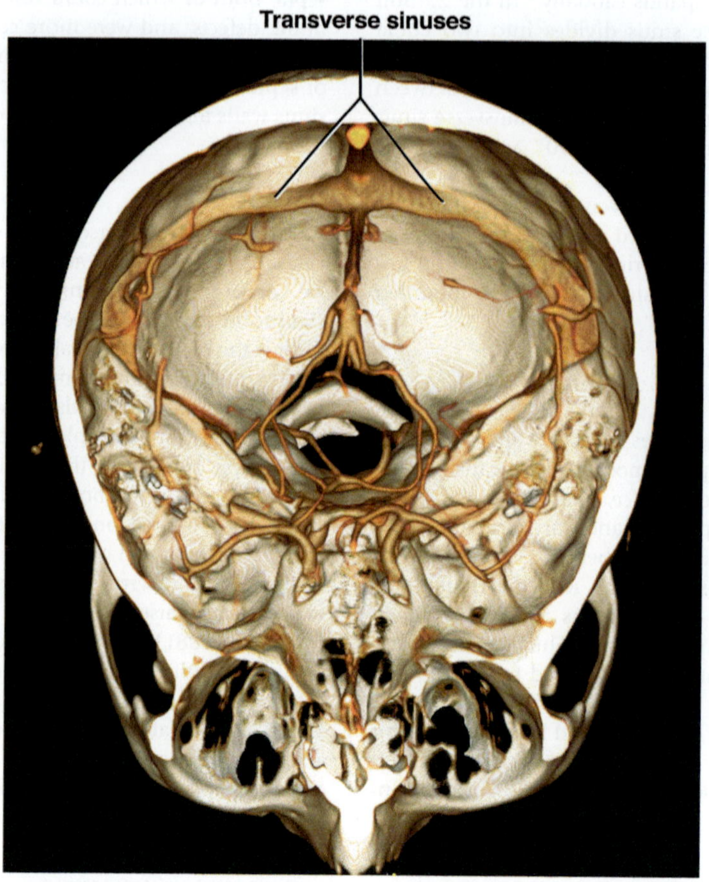

FIG. 4.2 3D reconstruction CT illustrating the transverse sinuses. (Courtesy Dr. Joel Curé.)

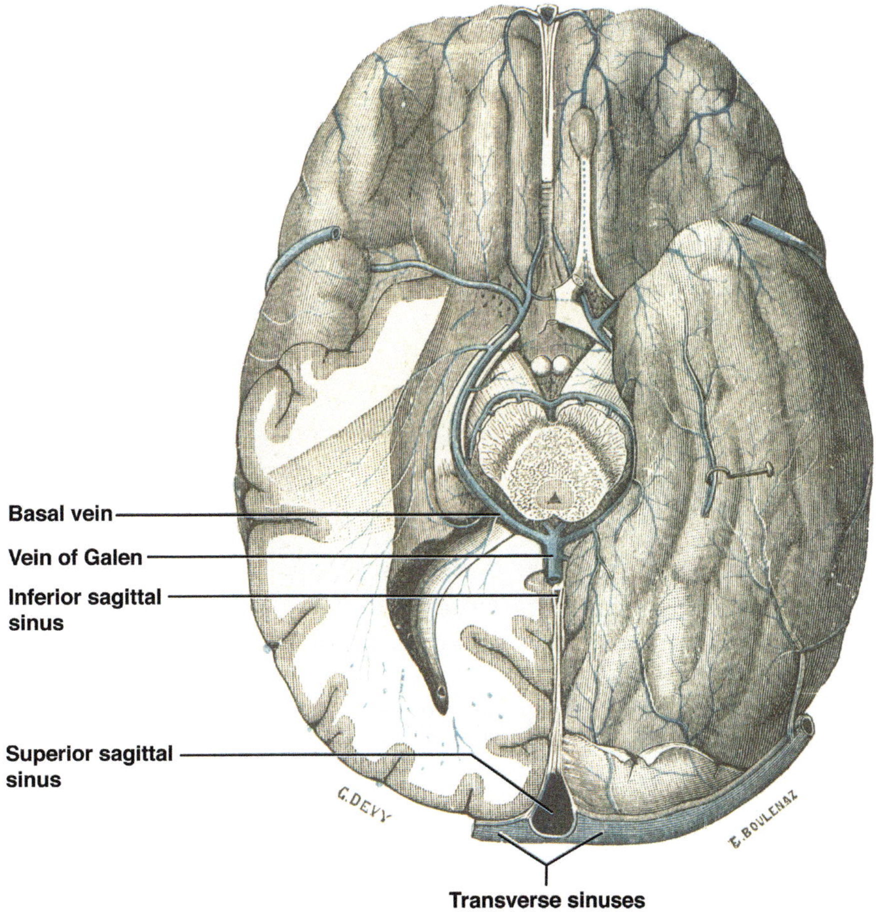

FIG. 4.3 Bridging veins draining the occipital lobe into the transverse sinus. (After Testut.)

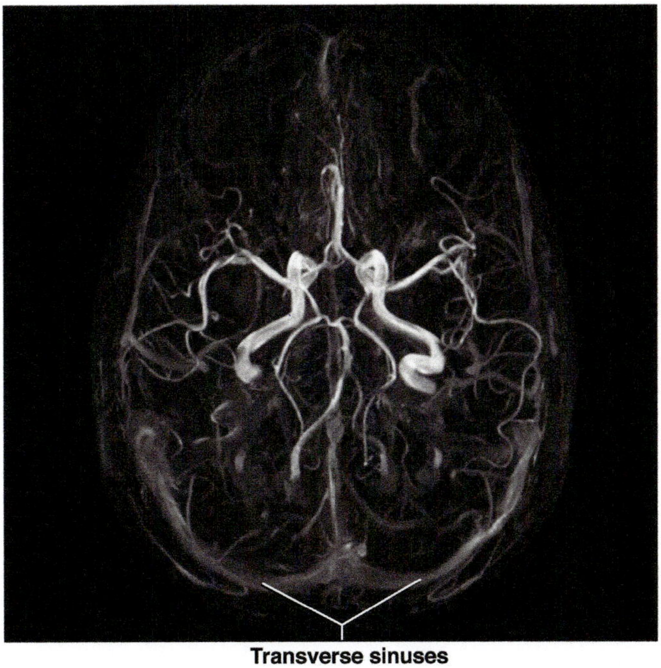

FIG. 4.4 MR angiography noting the circle of Willis and transverse sinuses.

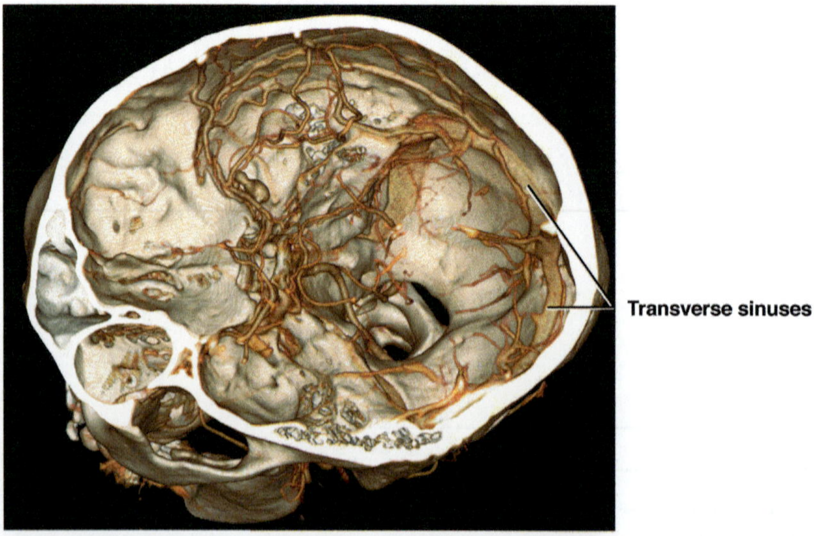

FIG. 4.5 3D reconstruction CT illustrating the transverse sinuses. (Courtesy Dr. Joel Curé.)

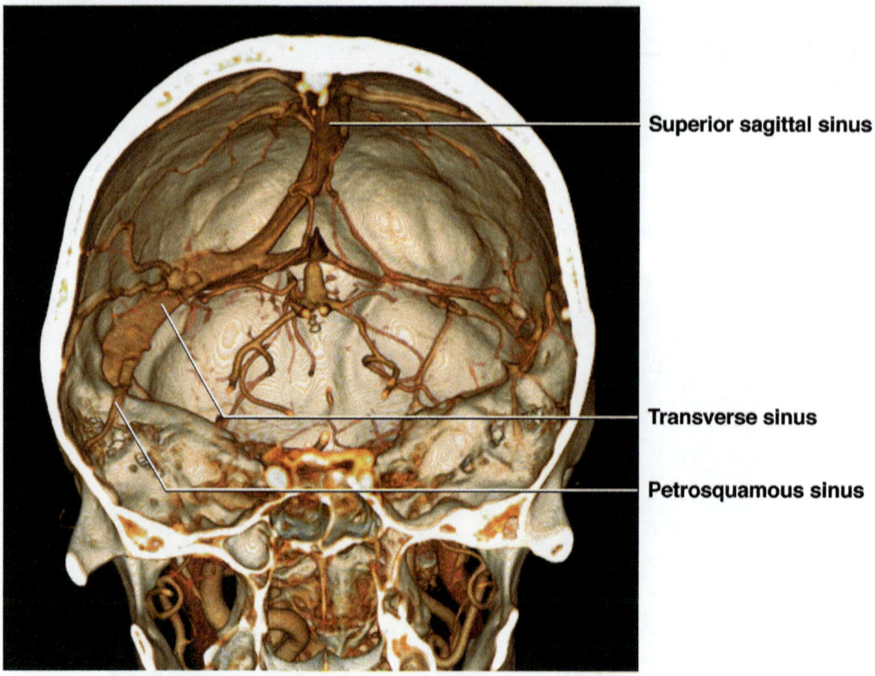

FIG. 4.6 3D reconstruction CT illustrating the transverse sinuses. Note the asymmetry between the left and right transverse sinuses. (Courtesy Dr. Joel Curé.)

longer than the right in some individuals[17] (Surendrababu et al., 2006).[36] Among the 31 cases that Woodhall examined (1936), 6 had a dominant transverse sinus on the right side, whereas 3 had a dominant sinus on the left. Browder et al.[14] studied 215 specimens and found that 33% showed right side dominance, 16% showed equal dominance (Figs. 4.7 and 4.8), 8% showed left side dominance, and the remainder had a variety of

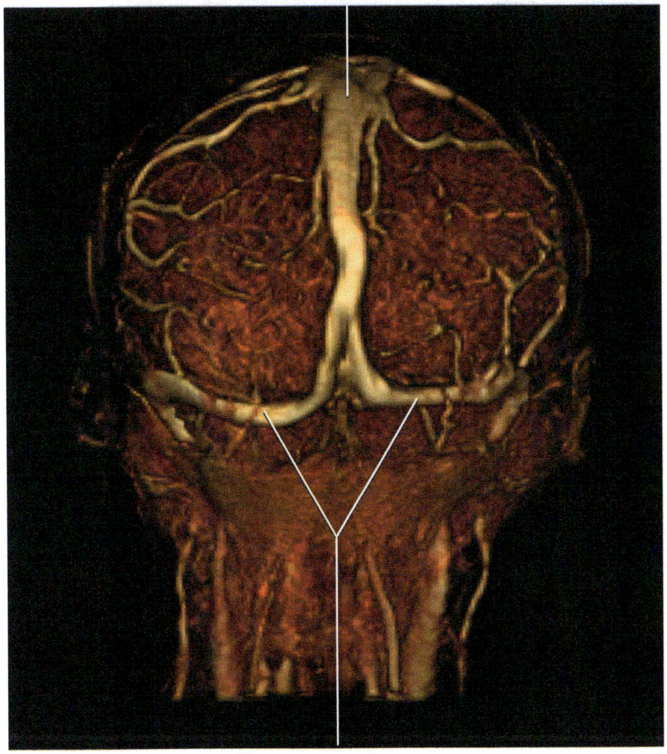

FIG. 4.7 3D reconstruction illustrating the transverse sinuses. (Courtesy Dr. Joel Curé.)

developmental aberrations. They observed that, in cases in which the distal 1–3 cm of the superior sagittal sinus was doubled, the smaller channel was the origin of the smaller transverse sinus. In some cases, they found that the lumen of the transverse sinus was narrowed by the presence of a vascular septum (Fig. 4.9). Another variation that Browder et al.[14] (1976) found was the presence of numerous connections joining the torcular Herophili to the transverse sinus: as many as five openings were observed in some specimens. In these cases, the transverse sinus usually was smaller on that side.

Hypoplasia of one transverse sinus may be seen.[8,18–21] Although uncommon, the transverse sinus may be completely absent.[14,15,22,23] Aplasias and hypoplasias are found most often on the left side. Lieutaud[23] recorded cases of complete absence of the left transverse sinus. Knott[22] and Browder and Kaplan (1976) described bilateral diminution of the transverse sinus, in which cases the majority of the blood terminated in the occipital and marginal sinuses. Hahn[24] and Streit[25] described duplication of the transverse sinus.

In transverse sinus aplasias overall, both the superior sagittal and straight sinuses usually drain into the contralateral transverse sinus, and in such cases, the superior petrosal sinus can continue directly into the sigmoid sinus.[8,26,27] The increased frequency of absent transverse sinuses on magnetic resonance venography (MRV) may be associated with increasing age. Rollins et al.[28] found that one transverse sinus was absent in 5% of patients who were less than 25 months old and in 13% of patients who were older than 25 months old. The authors suggested that this may be attributable to alterations in posterior cranial fossa venous flow patterns rather than structural involution of the transverse sinus. Rarely, the transverse sinus is severely hypoplastic and the contralateral transverse sinus is absent. In such cases, the superior sagittal and straight sinuses can both drain via an enlarged occipital sinus into the superior jugular bulbs.[29]

Developmental abnormalities of the proximal transverse sinus were observed in 13 of 422 specimens that Browder and Kaplan studied (1976). There was narrowing on the right side in five cases, on the left

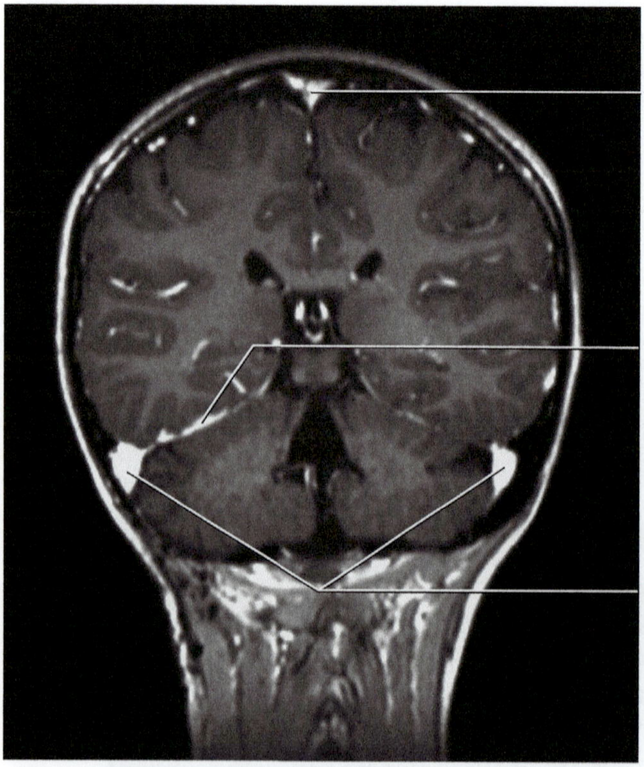

FIG. 4.8 Coronal, T1-weighted MRI with contrast noting the shape of typical transverse sinuses.

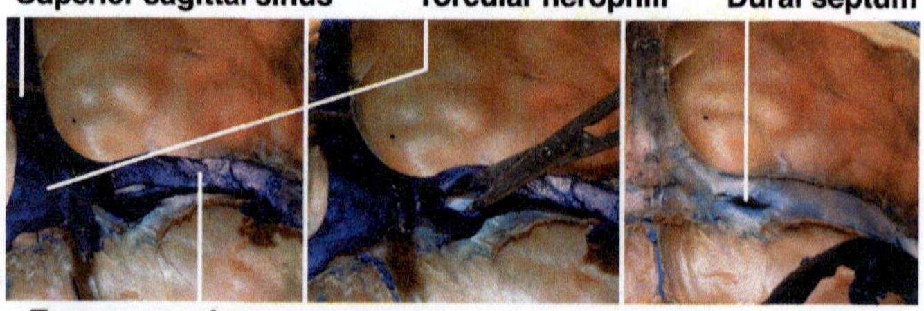

FIG. 4.9 Internal view of a cadaveric dissection of the posterior intracranial venous sinuses after the brain has been removed. Note the fenestrated proximal left transverse sinus and dural septum (far right).

in seven cases, and on both sides in one specimen. In the latter case, the superior sagittal sinus continued as a large occipital sinus that joined the marginal sinus and then the distal transverse sinuses at the jugular foramina. The authors also observed atresia of a segment of one transverse sinus in 11 (7 on the right and 4 on the left) of the 422 specimens studied and noted that part of the horizontal segment of the transverse sinus was doubled in 14 specimens (9 on the left and 5 on the right).

Barkow,[30] Hoople,[31] Knott,[22] Laff,[32] and Malacarne et al.[33] all described unusual cases in which most of the blood from the transverse sinus left the skull through the mastoid foramen. Hoople[31] found that the jugular foramen usually was contracted and the sigmoid sinus was reduced or absent when this occurred. In Knott's[22] cases, the transverse sinus was very small, measuring 1.5 mm in diameter. In the case of Malacarne et al., the mastoid foramen was enlarged, and a normal-sized lateral sinus exited through it. Laff[32] observed this as well, but also noted the presence of the following abnormalities: a small jugular foramen, absent superior jugular bulb, and an inferior petrosal sinus that emptied into a small internal jugular vein. Barkow[30] observed that, in addition to an enlarged mastoid foramen, the sigmoid sinus also was absent. Knott[22] described two instances of complete absence of the right transverse sinus with only a small venous channel terminating through the mastoid foramen. Woodhall[15] also found three similar cases. A case was reported in which the sigmoid sinus ended in a blind pouch and drained through the large mastoid foramen.[34]

Hoople[31] reported another variation in which the right transverse and sigmoid sinuses were small and the sigmoid sinus ended blindly at the jugular foramen with its drainage entering through the sinuses of the middle cranial fossa. Furstenberg[34] described a variation in the "lateral sinus" in which it was located in the soft tissues completely outside the skull. Finally, Williams[35] reported a "threadlike lateral sinus."

In the study of Ayanzen et al.,[18] 59% of the transverse sinuses observed were right dominant, 25% were left dominant, and 16% were codominant. Thirty-one percent of patients with normal magnetic resonance imaging (MRI) results had flow gaps. 90% had a nondominant transverse sinus, and 10% had a codominant sinus.[18] Surendrababu and Livingstone[36] made a similar observation. They investigated the variations in the cerebral venous anatomy of 100 patients and found that 59 had a right dominant transverse sinus, 30 had a left dominant sinus, and 10 had a codominant sinus. They also found that the right transverse sinus was hypoplastic in 13 patients, whereas the left was hypoplastic in 35. However, in one patient, the transverse sinus was absent on the left side.

Alper et al.[8] used time-of-flight MRV to observe the transverse sinuses in 105 people and found that 21 (20%) had aplasia of the left sinus, 41 (39%) had hypoplasia of the left sinus, 33 (31%) were symmetric, 6 (6%) had hypoplasia, and 4 (4%) had aplasia of the right sinus. In general, 62 (59%) had a larger right transverse sinus, and 10 (9.5%) had a larger left. Twenty-four percent had flow gaps (aplasia) in both transverse sinuses.

Overlapping lambdoidal sutures in infants may result in septation of the transverse sinus, usually at the proximal end. Hahn[24] and Streit[25] observed cases in which the transverse sinus was doubled, and in some, they observed that a fibrous septum of variable lengths, and sometimes a bony ridge, separated the channels (Fig. 4.9).

Some patients may have dilated distal end of the transverse sinus, sigmoid sinus, or the superior jugular bulb.[37] Duplication of the transverse sinus is more frequent than that of the sigmoid sinus.[27]

A stenosed jugular foramen with a small internal jugular vein is a rare phenomenon that affects the left side typically and is associated with significant enlargement of the contralateral vein. Occasionally, the affected side is associated with the absence of the transverse sinus, sigmoid sinus, or both.[27,38]

Ruttin[39] reported a case in which the superior petrosal sinus and a thin transverse sinus emptied into an enlarged sigmoid sinus through a small vein that then drained into the internal jugular vein. A 2-cm-long oblique sinus connecting the left and right transverse sinuses also has been reported.[17] Bergman et al.[40] reported that the transverse sinus can communicate occasionally with the cavernous sinus or ophthalmic veins through an aberrant vein.

PATHOLOGY

Transverse Sinus Thrombosis

Sinus thrombosis occurs in 3–4 people per 1,000,000, and estimated 86% of these cases involve the transverse sinuses.[41–43] Both the causes and patient presentations of transverse sinus thrombosis are highly variable.[44] However, transverse sinus venous thrombosis can be difficult to distinguish from other diagnoses because of its nonspecific clinical signs and MRV's lack of specificity.[45] The sigmoid notch sign is a simple and quick tool that is highly sensitive and specific, making it potentially useful, in conjunction with clinical judgment, for diagnosing transverse sinus venous thrombosis when dropout of flow is seen on MRV.[41] Both transverse and sigmoid sinus thromboses sometimes can complicate adjacent otitis and mastoiditis.[43]

Transverse-Sigmoid Sinus Dual Arteriovenous Fistulas and Embolization

Embolization (transarterial or transvenous), surgery, or a combination of both[46] may be used to treat transverse-sigmoid sinus dual arteriovenous fistulas with cortical venous drainage, which are associated with a high risk of hemorrhage (10%–40%) and significant morbidity and mortality.[46–48]

Arterial onyx embolization, which may be performed as an alternative to retrograde venous catheterization, is now used frequently as the first treatment for transverse sinus dural arteriovenous fistulas and can effect a complete cure. To prevent intracranial hemorrhage, a combination of arterial and venous surgery, as well as radiosurgery, should be considered if necessary.[49] Transvenous coil occlusion is a safe and effective treatment method in the large proportion of these fistulas.[50]

SURGERY

Identification of the Transverse Sinuses

To prevent injury of the transverse sinuses during surgery, incisions should be made at least 5 mm below the insertion of the musculus semispinalis capitis.[6] Both the superior nuchal line and inion are unreliable markers with which to locate the transverse sinus accurately,[51–53] and the semispinalis capitis, which is a more reliable anatomic structure than is the superior nuchal line, is used easily for intraoperative identification of the lower border of the medial segment of the transverse sinus[6] (Fig. 4.10). Considering that the width of the proximal transverse sinus is 6 mm on average, the first and most superior burr hole in the midline infratentorial supracerebellar approach can be placed safely approximately 1 cm below the inferior nuchal line.[54]

In cases of large petroclival meningioma surgery, indications for ligation and resection of the transverse sinus are controversial.[55] When large petroclival meningiomas require a wide operative field to be accessed, the transverse or sigmoid sinus often is ligated. However, some have reported immediate or delayed complications (24–48 h later) after sinus ligation and resection.

Venograms have been reviewed to identify relative tumor locations and the drainage patterns of the confluence of sinuses. Hwang et al.[55] classified the drainage patterns of the torcular Herophili into four types: type A (confluent and equal in both transverse sinuses); type B (confluent and nondominant on the tumor side); type C (confluent and dominant on the tumor side), and type D (unilateral only). Carotid angiographic studies have shown that 16.7% of individuals had an atretic or absent transverse sinus, an anomaly that is more common on the left than the right side. In these individuals, the vein of Labbé drains predominantly through the proximal sigmoid sinus. Sacrificing the sigmoid sinus may spare parts of the temporal lobe, with venous outflow supplied by the vein of Labbé.[56]

Intraoperative stimulation of the transverse sinuses during awake craniotomy has provided interesting results (Fig. 4.11). Stimulation of the inferior surface of the transverse sinus resulted in pain referred to the area near the asterion and mastoid process. Stimulation of the superior surface of the transverse sinus resulted in orbital and supraorbital pain.

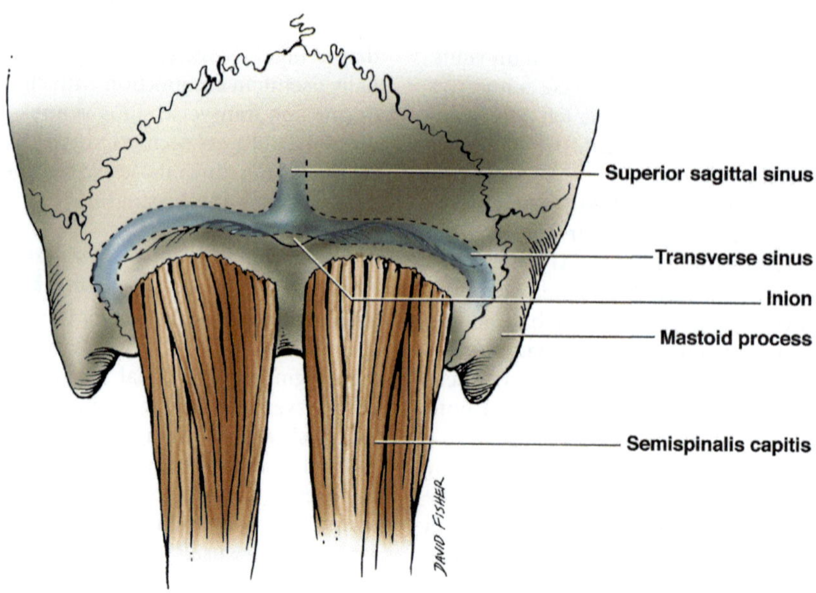

FIG. 4.10 Schematic drawing of the relationships of the transverse sinuses and the superior nuchal line and inion.

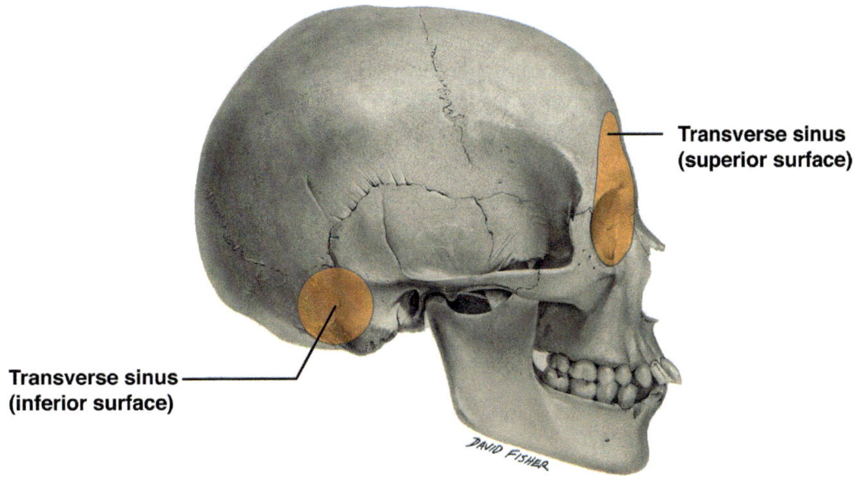

FIG. 4.11 Schematic drawing of referred pain sites following intraoperative stimulation of the transverse sinus during awake craniotomy.

REFERENCES

1. Streeter GL. The development of the venous sinuses of the dura mater in the human embryo. *Am J Anat.* 1915;18:145–178.
2. Butler H. The development of certain human dural venous sinuses. *J Anat.* 1957;91:510–526.
3. Senat MV, Schwarzler P, Alcais A, Ville Y. Longitudinal changes in the ductus venosus, cerebral transverse sinus and cardiotocogram in fetal growth restriction. *Ultrasound Obstet Gynecol.* 2000;16:19–24.
4. Laurichesse-Delmas H, Grimaud O, Moscoso G, Ville Y. Color Doppler study of the venous circulation in the fetal brain and hemodynamic study of the cerebral transverse sinus. *Ultrasound Obstet Gynecol.* 1999;13:34–42.
5. Ebraheim NA, Lu J, Biyani A, Brown JA, Yeasting RA. An anatomic study of the thickness of the occipital bone. Implications for occipitocervical instrumentation. *Spine.* 1996;(21):1725–1729; discussion 1729–1730.
6. Tubbs RS, Salter G, Oakes WJ. Superficial surgical landmarks for the transverse sinus and torcular herophili. *J Neurosurg.* 2000;93:279–281.
7. Zipnick RI, Merola AA, Gorup J, et al. Occipital morphology. An anatomic guide to internal fixation. *Spine.* 1996;21:1719–1724; discussion 1729–1730.
8. Alper F, Kantarci M, Dane S, Gumustekin K, Onbas O, Durur I. Importance of anatomical asymmetries of transverse sinuses: an MR venographic study. *Cerebrovasc Dis.* 2004;18:236–239.
9. Fofi L, Giugni E, Vadala R, et al. Cerebral transverse sinus morphology as detected by MR venography in patients with chronic migraine. *Headache.* 2012;52:1254–1261.
10. Han K, Chao AC, Chang FC, et al. Diagnosis of transverse sinus hypoplasia in magnetic resonance venography: new insights based on magnetic resonance imaging in combined dataset of venous outflow impairment case-control studies: post hoc case-control study. *Medicine.* 2016;95:e2862.
11. Strydom MA, Briers N, Bosman MC, Steyn S. The anatomical basis of venographic filling defects of the transverse sinus. *Clin Anat.* 2010;23:153–159.
12. Hollinshead W. *Anatomy for Surgeons.* 2nd ed. Philadelphia: Harper & Row; 1968.
13. Singh M, Nagashima M, Inoue Y. Anatomical variations of occipital bone impressions for dural venous sinuses around the torcular Herophili, with special reference to the consideration of clinical significance. *Surg Radiol Anat.* 2004;26:480–487.
14. Browder J, Kaplan HA, Krieger AJ. Anatomical features of the straight sinus and its tributaries. *J Neurosurg.* 1976;44:55–61.
15. Woodhall B. Variations of the cranial venous sinuses in the region of the torcular Herophili. *Arch Surg.* 1936;33:297.
16. Fukusumi A, Okudera T, Takahashi S, et al. Anatomical evaluation of the dural sinuses in the region of the torcular herophili using three dimensional CT venography. *Acad Radiol.* 2010;17:1103–1111.
17. Srijit D, Shipra P. Unusual venous sinuses. *Bratisl Lek Listy.* 2007;108:104–106.
18. Ayanzen R, Bird C, Keller P, McCully F, Theobald M, Heiserman J. Cerebral MR venography: normal anatomy and potential diagnostic pitfalls. *Am J Neuroradiol.* 2000;21:74–78.
19. Bykal L, Ceylan S, Akturk F, et al. Unilateral transverse sinus aplasia: a case report. *Turkish Neurosurg.* 1995;5:73–75.
20. Das AC, Hasan M. The occipital sinus. *J Neurosurg.* 1970;33:307–311.
21. Hacker H. Normal supratentorial veins and dural sinuses. In: Newton T, Potts D, eds. *Radiology of the Skull and Brain: Angiography.* St Louis, MO: Mosby; 1974:1851–1862.

22. Knott J. On the cerebral sinuses and their variations. *J Anat Physiol.* 1881;16:27–42.
23. Lieutaud J. *Essais Anatomiques.* Paris, France: P. M. Huart; 1742.
24. Hahn R. Anomalie del seno laterale. *Arch Ital Otol.* 1914;25:203.
25. Streit H. Ueber otologisch wichtige anomalien der hirnsinus, über accessorische sinus und bedeutendere venenverbindungen. *Archiv für Ohrenheilkunde.* 1903;58:85–128.
26. Kopuz C, Aydin ME, Kale A, Demir MT, Corumlu U, Kaya AH. The termination of superior sagittal sinus and drainage patterns of the lateral, occipital at confluens sinuum in newborns: clinical and embryological implications. *Surg Radiol Anat: SRA.* 2010;32:827–833.
27. Waltner JG. Anatomic variations of the lateral and sigmoid sinuses. *Arch Otolaryngol.* 1944;39:307–312.
28. Rollins N, Ison C, Booth T, Chia J. MR venography in the pediatric patient. *Am J Neuroradiol.* 2005;26:50–55.
29. Hamnett NT, Ogungbo B, Nahser H, Javadpour M. Anomalous cerebral venous sinus drainage. *Br J Neurosurg.* 2010;24:497–498.
30. Barkow JCL. Anatomische abhandlungen. *Breslau: F. Hirt.* 1851.
31. Hoople GD. LXXXI anomaly of the lateral sinus: report of a case. *Ann Otol Rhinol Laryngol.* 1936;45:1019–1028.
32. Laff HI. Unilateral absence of sigmoid sinus. *Arch Otolaryngol.* 1930;11:151–157.
33. Malacarne V, Bonnet C, Briolo G. *Encefalotomia Nuova Universale: Presso Giammichele Briolo;* 1780.
34. Furstenberg AC. Septic thrombophlebitis of the sigmoidsinus. *Trans Am Acad Ophthalmol.* 1937;42:424–431.
35. Williams HL. Apparent unilateral absence of the sigmoid sinus noted at operation. *Arch Otolaryngol.* 1930;12:339–341.
36. Surendrababu N, Livingstone R. Variations in the cerebral venous anatomy and pitfalls in the diagnosis of cerebral venous sinus thrombosis: low field MR experience. *Indian J Med Sci.* 2006;60:135.
37. Curé JK, Van Tassel P. Congenital and acquired abnormalities of the dural venous sinuses. *Semin Ultrasound CT MR.* 1994;15:520–539.
38. Manjunath KY. Anomalies of transverse and sigmoid sinuses associated with contracted jugular foramina. *Indian J Otolaryngol.* 2004;56:108–114.
39. Ruttin E. Kloaken- und blindsackbildung am sinus sigmoideus. *Acta Otolaryng.* 1926;9:217–220.
40. Bergman R, Thompson SA, Afifi AK, Saadeh FA. Cardiovascular system. In: Bergman R, ed. *Compendium of Human Anatomic Variation.* Baltimore-Munich: Urban & Schwarzenberg; 1988:93.
41. Chik Y, Gottesman RF, Zeiler SR, Rosenberg J, Llinas RH. Differentiation of transverse sinus thrombosis from congenitally atretic cerebral transverse sinus with CT. *Stroke.* 2012;43:1968–1970.
42. Ferro JM, Canhao P, Stam J, Bousser MG, Barinagarrementeria F, Investigators I. Prognosis of cerebral vein and dural sinus thrombosis: results of the International study on cerebral vein and dural sinus thrombosis (ISCVT). *Stroke.* 2004;35:664–670.
43. Stam J. Thrombosis of the cerebral veins and sinuses. *N Engl J Med.* 2005;352:1791–1798.
44. Kubiak BD, Albert SP, Tandoh MA, Fortune JB, Cunningham PR. Transverse sinus thrombosis after internal jugular vein ligation. *J Emerg Med.* 2012;43:e5–e9.
45. Leach JL, Fortuna RB, Jones BV, Gaskill-Shipley MF. Imaging of cerebral venous thrombosis: current techniques, spectrum of findings, and diagnostic pitfalls. *Radiographics.* 2006;26(suppl 1):S19–S41; discussion S42–13.
46. Wong GK, Poon WS, Yu SC, Zhu CX. Transvenous embolization for dural transverse sinus fistulas with occluded sigmoid sinus. *Acta Neurochir.* 2007;149:929–935; discussion 935–926.
47. Cognard C, Gobin YP, Pierot L, et al. Cerebral dural arteriovenous fistulas: clinical and angiographic correlation with a revised classification of venous drainage. *Radiology.* 1995;194:671–680.
48. Duffau H, Lopes M, Janosevic V, et al. Early rebleeding from intracranial dural arteriovenous fistulas: report of 20 cases and review of the literature. *J Neurosurg.* 1999;90:78–84.
49. Lv X, Jiang C, Li Y, Yang X, Wu Z. Intraarterial and intravenous treatment of transverse/sigmoid sinus dural arteriovenous fistulas. *Intervent Neuroradiol.* 2009;15:291–300.
50. Kirsch M, Liebig T, Kuhne D, Henkes H. Endovascular management of dural arteriovenous fistulas of the transverse and sigmoid sinus in 150 patients. *Neuroradiology.* 2009;51:477–483.
51. Fukui M, Natori Y, Matsushima T, Nishio S, Ikezaki K. Operative approaches to the pineal region tumors. *Child's Nerv Syst.* 1998;14:49–52.
52. Reid WS, Clark WK. Comparison of the infratentorial and transtentorial approaches to the pineal region. *Neurosurgery.* 1978;3:1–8.
53. Roberts DA, Doherty BJ, Heggeness MH. Quantitative anatomy of the occiput and the biomechanics of occipital screw fixation. *Spine.* 1998;23:1100–1107; discussion 1107–1108.
54. Suslu HT, Bozbuga M, Ozturk A, Sahinoglu K. Surface anatomy of the transverse sinus for the midline infratentorial supracerebellar approach. *Turk Neurosurg.* 2010;20:39–42.
55. Hwang SK, Gwak HS, Paek SH, Kim DG, Jung HW. Guidelines for the ligation of the sigmoid or transverse sinus during large petroclival meningioma surgery. *Skull Base.* 2004;14:21–28; discussion 29.
56. Bigelow DC, Hoffer ME, Schlakman B, Hurst RW, Smith PG. Angiographic assessment of the transverse sinus and vein of Labbé to avoid complications in skull base surgery. *Skull Base Surg.* 1993;3:217–222.

CHAPTER 5

The Sigmoid Sinus

ISLAM ALY • R. SHANE TUBBS

ANATOMY

The sigmoid sinus is a continuation of the transverse sinus and becomes the sigmoid sinus where the tentorium cerebelli ends (Figs. 5.1–5.3). It begins inferior to the temporal bone, posteromedial to the mastoid cells, and runs to the jugular foramen, extending through an S-shaped groove, where it meets the superior jugular bulb (Figs. 5.4–5.9). Inconstant veins that drain into the sigmoid sinus include veins from the pons and medulla oblongata. The sigmoid sinus has anastomoses with the mastoid emissary and condylar emissary veins routinely.

According to Dai et al.,[1] the sigmoid sinus in males is situated more posterior and lateral compared with that in females. This probably is attributable to the difference in cranial size base between the sexes. When comparing either side, regardless of cranial width, the sigmoid sinus on the right side protrudes deeper, covering a greater cross-sectional area, and is situated more laterally. This may be correlated with the fact that the right side is the dominant side for venous sinus drainage. Dai et al.[1] also found that males have a right sigmoid sinus positioned more anteriorly compared with their left.

The asterion is one landmark that has become a reference point used commonly (Fig. 5.6). The asterion is the convergence point of the lambdoid, occipitomastoid, and parietomastoid sutures and is used because it overlays the region of the transverse-sigmoid junction. However, many authors have found that the asterion is not a useful landmark because of its anatomic variability as well as the difficulty of identifying it. A study that Raso and Gusmão[2] conducted described a new craniometric point to demarcate the sigmoid sinus, the digastric point, which is located at the superior aspect of the mastoid notch or immediately above the posterior belly of the digastric muscle.

Of note, when reading the older literature, some writers use the term lateral sinus to describe the combined sigmoid and transverse sinuses. However, some have used lateral sinus to describe the transverse sinus

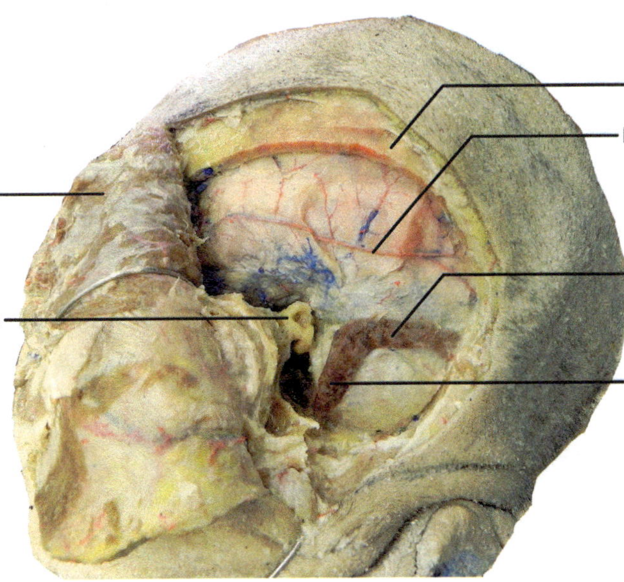

FIG. 5.1 Left anterior and posterior petrosectomy craniotomy demonstrating the sigmoid sinus from an extradural perspective.

Anatomy, Imaging and Surgery of the Intracranial Dural Venous Sinuses. https://doi.org/10.1016/B978-0-323-65377-0.00005-2

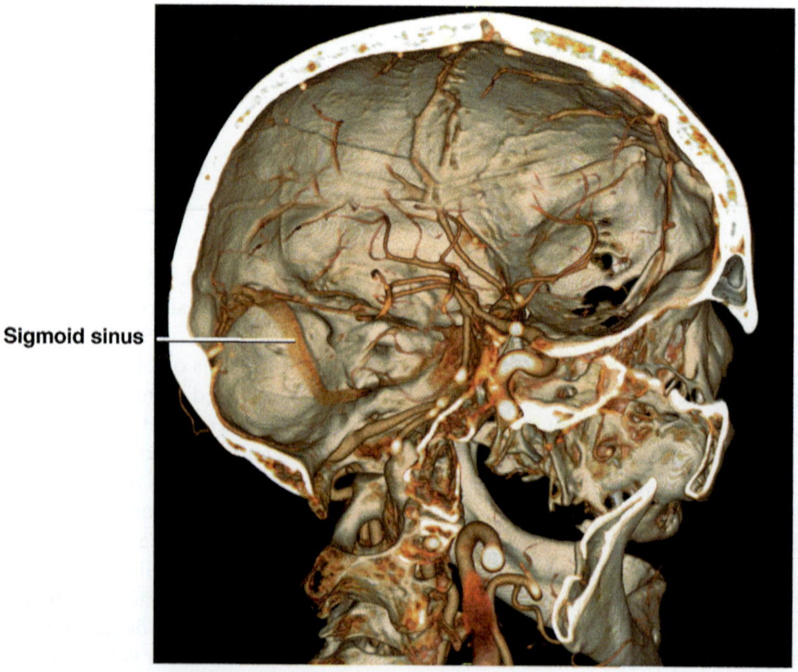

FIG. 5.2 Parasagittal 3D CTA noting the left sigmoid sinus. (Courtesy Dr. Joel Curé.)

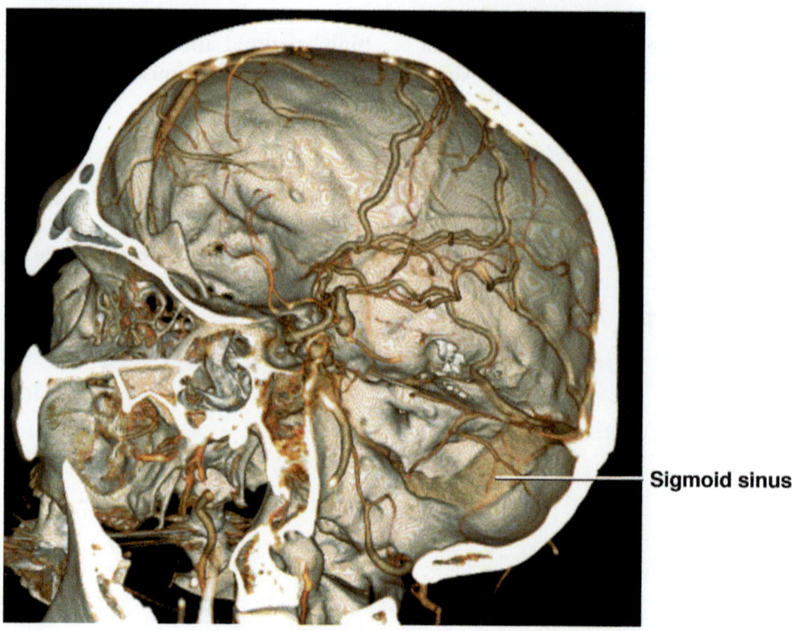

FIG. 5.3 Parasagittal 3D CTA noting the right sinus, which is larger in size than normal. (Courtesy Dr. Joel Curé.)

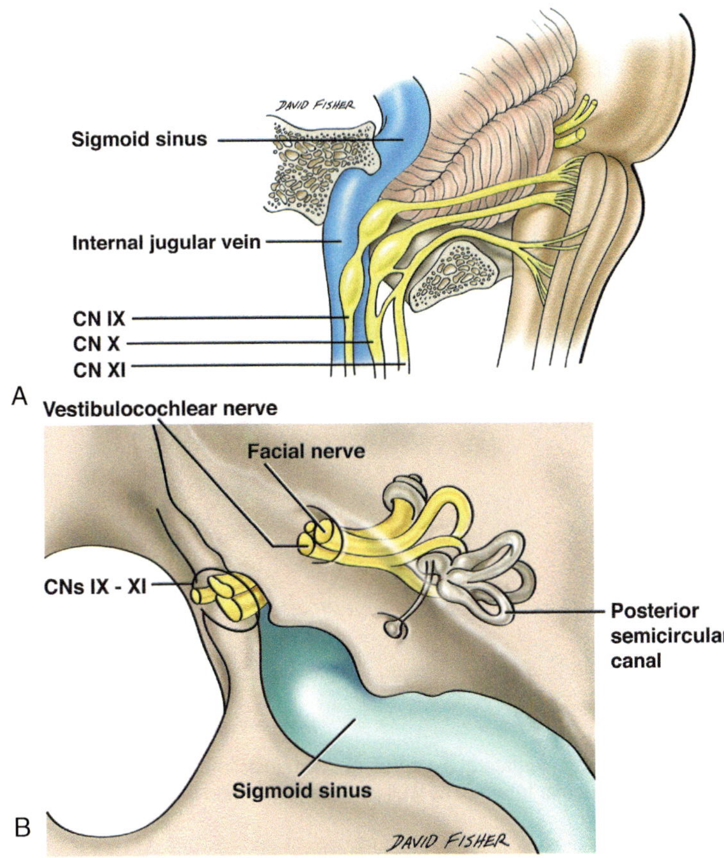

FIG. 5.4 **(A)** Drawing showing the general arrangement of the contents of the jugular foramen and the sigmoid sinus and its regional anatomy. Note the position of the endolymphatic sac above the sigmoid sinus. **(B)** Parasagittal schematic drawing of the junction between the sigmoid sinus and superior jugular bulb and noting the contents of the jugular foramen.

specifically. To confuse the matter more, some writers have used the term transverse sinus to refer to both the transverse and sigmoid sinuses.

EMBRYOLOGY

Development of the dural venous sinuses is related to that of the cerebral vesicles (prosencephalon, mesencephalon, rhombencephalon), the skull, and the ventral cardinal veins. At approximately week 6 in embryonic development, three dural venous plexuses, referred to as the rostral, middle, and caudal, form within the cerebral vesicles mesenchyme. Their primary function is to drain into the vena capitis prima.

At the very beginning of the fetal stage, when the embryo is still 40 mm, changes occur in the configuration of the sinuses that establish many of the morphologic features that are present in the adult brain. The only definitive aspect of the adult transverse sinus at this point in development is the sigmoid segment. By the 60-mm and 80-mm stages, with the development of the cerebral hemispheres and the subsequent caudal swing of the transverse sinus, the caudal end of the tentorial sinus migrates cranially and ventrally toward the junction between the sigmoid and transverse sinuses.[3]

The end of the second month of embryogenesis is a hallmark period for the development of the dural venous sinuses, particularly the sigmoid sinus. As the ventral portion of the lateral vein begins to regress backward, an anastomosis occurs between the caudal and middle plexuses. According to Butler,[4] this stage is marked by the sudden appearance of a large supraoptic anastomosis that allows a connection between the prooptic and posterior rhombencephalic veins. This anastomosis evolves into the sigmoid sinus. This area of anastomosis occurs above and behind the auditory vesicles. Coincidentally, the vena capitis prima transforms into the cavernous sinus.

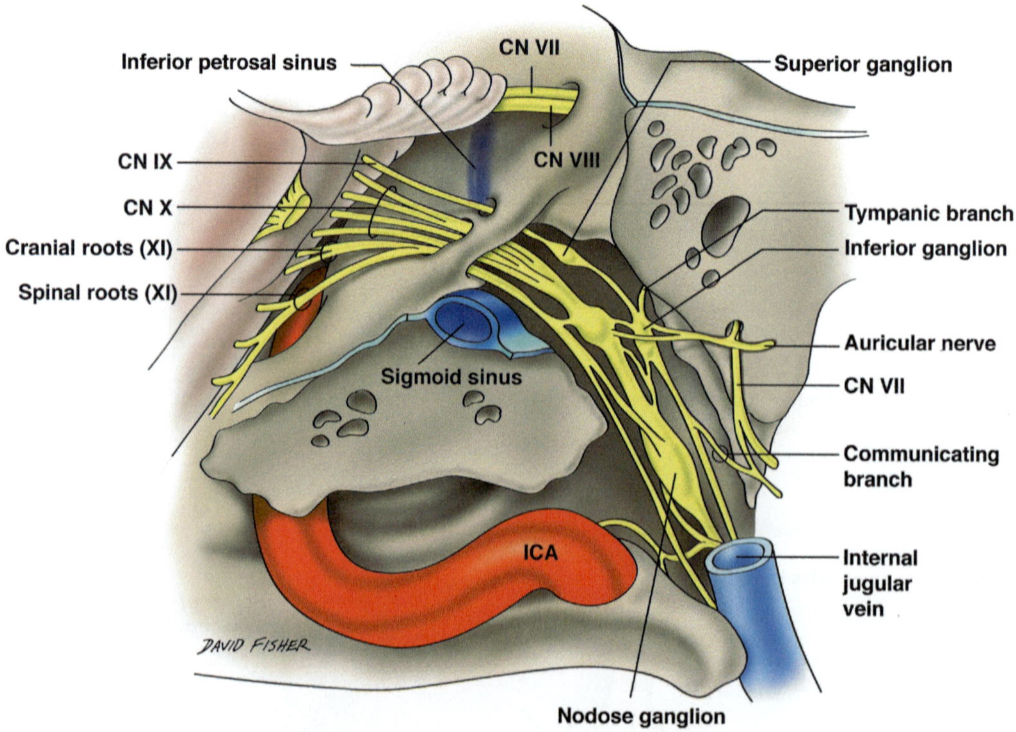

FIG. 5.5 Schematic drawing of a far lateral exposure of the jugular foramen and cerebellopontine angle. Note the relationships of the jugular foramen as well as the sigmoid and inferior petrosal sinuses.

The transverse sinus forms from the anterior cerebral vein, from the torcular to the entry of the lateral cerebral vein, as well as from an anastomosis between the prootic veins and anterior cerebral vein. Its original course is across the cavum epiptericum, but as the epiptericum decreases in size, it attaches to the margin of the tentorium cerebelli. As development continues, the transverse sinus rotates 180° secondary to the caudal expansion of the cerebral hemispheres, and its path extends from the sigmoid groove to the jugular foramen, thus forming the adult sigmoid sinus.

HISTOLOGY

Nishijima et al.[5] evaluated the normal sigmoid sinus closely and found that its interior surface is covered in a single layer of endothelial cells. Fascicles of connective tissue lay beneath the endothelium and are demarcated easily by the presence of the elastic lamina. The elastic laminae are uneven and do not run uniformly around the entire circumference of the sinus. The fascicles of connective tissue also are uneven, running randomly in various directions at angles formed by the fusion of the two dural leaves.

VARIATIONS

Knowledge of the anatomic variations of the sigmoid sinus is necessary not only for radiologic diagnosis but also when considering surgical or endovascular treatment of diseases at the skull base.[6] Unlike the transverse sinus, the sigmoid sinus has fewer variations.[7]

The study of Ramos-Junior et al.[8] compared both sides of 50 dry adult skulls through the use of transillumination with LASER. 78% of the cases had a larger sigmoid sinus width at the level of the sinodural angle on the right side, thus demonstrating that the sigmoid sinus is larger on that side. Another variation discovered in the same study was that the jugular foramen width also is not symmetrical in all skulls, as it was found that the width is greater on the right side in most skulls.

Williams has reported unilateral absence of the sigmoid sinus.[9,10]

Normally, the sigmoid receives blood from the transverse sinus and drains it into the internal jugular vein. These sinuses not only usually exhibit lateral dominance, more so on the right side, but also can be subject to segmental variations, with greater anatomic constancy found in the sigmoid sinus.[3] The drainage route also varies in cases in

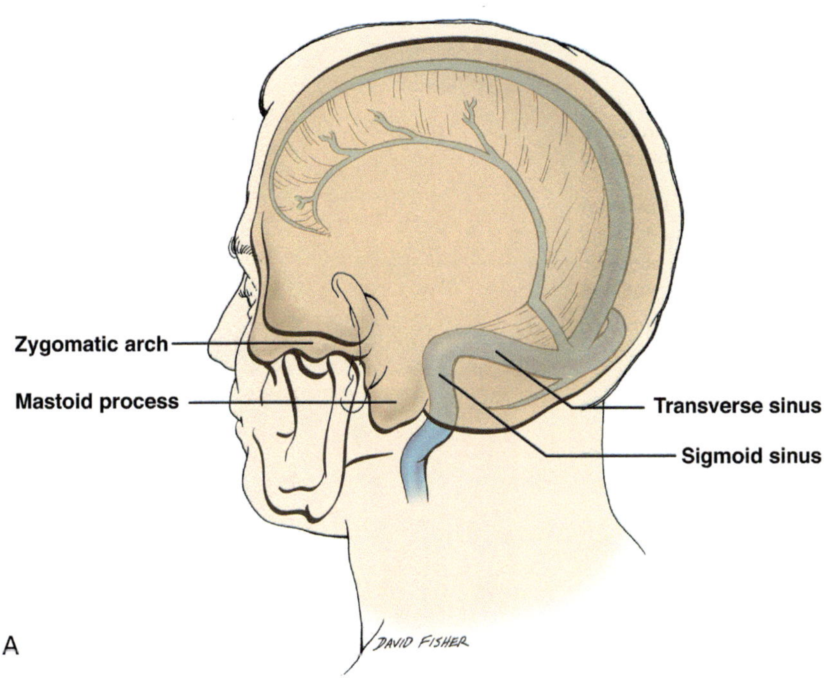

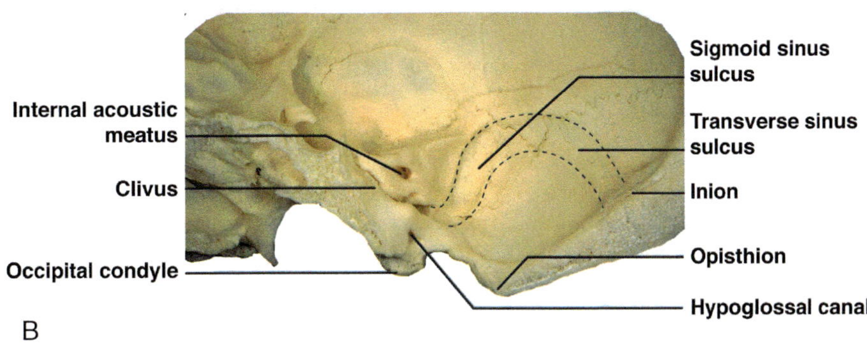

FIG. 5.6 **(A)** Schematic drawing of the course of the sigmoid sinus within the cranium. The junction between the transverse and sigmoid sinuses is most often found posterior to an imaginary line drawn through the mastoid notch. **(B)** Sagittal section through a dry skull specimen. The bony sulcus for the transverse and sigmoid sinuses is outlined.

which the sigmoid sinus is absent or hypoplastic. According to Surendrababu et al.,[11] hypoplasia of the sigmoid sinus is found most commonly on the left side. When this is the case, the transverse sinus drains into a mastoid emissary vein rather than the sigmoid sinus, and the inferior petrosal sinus empties into a small internal jugular vein. This has been reported in association with the underdevelopment of the petrous part of the temporal bone.[10,12]

In cases of transverse sinus atresia, or any form of malformation of the transverse sinus, the sigmoid sinus fills through the vein of Labbé or small, irregular intradural venous channels.[13] Collateral venous drainage also can occur through the emissary veins, occipital sinus, or vertebral venous system. When both the transverse and sigmoid sinuses are hypoplastic or absent, then drainage occurs through a large superior petrosal sinus, which passes through the mastoid foramen.[9,10]

Rutting observed a diverticulum on the superior surface of the sigmoid sinus. These luminal outpouches may lead to erosion into the internal acoustic meatus and cause tinnitus and sensorineural hearing loss. Sometimes, the sigmoid sinus can appear to be hugely dilated.

Sarmiento and Eslait[14] conducted a study to help develop surgical classifications of the sigmoid sinus'

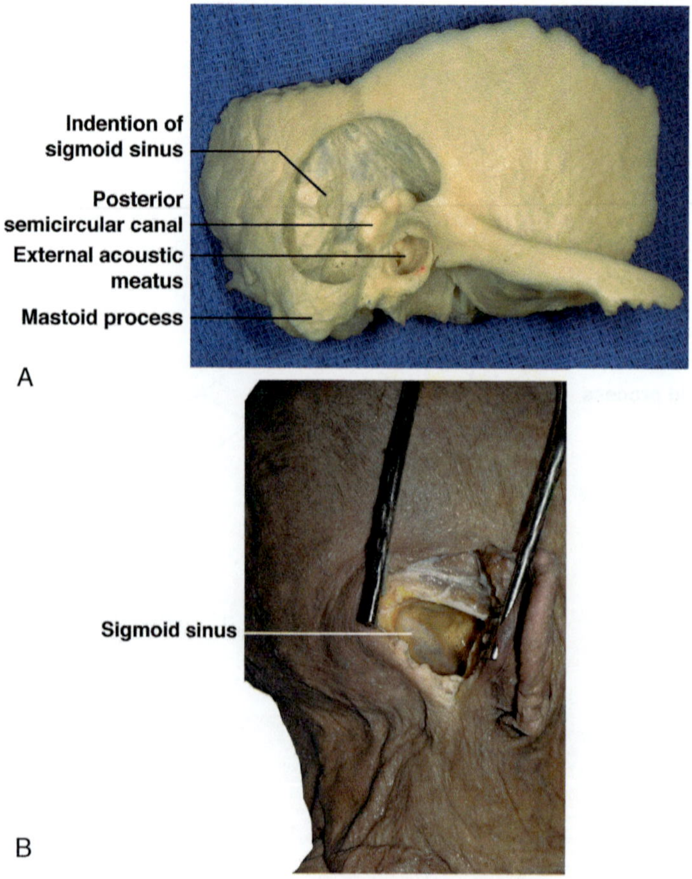

FIG. 5.7 **(A)** Right temporal bone following surgical drilling for a transmastoid approach. Note the indentation of the sigmoid sinus. **(B)** Cadaveric surgical exposure illustrating a transmastoid approach. Note the sigmoid sinus seen through a thin shell of bone and compare with Fig. 5.7A.

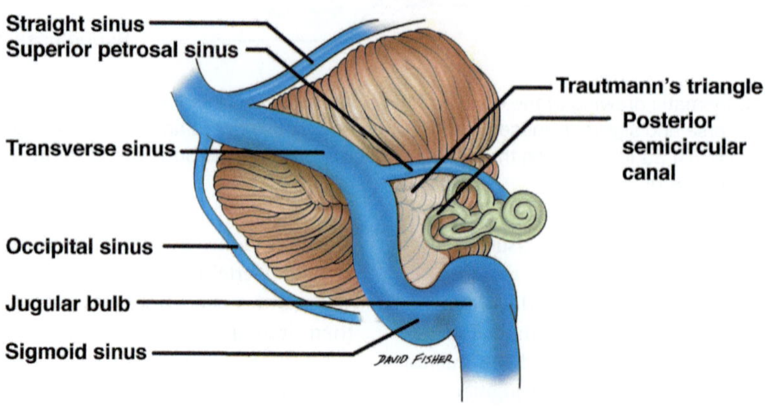

FIG. 5.8 Schematic drawing illustrating Trautmann's triangle and its borders.

variations. They examined 96 temporal bones and concluded that they differed in the approximate location of the sigmoid sinus in relation to the mastoid region. Their classification included three types with respect to Trautmann's triangle (Figs. 5.8 and 5.9). Trautmann's triangle is defined as the area bounded posteriorly by the anterior border of the sigmoid sinus, anteriorly by the posterior semicircular canal, and superiorly by

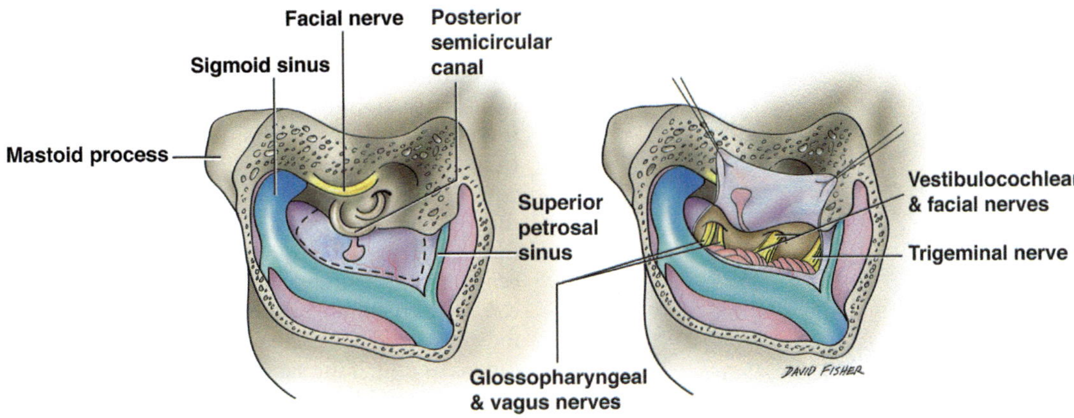

FIG. 5.9 Trautmann's triangle (left) and following opening of the dura mater (right). Note the endolymphatic duct centered on the dura mater in both images.

the superior petrosal sinus.[15] The classification is as follows:

- Type 1: Posterior sigmoid sinus causes an increase in the size of Trautmann's triangle (22.3%).
- Type 2: Anterior sigmoid sinus causes reduction of the area of Trautmann's triangle (57.5%).
- Type 3: Medial displacement of the sigmoid sinus causes reduction of the area of Trautmann's triangle (20.2%).

A controversial issue in anatomic variation is the relation between the distance of the sigmoid sinus from the posterior border of the external acoustic meatus and the degree of pneumatization of the mastoid process.[1,16–18] The literature indicates largely that the distance is shorter in a well-pneumatized temporal bone. In these cases, the sigmoid sinus typically is situated medially.[1,16,18] Occasionally, the sigmoid sinus may follow an unusual path, coursing anteriorly and approaching the external acoustic meatus at its posterior wall.[19]

The transverse sinus is duplicated more frequently than is the sigmoid sinus. This occurs through the formation of two channels separated by a bony ridge or fibrous septum.[7] Jugular foramen stenosis with a small internal jugular vein typically occurs on the left side and is associated with enlargement of the contralateral vein. The side affected is associated occasionally with an absent sigmoid sinus, transverse sinus, or both.[7,12]

IMAGING

Various imaging techniques have been used to visualize the dural venous sinuses (Fig. 5.10). Some modalities are more useful than are others depending on the disease pattern that is being examined. Imaging modalities that have been used include angiography, intravenous digital subtraction angiography, CT, MRI, and MR angiography. The use of multidetector row CT (MDCT) has allowed proper evaluation of the posterior cranial fossa with thin-sectional axial images and/or 3D-reconstructed images. This type of imaging also provides higher spatial and temporal resolution.

According to Curé et al.,[13] the gold standard for radiologic diagnosis of the dural venous sinus diseases is conventional angiography. Conventional angiogram can be less helpful in certain diseases, such as detecting the absence of a dural venous sinus, because it cannot differentiate between thrombosis and aplasia, which occurs most frequently at the transverse sinus.

MRI is a noninvasive imagining modality, which makes it more appealing, but it is not the best technique with which to visualize diseases of the dural venous sinus. With MRI, a dural venous sinus can be visualized through the use of a flow signal only if it is patent. If patency is compromised, as in cases of thrombosis, it may be absent in MRI images. There is speculation that a thrombus that consists of methemoglobin, which should appear white on T1-weighted images, might be confused with flow on 2D gradient-echo sequences and lead to the conclusion that a sinus is patent when, in fact, it is not.

PATHOLOGY

Nishijima et al.[5] studied the case of a 58-year-old woman with an AV malformation of the lateral and sigmoid sinuses with occlusion of the sigmoid, and their close observations of the malformation's histology revealed remarkable findings. The intima of the sinus was thickened, and the

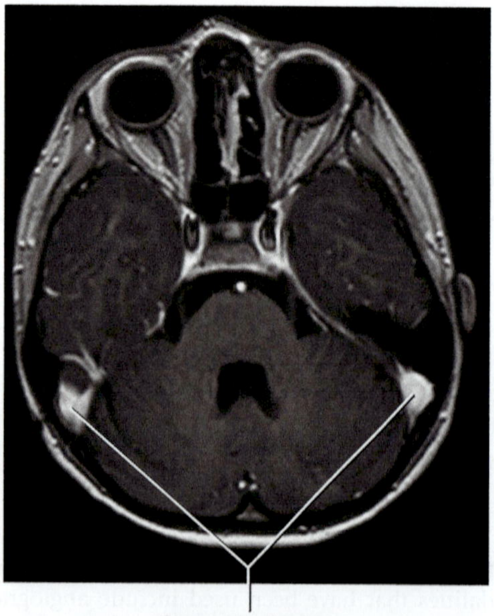

FIG. 5.10 Axial T1-weighted MRI of the brain noting the sigmoid sinuses.

elastic laminae were both thick and interrupted. Streeter[20] speculated that this disease may have been secondary to the enlargement of intradural arteriovenous shunts that may have occurred during embryonic development. After thorough examination of AV fistulas of the dural sinuses, Nishijima et al.[5] speculated that the cause is secondary to an increase in the blood flow that causes the fistula to form. Once this occurs, the dural arteries' intimal layer thickens, which leads to a dilation of the dural veins attributable to the influx of arterial blood that can lead to thrombogenesis and further damage to the intima.

Various authors have explored the pathogenesis of dural arteriovenous fistulas. Sakaki et al.[21] followed five cases that described the development of an AV fistula in the transverse-sigmoid sinus after removal of the sigmoid sinus. In the cases reported, a dural AV fistula developed several years (2–6) after surgical occlusion of the sigmoid sinus. In each of the patients, all that remained of the sinus postsurgery was a small stump on the retrosigmoid sinus portion. Histologic examination of all the resected sinuses and AV fistulas depicted a dural wall with subintimal fibrous thickening as well as hypertrophic changes in the sinus wall. The wall also contained numerous vessels with clots. The authors concluded that the dural arteriovenous fistulas that formed after surgery were secondary to thrombosis or thrombophlebitis. They also stated that development might be secondary to late sinus hypertension following resection of the sigmoid sinus.

Wang et al.[22] studied two pathologic anomalies of the sigmoid sinus, diverticulum and wall dehiscence. These two have been found to be the main culprits in pulsatile tinnitus, which occurs secondary to malformation of the vascular structures near the ear. Typically, the rhythm of pulsatile tinnitus is synchronous with the person's heartbeat. The pulsations occur from the vibrations of an uncovered sinus as blood flows through. These vibrations can resonate with the adjacent mastoid air cells and then be transmitted to the ear. A diverticulum of the sigmoid sinus forms when the sinus erodes into the adjacent mastoid cells. This can occur only if the sigmoid sinus wall is dehiscent or weak. A sigmoid sinus wall dehiscence is a defect of the mastoid part of the temporal bone at the area covering the sigmoid sinus, in which the mastoid cells enclose and constrict the sinus. Although these two anomalies seem to be associated, they can occur independently. The study of Wang et al.[22] followed 28 patients with one or both anomalies. Through the use of CT angiogram and digital subtraction angiograms, they concluded that a sigmoid sinus diverticulum is merely a focal pouch that extrudes into the adjacent mastoid region, whereas sigmoid sinus wall dehiscence is an osseous defect of the bone without the presence of a diverticulum. The authors found a correlation between these defects and gender in which there was a marked female predominance. The increased prevalence in women was attributed to a change in their hormonal balance as they age. The authors proposed that the occurrence of sigmoid sinus diverticulum might be an early sign of osteoporosis secondary to a decrease in the estrogen and progesterone levels in the premenopausal period.

Meningiomas involving the sigmoid sinus are quite uncommon, representing only 10% of all meningiomas. Normally, patients who have a meningioma involving the sigmoid sinus usually are symptomatic, presenting with dizziness, headache, ataxia, and papilledema. According to Mazur et al.,[23] a meningioma arises from arachnoid cap cells within the arachnoid granulations and can penetrate into the walls of the dural sinus. The meningiomas they reported in their study were predominantly grade I, in accordance with the WHO criteria. Typically, these tumors are attached to the dura and composed of a sheetlike growth pattern circumscribed well, prominent nucleoli, and potentially, psammoma bodies. Psammoma bodies are concentric lamellated calcifications that may be present in some, but not all, meningiomas. Grade I usually are localized and may not harm surrounding structures, but grades II and III can expand, spread into the dural sinuses, and occlude them.

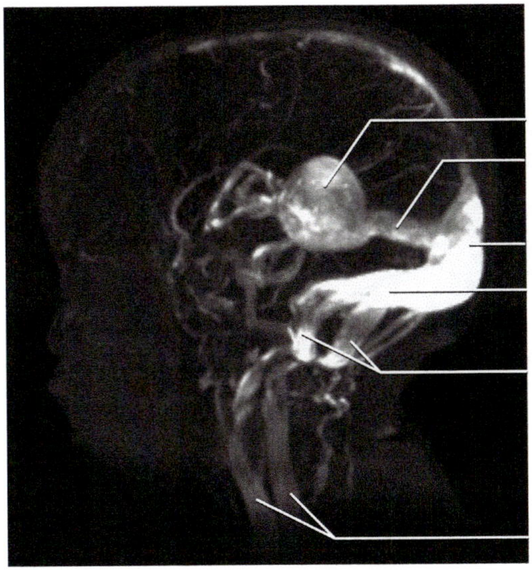

FIG. 5.11 MRV of a child with a vein of Galen malformation and engorgement of the straight, sigmoid, and transverse sinuses.

Vein of Galen aneurysms can result in tremendous enlargement of the dural venous sinuses (Fig. 5.11). Lastly, with skull base fractures, involvement of the sigmoid sinus can result in subcutaneous bleeding over the mastoid region, i.e., Battle sign (Fig. 5.12).

SURGERY

According to Sundt and Piepgras,[24] the preferred surgical treatment for arteriovenous malformations involving the sigmoid sinus is complete sinus excision. The surgical approach the authors described emphasized that the surgeon must have an access point to the region between the inion and the mastoid process for better exposure. First, a scalp flap is created to expose the mastoid process. Second, the soft tissue is dissected by incising the deep cervical fascia and nuchal musculature to expose the cranium better. Each surgeon has his or her own preferred technique for drilling during a craniotomy. Sundt and Piepgras[24] stated that the air drill should be held at a 30-degree angle vertical to the bone, as it allows better visualization. Risk of a dural tear is reduced by switching the drill tip as the drilling penetrates deeper. Once the sinus is exposed, and adequate hemostasis is achieved, the sinus can be ligated. According to the authors, the best way to do this is by placing two hemostats 1.5 cm across the sinus to occlude flow and then cutting the ligated portion. Once this is accomplished, the medial part of the sinus can be closed with a running suture. After the sinus is ligated, it should be simpler to find the area of the AV malformation, which usually is at the junction between the transverse and sigmoid sinuses, and then excise it.

The transverse-sigmoid junction is the most common location for dural arteriovenous fistulas, and therefore, it is no surprise that there are various surgical techniques for their treatment. According to Kakarla et al.,[25] two types of dural AV fistulas are found at this junction: one that has a single leptomeningeal vein along the tentorium in the supratentorial compartment and one that involves the entire sinus. Surgical treatment depends on the type of fistula involved. The surgical technique described in their study involved obliteration of the draining vein with bipolar cauterization or clip ligation. Although most dural AV fistulas can be treated by embolization techniques, some are torturous and, therefore, require surgical exposure.

Before transecting the sinus, the sinus pressure is assessed by clamping it to evaluate contralateral venous drainage. If the pressure is greater than 10 mm Hg after it has been clamped for 30 min, then the sinus should not be ligated. It is important to determine whether it should be excised or not, because ligation can lead to serious complications, including infarction and hemorrhage. Hwang et al.[26] suggested that before the sinus is ligated, it is best to determine whether the contralateral sinus is patent; if both sinuses are patent, then the relative size of the sinuses should be assessed via CT or venography, and the smaller of the two sinuses should be ligated.

Landmarks are very important in surgical procedures, and superficial landmarks on the occipital and

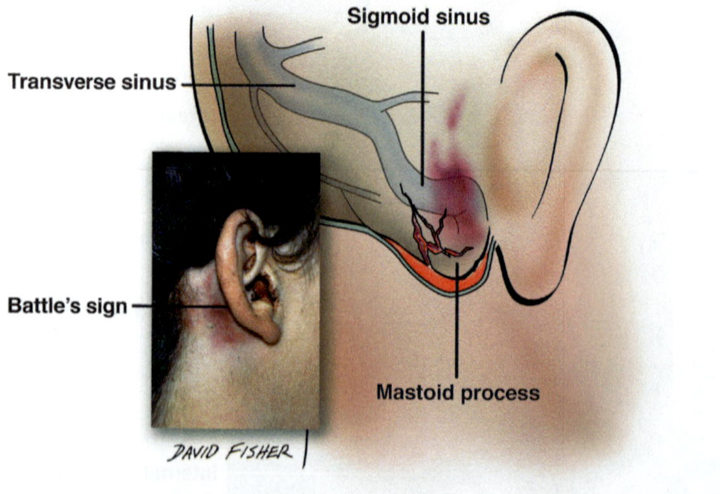

FIG. 5.12 Combined clinical case and schematic drawing of Battle sign noting the fracture through the mastoid part of the temporal bone and hemorrhage from the sigmoid sinus into the surrounding subcutaneous tissues.

temporal bones can be helpful in craniotomies. Raso and Gusmão[2] used the asterion as the upper landmark and the digastric point as the lower landmark to help expose the border of the sigmoid using a suboccipital approach. By drilling between these two landmarks, one can expose the entire lateral border of the sigmoid better and decrease the risk of damaging the sinus wall. A craniectomy should be considered for complex lesions, such as those with significant dural and osseous feeders.[25] A surgeon should be aware that during such a procedure, the scalp, transosseous, and dural feeders might be enlarged, thus increasing the complexity of exposure.[25] In 1905, Bochardt reported that dividing the sigmoid sinus can help expose cerebellopontine tumors.[26] Surgical management of tumors is rather complex, especially if the tumor has invaded surrounding structures, and radical resection of a meningioma is controversial. When a meningioma occludes a venous sinus completely, a gross, total resection of the intravascular portion usually is the technique preferred.[23]

As Mazur et al.[23] described, conservative management consists of debulking the tumor from the walls of the sinus and then resecting it from the brain. This technique is considered conservative, because the sinus is not opened, the dissection is purely extravascular, and any remnants of the tumor are treated by radiation therapy. Aggressive management involves opening the sinus and resecting the intravascular portion of the tumor. In this situation, venous reconstruction is necessary. Aggressive management is thought to be the treatment of choice only when the sinus is occluded completely. After the tumor is removed, the sinus must be reconstructed by sewing a dural flap. According to Mazur et al.,[23] the sigmoid sinus can be scarified at any point distal to the superior petrosal sinus and vein of Labbé. Once the sinus is ligated, then the ipsilateral vein of Labbé can be used to drain the sinus. The larger the meningioma, the more likely it will need to be resected. Usually tumors that are larger than 3 cm, or those with symptomatic mass effect, require resection.

Management of a meningioma of the sigmoid sinus varies by case. Treatment options can range from radical resection with reconstruction of the sinus to subtotal resection followed by radiation therapy to eradicate the remainder of the tumor. Commonly, the Simpson Grading system is used to assess the removal of a meningioma.[23] The system is as follows:

- I → macroscopic complete removal of the tumor with excision of its dural attachment as well as removal of any abnormal bone. This includes resection of the venous sinus involved.
- II → macroscopic complete removal of the tumor and any visible extensions with coagulation of its dural attachment.
- III → macroscopic complete removal of the intradural tumor without resection of coagulation of its dural attachment or its extradural extension.
- IV → potential removal.
- V → decompression of the tumor, with or without biopsy.

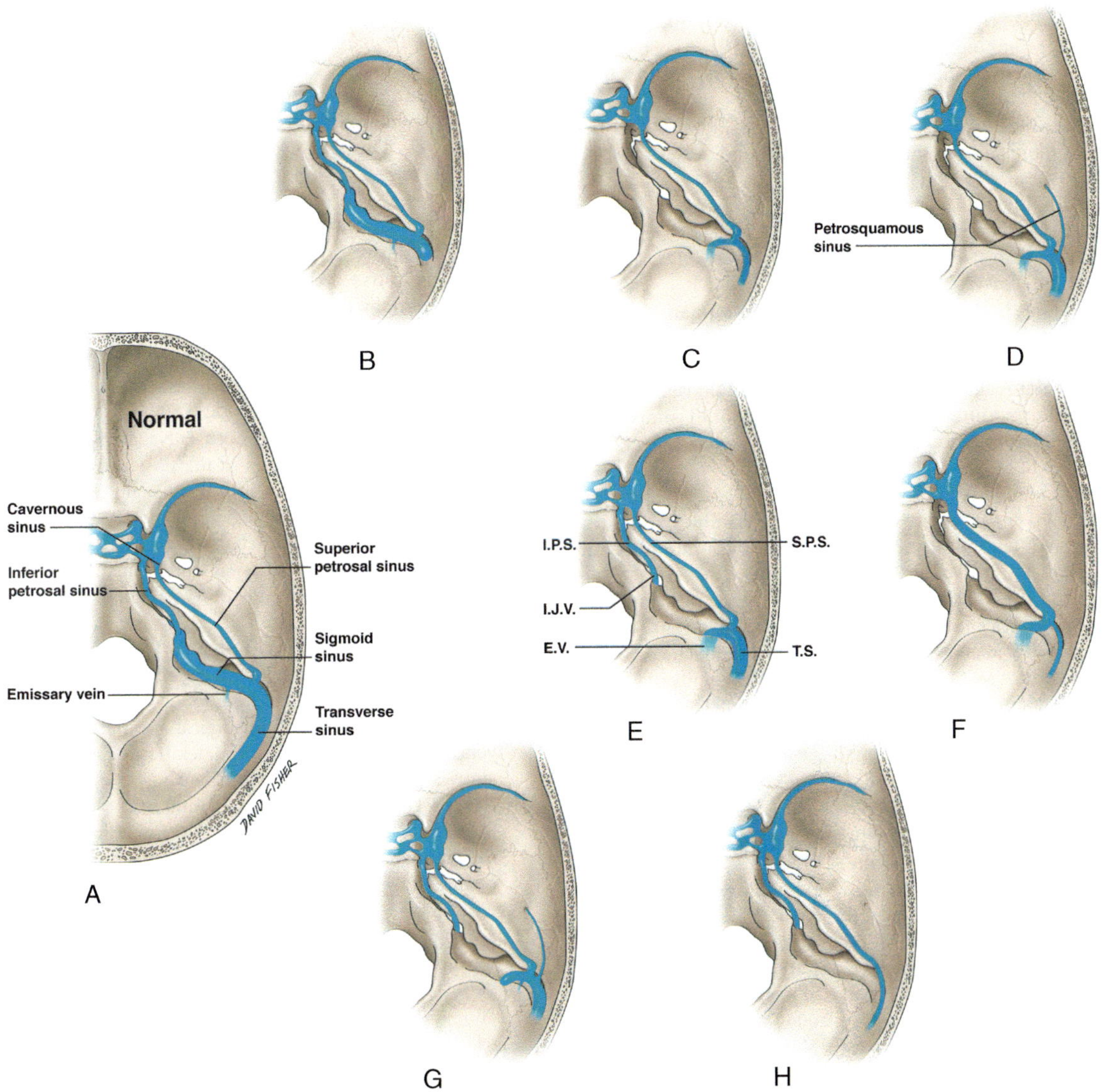

FIG. 5.13 Variations of the sigmoid sinuses after Waltner JG. 1944. **(A)** Common configuration of the sigmoid sinus. **(B)** Almost complete agenesis of the transverse sinus and absence of the inferior petrosal sinus. **(C)** Agenesis of the sigmoid sinus with partial absence of most of the proximal transverse sinus, enlarged emissary vein, and absence of the inferior petrosal sinus. **(D)** Configuration seen in C with addition of persistent petrosquamous sinus. **(E)** Configuration seen in C but with increased size of emissary vein (E.V.). Also note the superior petrosal sinus (S.P.S.), transverse sinus (T.S.), emissary vein (E.V.), internal jugular vein (I.J.V.), and inferior petrosal sinus (I.P.S.). **(F)** Configuration of E but with enlarged superior petrosal sinus. **(G)** Absence of majority of sigmoid sinus but presence of petrosquamous sinus. **(H)** Configuration of G but with complete absence of sigmoid sinus and absence of petrosquamous sinus.

Before any form of surgical procedure is selected, a thorough diagnostic evaluation should be conducted to assess the extent of malformation and whether it is an arteriovenous fistula or a tumor. Surgery depends on the degree of the malformation, extent of tumor invasion, sinus patency, the patient's age, as well as the surgeon's experience, all of which must be considered before resorting to surgery. Anatomic variations of the sigmoid sinus must be considered during such surgeries (Fig. 5.13).

REFERENCES

1. Dai PD, Zhang HQ, Wang ZM, Sha Y, Wang KQ, Zhang TY. Morphological and positional relationships between the sigmoid sinus and the jugular bulb. *Surg Radiol Anat.* 2007;29:643–651.
2. Raso JL, Gusmão SNS. A new landmark for finding the sigmoid sinus in suboccipital craniotomies. *Neurosurgery.* 2011;68:1–6.
3. San Millán Ruíz D. *Systèmes Veineux De La Base Du Crâne Et De La Jonction Cranio-Cervicale: Anatomie Macroscopique Et Radiologique Et Implications Cliniques. Thèse De Doctorat.* Univ. Genève; 2006.
4. Butler H. The development of certain human dural venous sinuses. *J Anat.* 1957;91:510–526.
5. Nishijima M, Endo S, Koizumi F, Kuwayama N, Owada K, Takaku A. Etiological evaluation of dural arteriovenous malformations of the lateral and sigmoid sinuses on histopathological examinations. *J Neurosurg.* 1992;76:600–606.
6. Tanoue S, Hori Y, Kashiwagi J, Kiyosue H, Mori H, Okahara M. Venous structures at the craniocervical junction (anatomical variations evaluated by multidetector row CT). *Br J Radiol.* 2010;83:831–840.
7. Waltner J. Anatomic variations of the lateral and sigmoid sinuses. *Arch Otolaryngol Head Neck Surg.* 1944;39:307–312.
8. Ramos Jr SP, Caetano IM, Gusmão SNS, Nicolata AA, Raso JL, Santos M. Comparative morphometric study of the sigmoid sinus sulcus and the jugular foramen. *Arq Neuropsiquiatr.* 2014;72:694–698.
9. Williams HL. Apparent unilateral absence of sigmoid sinus noted at operation. *Arch Otolaryngol.* 1930;12:339–341.
10. Williams HL, Hallberg OE. Congenital absence of cranial venous sinuses on the right. *Arch Otolaryngol.* 1941;33:78.
11. Surendrababu N, Subathira, Livingstone RS. Variations in the cerebral venous anatomy and pitfalls in the diagnosis of cerebral venous sinus thrombosis: low field MR experience. *Indian J Med Sci.* 2006;60:135–142.
12. Manjunath KY. Anomalies of transverse and sigmoid sinuses associated with contracted jugular foramina. *Indian J Otolaryngol Head Neck Surg.* 2004;56:108–114.
13. Curé JK, Smith T, Van Tassel P. Normal and variant anatomy of the dural venous sinuses. *Semin Ultrasound CT MR.* 1994;15:499–519.
14. Sarmiento PB, Eslait FG. Surgical classification of variations in the anatomy of the sigmoid sinus. *Otolaryngol Head Neck Surg.* 2004;131:192–199.
15. Reis CVC, Zabramski JM, Safavi-Abassi S, Deshmukh P, Spetzler RF, Preul MC. Trautmann's triangle and the transpetrosal approaches: an anatomical study. *Skull Base.* 2007;17:79.
16. Shatz A, Sade J. Correlation between mastoid pneumatization and position of the lateral sinus. *Ann Otol Rhinol Laryngol.* 1990;99:142–145.
17. Turgut S, Tos M. Correlation between temporal bone pneumatization, location of lateral sinus and length of the mastoid process. *J Laryngol Otol.* 1992;106:485–489.
18. Ichijo H, Hosokawa M, Shinkawa H. The relationship between mastoid pneumatization and the position of the sigmoid sinus. *Eur Arch Oto-Rhino-Laryngol.* 1996;253:421–424.
19. Gangopadhyay K, McArthur PD, Larsson SG. Unusual anterior course of the sigmoid sinus: report of a case and review of the literature. *J Laryngol Otol.* 1996;110:984–986.
20. Streeter GL. The development alterations in the vascular system of the brain of the human embryo. *Contributions to Embryology.* Johnson. 1918:5–38.
21. Sakaki T, Kakizaki T, Morimoto T, Nagata K, Nakase H. Dural arteriorvenous fistula of the posterior fossa developing after surgical occlusion of the sigmoid sinus (Report of five cases). *J Neurosurg.* 1996;84:113–118.
22. Wang G, Gong S, Liang X, et al. Clinical characteristics of pulsatile tinnitus caused by sigmoid sinus diverticulum and wall dehiscence (a study of 54 patients). *Acta Otolaryngol.* 2014;134:7–13.
23. Mazur MD, Couldwell W, Cutler A, Taussky P. Management of meningiomas involving the transverse or sigmoid sinus. *Neurosurg Focus.* 2013;35:9.
24. Sundt TM, Piepgras D. The surgical approach to arteriovenous malformations of the lateral and sigmoid dural sinuses. *J Neurosurg.* 1983;59:32–39.
25. Kakarla U, Albuquerque F, Deshmukh V, McDougall C, Spetzler R, Zabramski J. Surgical treatment of high-risk intercranial dural arteriovenous fistulae: clinical outcomes and avoidance of complications. *Neurosurgery.* 2007;61:447–459.
26. Hwang S, Gwak H, Kim D, Jung H, Paek S. Guidelines for the ligation of the sigmoid or transverse sinus during large petroclival meningioma surgery. *Skull Base.* 2004;14:21–28.

FURTHER READING

1. Rutting E. Kloaken und blindsackbildung am sinus sigmoideus. *Acta Otolaryngol.* 1926;9:217–220.
2. Scarrow AM, Jungreis C, Scarrow M, Williams RL, Yonas H. Removal of a thrombus from the sigmoid and transverse sinuses with a rheolytic thrombectomy catheter. *AJNR Am J Neuroradiol.* 1999;20:1467–1469.

CHAPTER 6

The Occipital Sinus

PAMELA YOUSSEF • R. SHANE TUBBS

The dural venous sinuses are divided into superior and inferior groups; the superior drains the majority of the brain and the skull, whereas the inferior drains the sylvian veins, the basal and medial parts of the undersurface of the brain, the orbits, and the sphenoparietal sinus.[1] Together with the superior and inferior sagittal sinuses, and the straight, transverse, and sigmoid sinuses, the occipital sinus constitutes a part of the superior group.

Among the dural venous sinuses, the occipital sinus is one of those studied least (Figs. 6.1–6.5). One reason for this might be its absence in a significant number of people with no clinical sequelae; another reason may be the high degree of variation that it exhibits, which is discussed later. Multiple anatomic studies have mentioned the occipital sinus, but the research on it showed that it is present in 65%[2] and 75% of cadavers.[3]

ANATOMY

The normal occipital sinus lies on the midline[4] and is positioned primarily at the base of the falx cerebelli.[5] It descends to the margins of the foramen magnum[6] and extends from the foramen magnum up to the torcular Herophili.[4] Drainage toward the foramen magnum or into the jugular fossa or suboccipital veins also is possible[4] It also may deviate to one side, serve as a collateral channel for a small transverse sinus[3] or replace an aplastic transverse sinus,[1] which is discussed further in the variations section.

The occipital sinus is an ellipsoid structure and usually is a single channel, the size of which can range from 1 to 4 mm.[3] It has been noted to be larger close to the confluence of sinuses, after which the breadth narrows as the sinus approaches the margins of the foramen magnum.[5] Its length can vary between 15 and 70 mm, with an average length of 35 mm.[2] The inner diameter measures between 0.33 and 7.06 mm at the midpoint, and the perimeter ranges from 0.77 to 17.61 mm.[5]

The inner wall of the occipital sinus consists of a connection of fibrous bands, bridges, and septae that become denser as the sinus approaches the torcular Herophili. In cases in which multiple occipital sinus channels are present, they have been found to be close to each other and at the midline.[5] The presence of multiple sinuses does not imply a larger size or diameter.

Histological studies show elastic fibers in the tunica intima under the endothelium. Nerve fibers were not observed in these sections. In addition, bundles of collagen fibers also can be seen with staining. These two histologic characteristics contribute to the occipital sinus' resistance to stretching and reflect more effective blood drainage.[5]

EMBRYOLOGY

To understand the embryologic origin of the occipital sinus, a short general explanation of the origination of the venous system must be provided first. Basically, the cerebral venous system begins as a single primary head vein observed first in 4-mm embryos. A single layer of endothelial cells forms this structure that later acquires three tributaries. In the 14-mm embryo, after the dura mater veins become distinct from the cerebral veins, the primary head vein drains three plexiform groups newly formed: the anterior, medial, and posterior dural plexuses.[7,8] The posterior dural plexus is the embryonic structure that becomes the occipital sinus in the adult.[8] Streeter[8] reported further that the posterior venous plexus undergoes minor variations through the different embryologic stages, unlike the anterior and middle venous plexuses.

Although the posterior venous plexus, which gives rise to the occipital sinus, begins to become distinct in the 14-mm embryo stage,[9,10] the occipital sinus can only be identified later. It also is a secondary embryonic anastomosis, as it is continuous with the posterior internal vertebral venous plexus. This anastomosis lasts until after the 80-mm embryo, when the cerebellar lobes form.[9]

Okudera et al.[11] reported that rather than a single occipital sinus, it is instead a collection of 3–7

Anatomy, Imaging and Surgery of the Intracranial Dural Venous Sinuses. https://doi.org/10.1016/B978-0-323-65377-0.00006-4

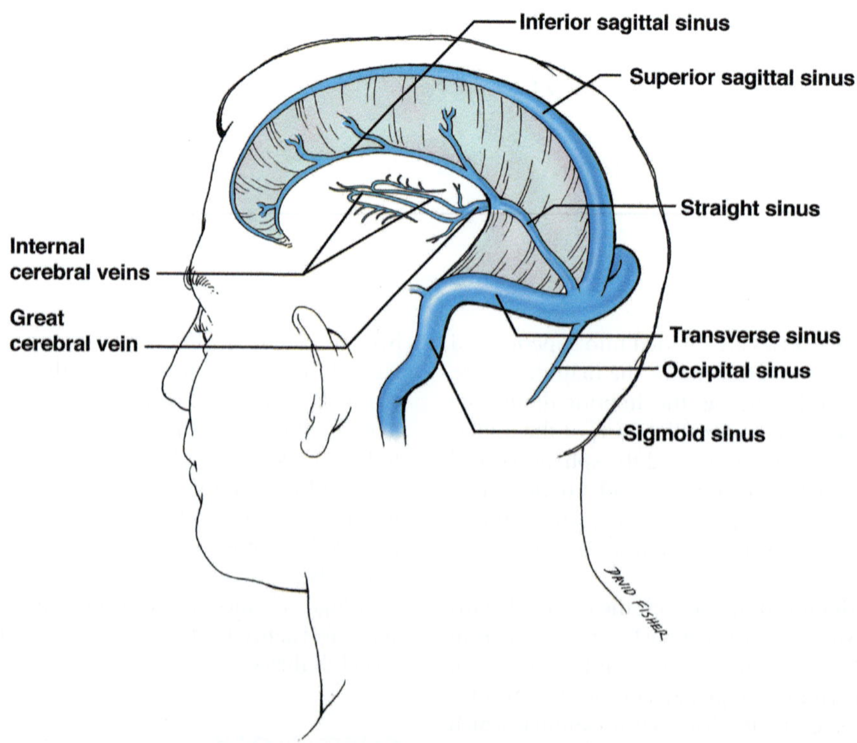

FIG. 6.1 Schematic drawing of the occipital sinus and related dural venous sinuses.

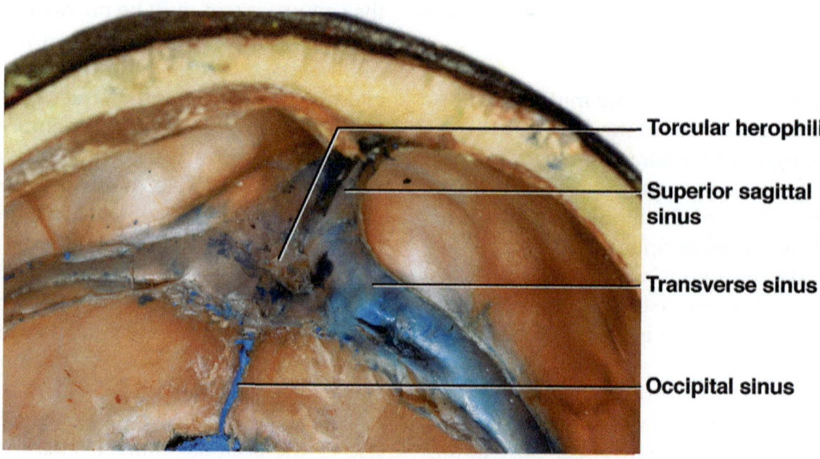

FIG. 6.2 Anterior view of a dissected occipital sinus.

plexiform venous channels that originate from the torcular plexus. These venous channels are not visible until the age of 3 fetal months, which corresponds to the 65-mm embryo stage[11] or 4[12] fetal months. Padget[9] was unable to identify them until the 80-mm embryo stage. The occipital channels originate in the torcular plexus and grow downward toward the marginal sinuses around the foramen magnum. These channels undergo a rapid growth phase followed by a rapid regression phase. The greatest growth and development phase is at approximately 4 or 5 months of fetal age. This is followed by regression through diminution and union in

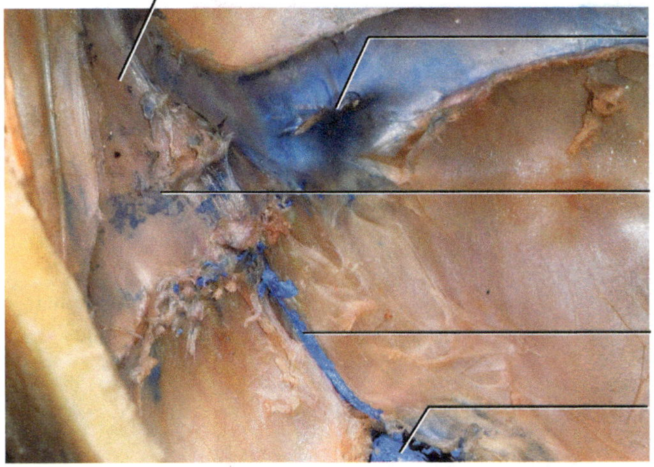

FIG. 6.3 Anterolateral view of a dissected occipital sinus.

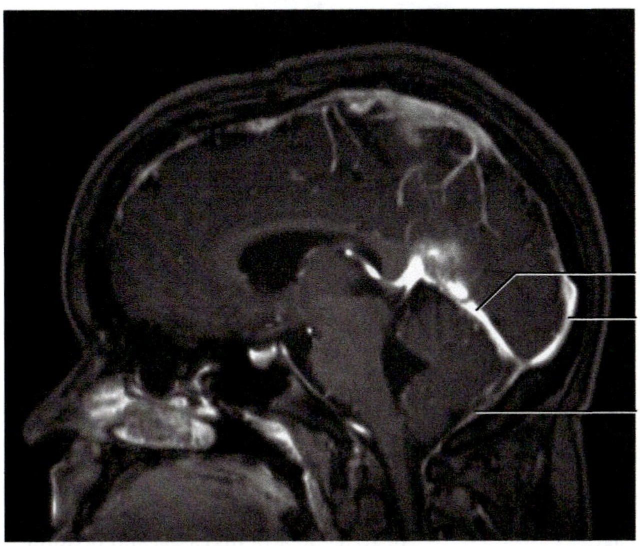

FIG. 6.4 Sagittal T1-weighted MRI noting the occipital sinus.

the months that follow, and only a few of them remain at 6 or 7 months. These remaining few venous channels connect the transverse sinuses to the marginal or sigmoid sinuses.[11] This change occurs simultaneously with a physiologic response to a change that corresponds to increased venous drainage from the intracranial to the extracranial spaces.[11]

Many studies have shown that the occipital sinus is more prominent in neonates[13] and relatively narrower in adults.[14] Widjaja and Griffiths[15] found a statistically significant correlation between the presence of the occipital sinus and age. In their study, they reported the presence of the occipital sinus predominantly in patients less than 2 years, and not more than 9 years of age. Similarly, Rollins et al.[16] reported the presence of the occipital sinus predominantly in children less than 25 months, but not more than 5 years. The explanation they provided for their findings are consistent with Okudera et al.'s[11] hypothesis. The increased venous drainage into the vertebral venous plexus becomes much more prominent that into the internal jugular vein as the child learns to walk and leads to the

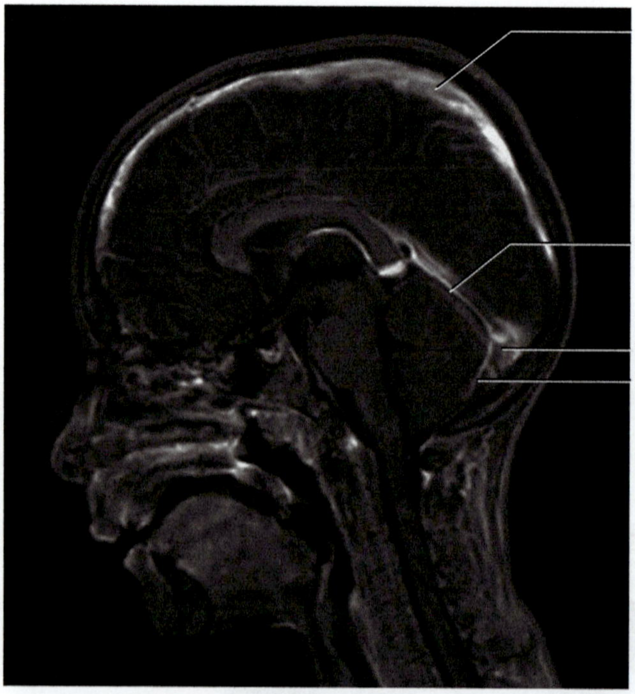

FIG. 6.5 Sagittal T1-weighted MRI noting the occipital sinus.

reduction in the size and number of occipital sinuses in older children and adults.[15] Other factors also should be considered to determine the presence or absence of the occipital sinus, such as imaging modalities that are discussed in a separate section.

VARIATIONS

The inconsistency between different studies that have attempted to study the occipital sinus is attributable to the large number of variations this structure exhibits, including the presence, location, size, drainage, morphology, termination, and relation to age.

Although numerous anatomic studies have reported and proved the dominant presence of the occipital sinus,[2,3,6,9,13,17–21] others have found that the occipital sinus predominantly was absent.[15,22]

Das and Hasan[2] detected its presence in 129 of their 200 adult specimens, whereas Knott[6] found it in 42 of his 44 specimens. Browder et al.[3] noted its presence in 85% of their specimens, and Tanoue et al.[23] detected its presence in 18 of their 50 patients. This latter study used contrast-enhanced computed tomography (CT) with a multidetector scanner.

With respect to morphology and location, a single occipital sinus may be positioned at the midline, or on the right or left side. It also may divide occasionally into two or more divisions caudally or cranially.[2,24,25] Of the 42 occipital sinuses found in Knott's[6] studies, 33 had a single and 9 a bilateral occipital sinus. Browder et al.[3] found a single occipital sinus in 75% of their specimens, a paired sinus in 8%, and the remaining 2% showed occipital sinuses that served as a major drainage pathway. Among the 200 specimens Das and Hasan[2] studied, a single midline occipital sinus was found in 35% of the specimens, a double sinus in 22.5%, a single left-sided sinus in 4%, and a single right-sided sinus in 3%. Baker[26] reported a double occipital sinus in 25%–30% of his cases, and possible absence in up to 3%. D'Costa et al.[27] reported 15.4% cases with duplicated falx cerebelli and duplicated occipital sinuses in 52 cadavers of South Indian origin (Fig. 6.6).

With respect to location, in 33 of the 42 specimens in Knott's[6] study that had a single occipital sinus, it originated above the torcular Herophili; seven had a sinus that opened into the left lateral sinus; five had a sinus that opened into the right lateral sinus, and three were connected with the straight sinus a quarter of an inch in front of the torcular Herophili. In one of the nine cases with a bilateral occipital sinus, the sinus was found beneath the dura mater on both sides of the internal occipital crest. In two other cases among the

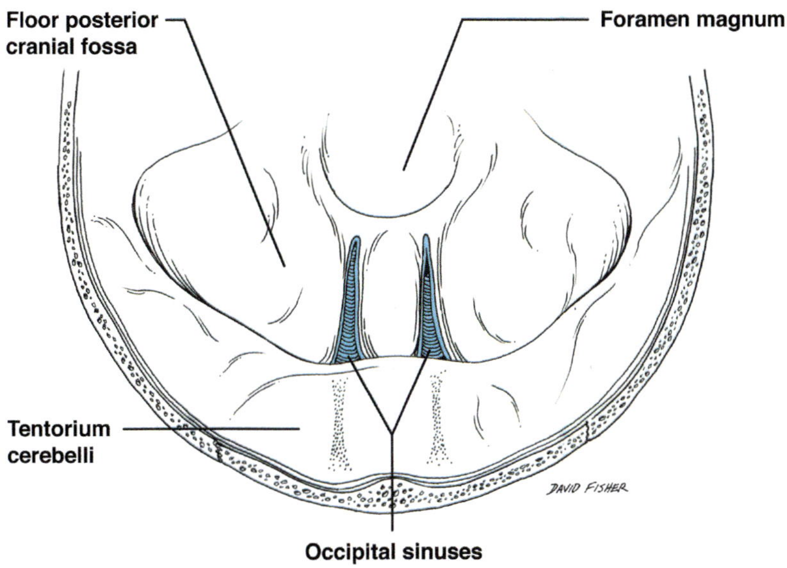

FIG. 6.6 Schematic drawing of duplicated occipital sinuses.

nine specimens with a bilateral occipital sinus, the left occipital sinus continued to form the marginal sinus that joins the lateral sinus at the jugular foramen, and then connected to the veins of the spinal canal. Another three of these nine cases had very small occipital sinuses that ended below the anastomosing network on the posterior lip of the margin of the foramen magnum. A triple occipital sinus is a rare finding in anatomical studies[14] that was found to be composed of a mesh of venous collaterals in some cases.[16] In other conditions, rather than passing at the midline, the occipital sinus deviates to one side occasionally and merges with the sigmoid sinus as it passes through the jugular foramen.[28]

The length, width, diameter, and drainage of the occipital sinus also have shown high variability in different studies, which poses a challenge in posterior cranial fossa surgical approaches.[28] According to Das and Hasan,[2] the length ranges from 1.5 to 7 cm, and the width from 1 to 19 mm near its termination. Sometimes, the occipital sinus actually functions as the main drainage of the venous sinuses.[15,24,28] In these cases, also the marginal sinus is large, and the occipital sinus grows to the extent that it may replace the sigmoid sinus,[28] in which cases, the transverse sinus is absent. The occipital sinus also functions as the main drainage when the lateral sinus is rudimentary.[29]

Tanoue et al.[23] found a "prominent type" of occipital sinus in 4 of the 18 cases in which they found an occipital sinus. Three of these cases drained into the sigmoid sinus, whereas seven others drained into the marginal sinus. Others have reported a normal, hypoplastic, or absent transverse and sigmoid sinus associated with the occipital sinus draining into the superior bulb of the internal jugular vein.[30]

In 2% of the cases Baker[26] studied, he described a huge occipital sinus that received drainage from the straight and superior sagittal sinuses. Tubbs et al.[31] also reported an unusually large occipital sinus (1.5 cm × 6 cm) that, rather than draining into the marginal sinus as is typical, drained directly into the jugular foramen and subsequently into the internal jugular vein.

Another variation in the drainage pattern detected is an occipital sinus that drains into the sigmoid sinus,[14] which has been referred to as an oblique occipital sinus[29] (Figs. 6.7–6.14). Another oblique occipital sinus also was reported that terminated in the straight sinus, where it functioned as the main drainage in the case of a rudimentary transverse sinus.[29] These authors also reported another variation in which the occipital sinus drains directly into the bulb of the left lateral sinus, with no drainage into the right. Kobayashi et al. in an imaging study of 555 patients found that the occipital sinus had communication with the sigmoid sinus in 11.9%. Interestingly, one reported variant of the superior sagittal sinus is direct drainage into the jugular bulb. We believe that such a report might actually be a description of an oblique occipital sinus.

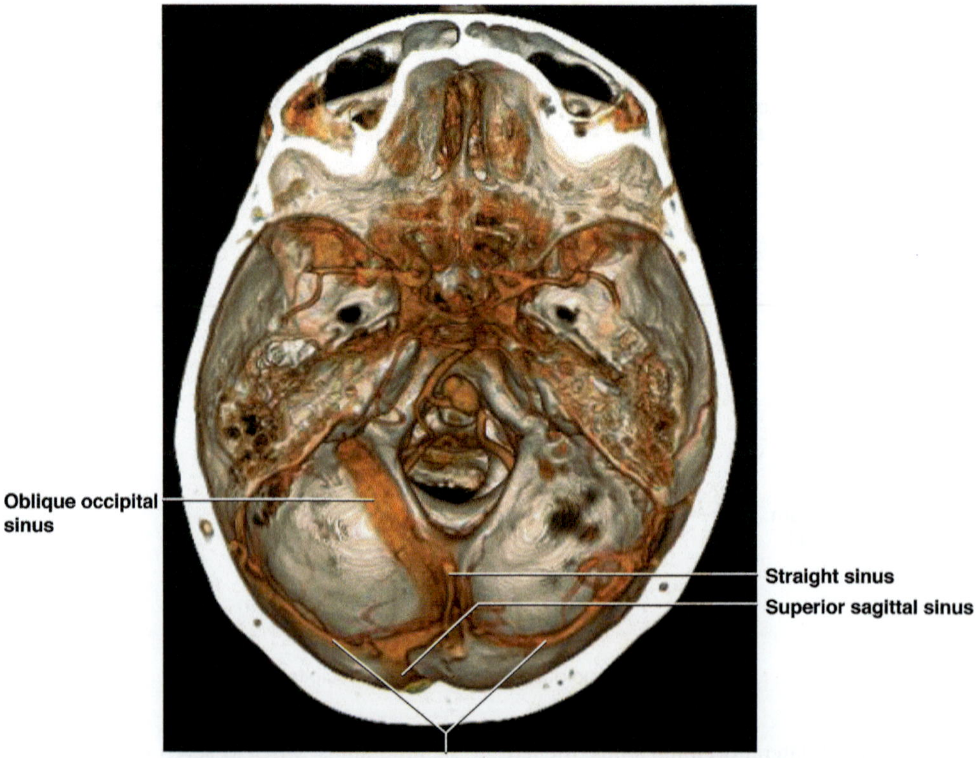

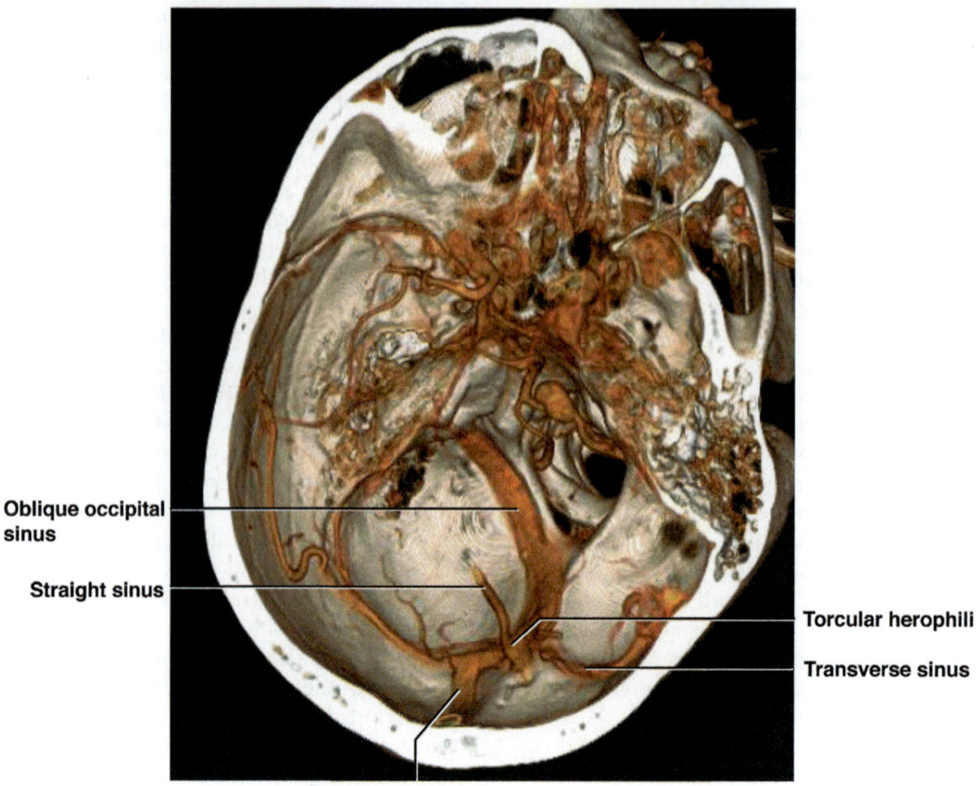

FIGS. 6.7–6.10 3D CTA noting oblique occipital sinuses. (Courtesy Dr. Joel Curé.)

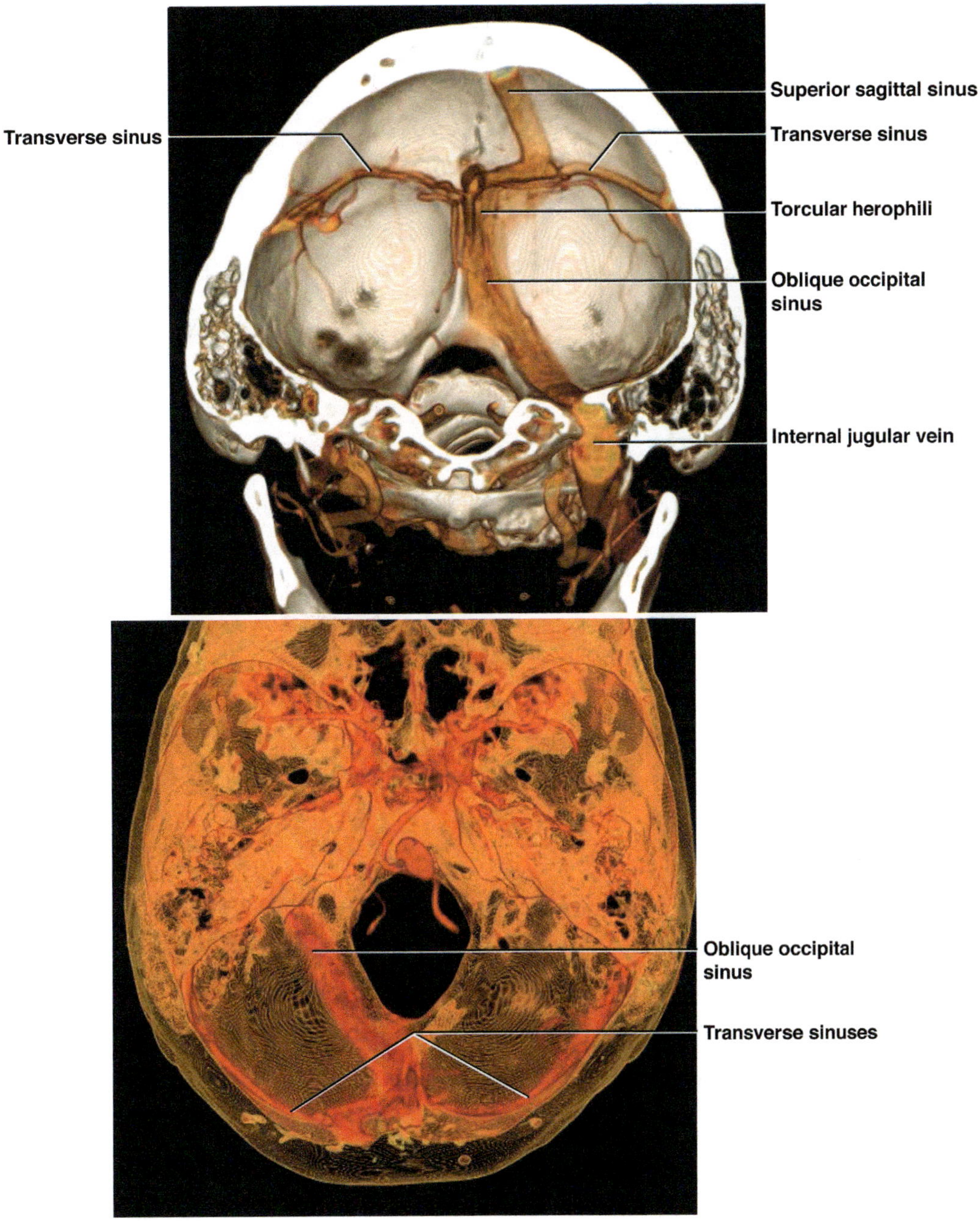

FIGS. 6.7–6.10, cont'd

In addition to an oblique occipital sinus, Shoja et al.[32] also reported a duplicated falx cerebelli. The marginal sinus was absent, and in addition to the 2.5-mm occipital sinus found near the posterolateral rim of the foramen magnum, there was an additional sinus on the right side to which they referred as the "lateral occipital sinus." This sinus included one medial branch that connected the right sigmoid sinus to the occipital sinus, and two lateral branches that connected the right transverse sinuses. Shoja et al.[32] also reported another case of an oblique occipital sinus that was found posterolateral to the foramen magnum coursing superiorly and posteromedially

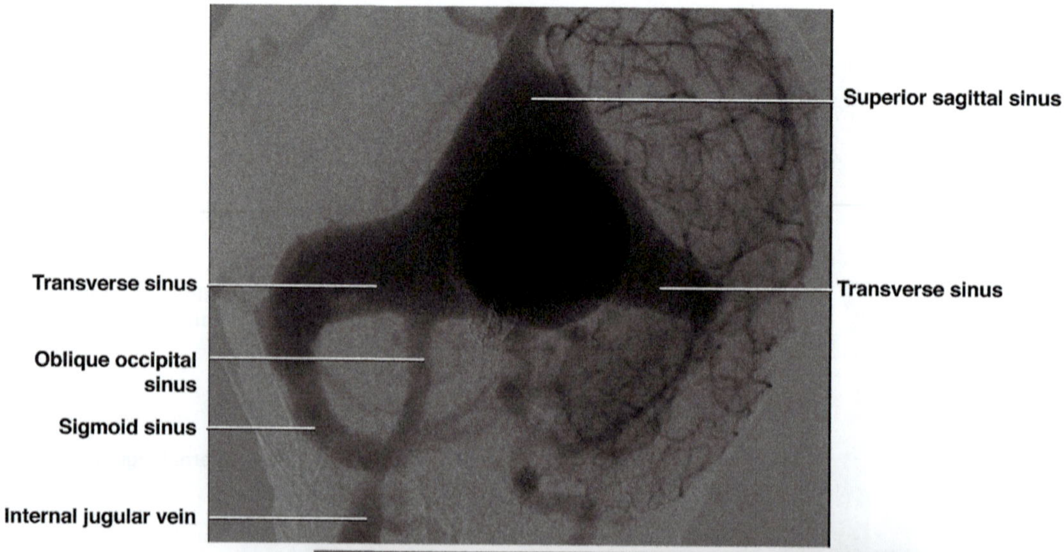

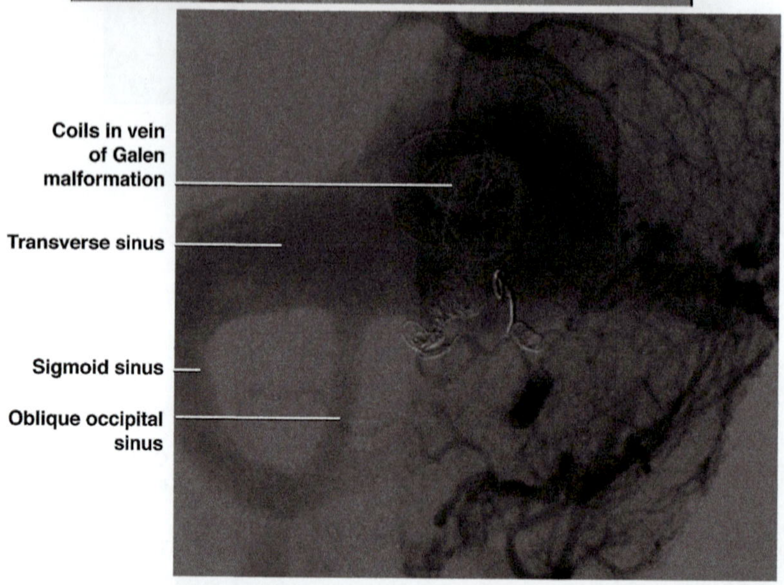

FIGS. 6.11 AND 6.12 Oblique occipital sinuses noted in a patient with vein of Galen malformation.

and connecting the terminal portion of the right sigmoid sinus to the occipital and right transverse sinuses via one medial and two lateral branches, respectively.

The most common termination site of the occipital sinus is the torcular Herophili, but the transverse, superior sagittal, or straight sinus are also other reported termination sites.[2] Kopuz et al.[24] provided a more detailed classification of the termination of the occipital sinus in neonates. They identified six types of termination in the region of the torcular. In type 1, two occipital sinuses open to the confluence while the superior sagittal sinus is continuous with the right transverse sinus. In type 2, more than two occipital sinuses open to the confluence, while the transverse and sagittal sinuses exhibit the same pattern as in type 1. Type 3 is similar to type 1, except that the superior sagittal sinus is continuous with the left transverse sinus. Type 4 is similar to type 2, with the same exception. In type 5, the superior sagittal sinus drains into the confluence to which both the transverse sinus and two occipital sinuses are connected. In type 6, the superior sagittal sinus bifurcates before joining the transverse sinus.

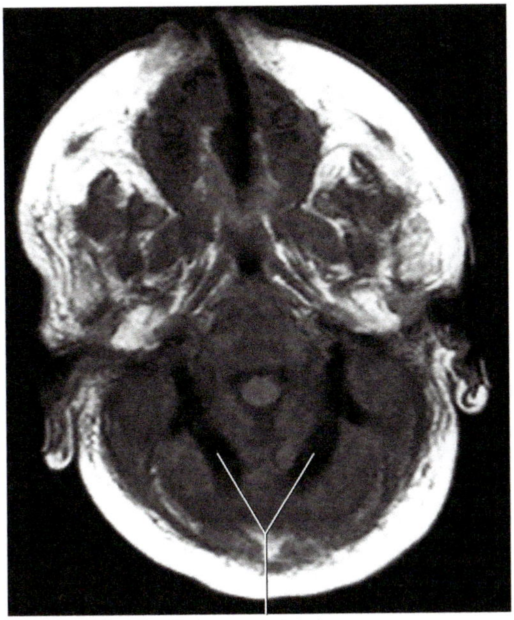

FIG. 6.13 Axial T1-weighted MRI in a patient with bilateral oblique occipital sinuses. (Courtesy Dr. Joel Curé.)

Finally, with respect to the relation with age, various anatomic studies have shown different outcomes. Widjaja and Griffiths[15] and Kopuz et al.[24] reported that the occipital sinus is relatively wider in neonates compared with adults. In addition, Rollins et al.[16] reported a possible age-related regression of the occipital sinus because their magnetic resonance venography (MRV) study showed its presence in 13% of 25-month-old patients, but in only 2% of patients older than 5 years.

IMAGING

Multiple imaging techniques that can be classified primarily as invasive or noninvasive have been used to study the cerebral venous system. Catheter-based digital subtraction angiography (DSA), a more invasive method, was used traditionally in the past. Less invasive techniques have replaced this method largely, such as computed tomography venography and different types of cerebral MRV.[33]

Although DSA visualizes the vein of Galen and the superior sagittal, straight, and the transverse sinuses reliably, the occipital sinus cannot be visualized effectively with this technique.[34] In addition, CT lacks the anatomic delineation that would allow detection of such a structure as the occipital sinus.[34]

With respect to the venography technique, in a study of MR venography in children, only 18% of cases were found to have an occipital sinus.[15] This finding is inconsistent with other anatomic studies mentioned previously, where the occipital sinus was found in many more specimens.[2] One of the reasons for this inconsistency might be that the occipital sinus was collapsed, or exhibited slow flow, as in both cases, 2D time-of-flight venography would be unable to visualize it.[15]

PATHOLOGY

The occipital sinus is believed to play a minimal role in venous outflow, as it is usually small or absent.[5] As a consequence, occlusion of this sinus has not been shown to produce any significant recognizable disturbances in cerebral venous drainage. Enlargement of the sinus is often seen in dural venous fistulas or vein of Galen malformations. Therefore, in these pathologies, care must be taken when opening the dura mater during surgical exposure.

SURGERY

As mentioned earlier, the occipital sinus shows a high degree of individual variation. In addition, it varies greatly between age groups, with infants and children generally having much larger occipital sinuses.[15,16] Therefore, avoiding injury to this structure during surgery can be challenging. However, in the majority of people, the occipital sinus exhibits a midline path,[4] which allows the area that must be avoided to preserve the occipital sinus to be determined more easily.

Surgeries that pose a high risk of sacrificing the occipital sinus primarily are posterior cranial fossa surgeries. Yaşargil[35] described multiple surgeries performed with the median suboccipital approach that pose a high risk of injuring the occipital sinus. When present, the occipital sinus is sacrificed often during these procedures, with no reported clinical disturbances. However, efforts should be made to preserve this sinus, if possible.

Knowing the diameter, perimeter, and length of the occipital sinus can provide an approximation of the area that should be avoided in posterior cranial fossa surgery to preserve this structure. Balak et al.[5] estimated that the area of risk is up to 1 cm from the midline. A more careful evaluation should be performed in cases with an oblique occipital sinus.[29]

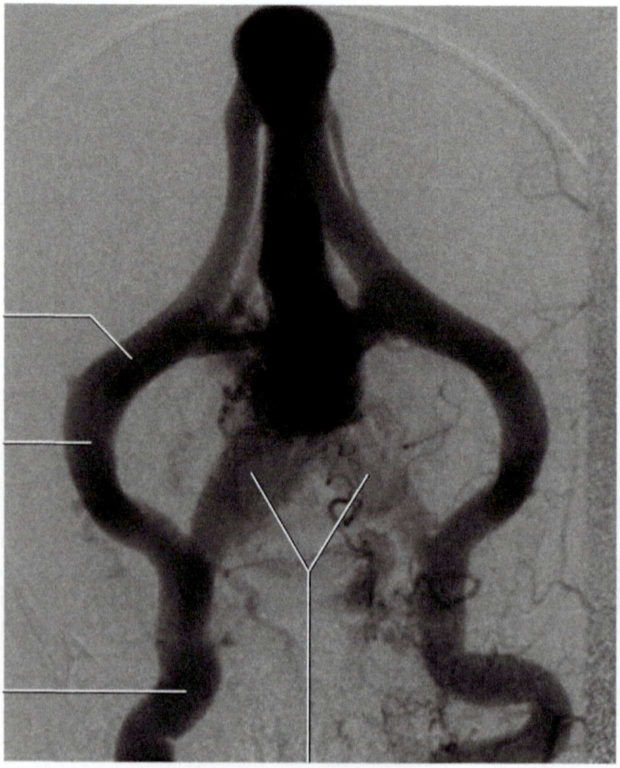

FIG. 6.14 Angiogram venous phase in a patient with vein of Galen malformation and bilateral oblique occipital sinuses.

REFERENCES

1. Curé JK, Tassel PV, Smith MT. Normal and variant anatomy of the dural venous sinuses. *Semin Ultrasound CT MR*. 1994;15:499–519.
2. Das AC, Hasan M. The occipital sinus. *J Neurosurg*. 1970;33:307–311.
3. Browder J, Kaplan HA, Krieger AJ. Anatomical features of the straight sinus and its tributaries. *J Neurosurg*. 1976;44:55–61.
4. Scott JN, Farb RI. Imaging and anatomy of the normal intracranial venous system. *Neuroimaging Clin N Am*. 2003;13:1–12.
5. Balak N, Ersoy G, Uslu U, et al. Microsurgical and histomorphometric study of the occipital sinus: quantitative measurements using a novel approach of stereology. *Clin Anat*. 2010;23:386–393.
6. Knott JF. On the cerebral sinuses and their variations. *J Anat Physiol*. 1881;16:27–42.
7. Mall FP. On the development of the blood vessels of the brain in the human embryo. *Am J Anat*. 1914;4:1–18.
8. Streeter GL. The development of alterations in the vascular system of the brain of the human embryo. *Contrib Embryol*. 1918;24:7–38.
9. Padget DH. Cranial venous system in man in reference to development of adult configuration and relation to arteries. *Am J Anat*. 1956;98:307–355.
10. Truwit CL. Embryology of the cerebral vasculature. *Neuroimaging Clin N Am*. 1994;4:663–689.
11. Okudera T, Huang YP, Ohta T, et al. Development of posterior fossa dural sinuses, emissary veins, and jugular bulb: morphological and radiologic study. *AJNR Am J Neuroradiol*. 1994;15:1871–1883.
12. Masaki S. Studies on the development of the dural sinuses of the human fetus. *Fukuoka Igaku Zasshi*. 1959;50:2769–2788. [in Japanese].
13. Woodhall B. Anatomy of the cranial blood sinuses with particular reference to the lateral. *Laryngoscope*. 1939;49:966–1010.
14. Lang J. *Clinical Anatomy of the Posterior Cranial Fossa and its Foramina*. New York, NY: Thieme; 1991:6–9.
15. Widjaja E, Griffiths PD. Intracranial MR venography in children: normal anatomy and variations. *AJNR Am J Neuroradiol*. 2004;25:1557–1562.
16. Rollins N, Ison C, Booth T, Chia J. MR venography in the pediatric patient. *AJNR Am J Neuroradiol*. 2005;26:50–55.

17. Gibbs E, Gibbs F. The cross section areas of the vessels that form the torcular and the manner in which flow is distributed to the right and to the left lateral sinus. *Anat Rec*. 1934;59:419–426.
18. Woodhall B. Variations of the cranial venous sinuses in the region of the torcular Herophili. *Arch Surg*. 1936;33:297.
19. Woodhall B, Seeds AE. Cranial venous sinuses, correlation between skull markings and roentgenograms of the occipital bone. *Arch Surg*. 1936;33:867–875.
20. Baló J. The dural venous sinuses. *Anat Rec*. 1950;106:319–324.
21. Browning H. The confluence of dural venous sinuses. *Am J Anat*. 1953;92:307–329.
22. San Millan Ruíz D, Gailloud P, Rufenacht DA, Delavelle J, Henry F, Fasel JH. The craniocervical venous system in relation to cerebral venous drainage. *AJNR Am J Neuroradiol*. 2002;23:1500–1508.
23. Tanoue S, Kiyosue H, Sagara Y, et al. Venous structures at the craniocervical junction: anatomical variations evaluated by multidetector row CT. *Br J Radiol*. 2010;83:831–840.
24. Kopuz C, Aydin ME, Kale A, Demir MT, Corumlu U, Kaya AH. The termination of superior sagittal sinus and drainage patterns of the lateral, occipital at confluens sinuum in newborns: clinical and embryological implications. *Surg Radiol Anat*. 2010;32:827–833.
25. Adeeb N, Mortazavi MM, Tubbs RS, Cohen-Gadol AA. The cranial dura mater: a review of its history, embryology, and anatomy. *Childs Nerv Syst*. 2012;28:827–837.
26. Baker AB. In: *Clinical Neurology*. Vol. 3. New York, NY: Hoeber-Harper; 1955:1686.
27. D'costa S, Krishnamurthy A, Nayak SR, et al. Duplication of falx cerebelli, occipital sinus, and internal occipital crest. *Rom J Morphol Embryol*. 2009;50:107–110.
28. Hollinshead WH. *Anatomy for Surgeons*. 2nd ed. Vol. 1. Philadelphia: Harper & Row; 1968:12–22. 83-85.
29. Tubbs RS, Bosmia AN, Shoja MM, Loukas M, Curé JK, Cohen-Gadol AA. The oblique occipital sinus: a review of anatomy and imaging characteristics. *Surg Radiol Anat*. 2011;33:747–749.
30. San Millan Ruíz D. *Systèmes veineux de la base du crâne et de la jonction cranio-cervicale: Anatomie macroscopique et radiologique et implications cliniques*. Universite de Geneve; 2006:1–90. Unpublished doctoral dissertation.
31. Tubbs RS, Shoja MM, Loukas M. An unusual finding of the posterior cranial fossa: one case report. *Ital J Anat Embryol*. 2008;113:83–86.
32. Shoja MM, Tubbs RS, Loukas M, Shokouhi G, Oakes WJ. A complex dural-venous variation in the posterior cranial fossa: a triplicate falx cerebelli and an aberrant venous sinus. *Folia Morphol (Warsz)*. 2007;66:148–151.
33. Agid R, Shelef I, Scott JN, Farb RI. Imaging of the intracranial venous system. *Neurol*. 2008;14:12–22.
34. Modic MT, Weinstein MA, Starnes DL, Kinney SE, Duchesneau PM. Intravenous digital subtraction angiography of the intracranial veins and dural sinuses. *Radiology*. 1983;146:383–389.
35. Yaşargil MG. *Microneurosurgery*. New York, NY: Thieme; 1996:29–68.

CHAPTER 7

The Torcular Herophili (Confluence of Sinuses)

ANDRE GRANGER • R. SHANE TUBBS

ANATOMY

The torcular Herophili (confluence of sinuses) is a highly variable structure that constitutes a vital part of the network of dural venous sinuses (Figs. 7.1–7.5). The torcular Herophili is defined historically as the intersection of the superior sagittal sinus (SSS), the straight sinus (StS), the occipital sinus (OS) and the two transverse sinuses (TS).[1,2] Its size varies and it is located inferior to the occipital lobes and posterosuperiomedially to the cerebellum.

As a general rule, and with the torcular Herophili as the point of reference, the SSS, OS, and the StS represent inflow tracts, while the two TS represent outflow tracts. The direction of flow observed in individual specimens depends heavily on the diameters of each of the sinuses, the specific variant of the torcular Herophili present, and the presence of an intraluminal septum in the vicinity of the torcular Herophili (Fig. 7.6). Park et al.[2] observed this intraluminal septum in 16.2% (5 of 31) of specimens and Ishizaka[3] in 13% (7 of 52) of specimens.

Lamina chordae, a special type of chordae Willisii, were observed in some specimens Shao et al.[4] examined, and separated the lumen into two channels.

The central aspect of the external occipital protuberance, or the inion, was believed previously to be a reliable external anatomical landmark with which to locate the torcular Herophili. However, Tubbs et al.[5] found that this marker was unreliable, and the internal occipital protuberance, which was located inferior to the inion in the majority (73.3%) of cases was a more reliable marker.[5,6] The concavity at the internal occipital protuberance that houses the torcular Herophili is known as the torcular fossula or fossa of Zoja.

EMBRYOLOGY

The primary arrangement for drainage of capillaries in the head of a human embryo consists of a primary head vein that begins in the region of the midbrain and runs caudally along the brain tube. Blood drains from the capillary network via this primary head vein, which serves as the starting point of venous drainage from the brain tube. The anastomosing venous loops stemming from the capillaries drain in the form of three plexuses, the anterior, middle, and the posterior dural.

As the forebrain continues to develop, the anterior plexus is displaced caudally by several proposed phenomena, leaving a segment of its anterior network behind. This portion represents the sagittal plexus. The SSS develops from the sagittal plexus at the midline. The StS also forms from a tributary that belonged originally to the anterior plexus. As the embryo matures, the anterior plexus loses much of its plexiform architecture. It fuses with the middle plexus and drains caudally, becoming a simplified remnant of its former self, and now functions as a point of intersection of the SSS, the StS, the OS, and the two TSs. This marks the birth of the torcular Herophili, the last trace of the anterior and middle dural plexuses.[7–9]

Flow in the region of the torcular Herophili may not always be unobstructed.[2,3,10] In some specimens obstructed in part, a circumferential thickening narrowed the lumen of the TS just lateral to the torcular Herophili. These meshes were thought to be the relics of the venous plexuses from which the torcular Herophili originated.[11–13]

HISTOLOGY

The torcular Herophili is a very simple structure under the microscope. It is lined by endothelial cells and lies between the tough, fibrous meningeal and periosteal layers of the dura.[10] In the connective tissue below these endothelial cells, smooth muscle cell layers may be visualized by light and electron microscopy. In some specimens, trabeculae also may be observed. The purpose of the smooth muscle cells and the trabeculae are

Anatomy, Imaging and Surgery of the Intracranial Dural Venous Sinuses. https://doi.org/10.1016/B978-0-323-65377-0.00007-6

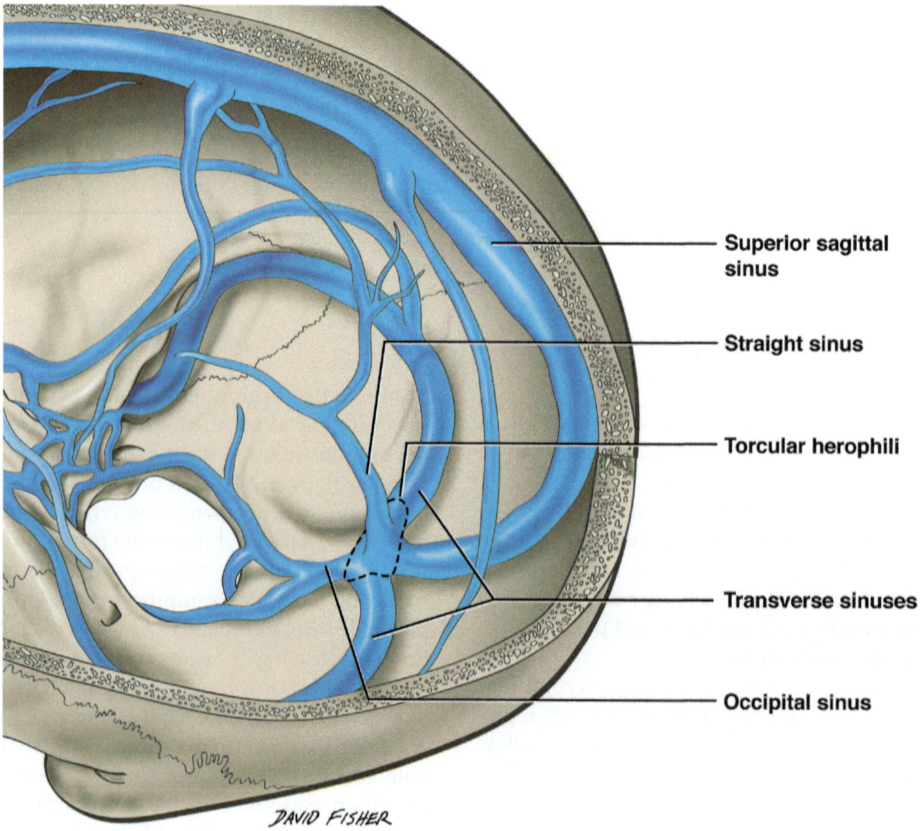

FIG. 7.1 Schematic drawing of the venous sinuses contributing to the torcular Herophili, which is outlined.

unclear, but some suggest that they may play a role in regulating blood flow in the area.[3]

The presence of fat in the intracranial cavity usually suggests a pathological process. However, a few cases of fat at the torcular Herophili in the absence of disease have been mentioned.[14,15] Although the prevalence is low, one should not immediately conclude that fat seen on histological specimens indicates an abnormality.

VARIATIONS

The torcular Herophili remains one of the most variable structures among the network of dural venous sinuses (Fig. 7.6). In this chapter, we adopt the variations Kobayashi et al.[9] described, which can be divided into nine groups, as follows:

1. Type 1–The SSS, StS, and the bilateral TS join at one point. Type 1 was observed in 32.7% (180 of 549) of patients.
2. Type 2–The StS branches into bilateral TSs.
   a. Type 2a, the SSS into the right TS, was observed in 31.5% (173 of 549) of patients.
   b. Type 2b, the SSS into the left sinus, was observed in 6.2% (34 of 549) of patients.
3. Type 3–The SSS and the StS branch into the bilateral TSs. Type 3 was observed in 18.9% (104 of 549) of patients.
4. Type 4–The SSS branches into bilateral TSs.
   a. Type 4a, the StS into the right TS, was observed in 3.1% (17 of 549) of patients.
   b. Type 4b, the StS into the left TS, was observed in 4.4% (24 of 549) of patients.
5. Type 5
   a. Type 5a, the StS into the OS, was observed in 0.5% (3 of 549) of patients.
   b. Type 5b, the StS communicates with veins other than the OS only via the small anastomotic veins, was observed in 0.4% (2 of 549) of patients.

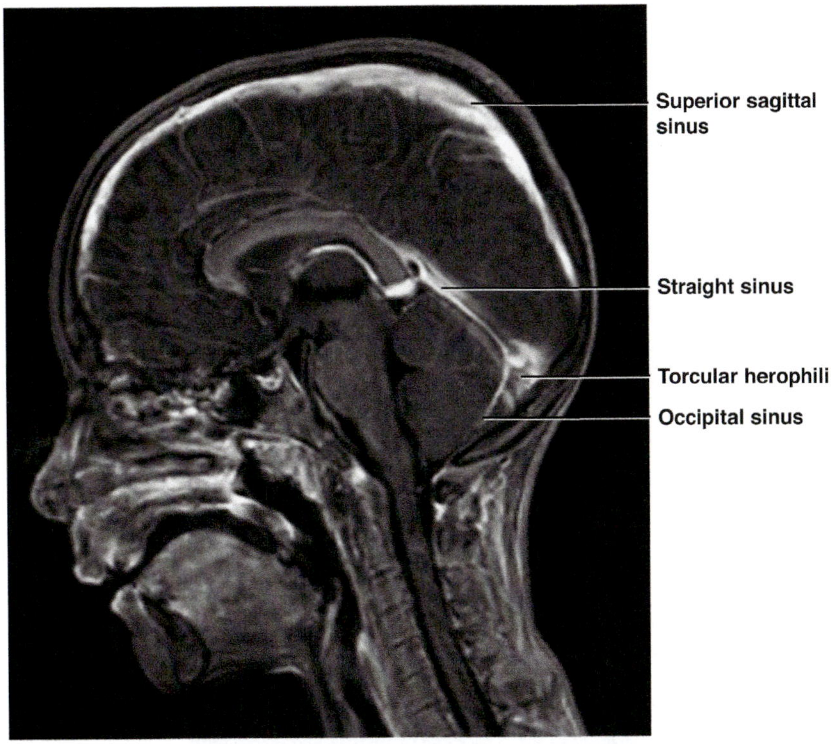

FIG. 7.2 Midsagittal T1-weighted MRI following contrast. Note the torcular Herophili

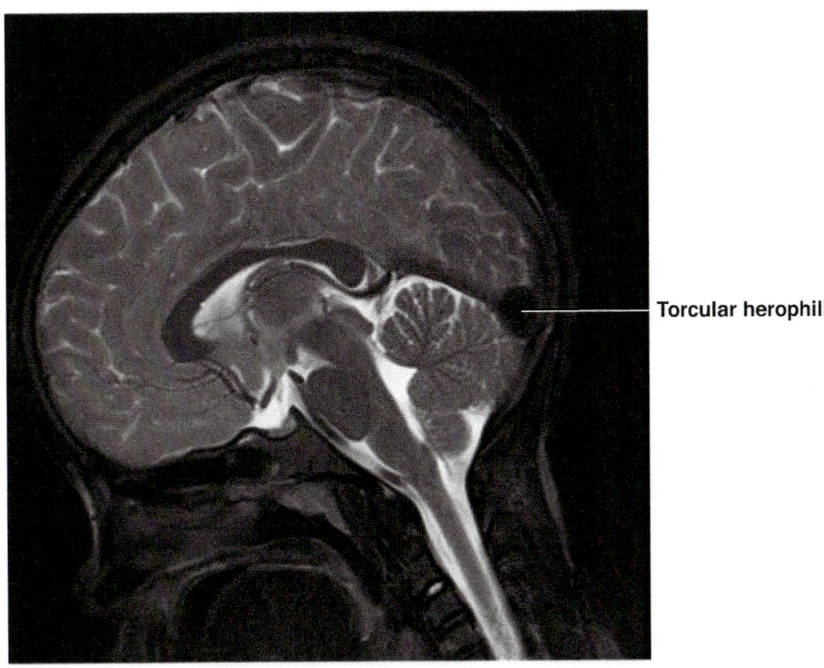

FIG. 7.3 Midsagittal T2-weighted MRI. Note the torcular Herophili

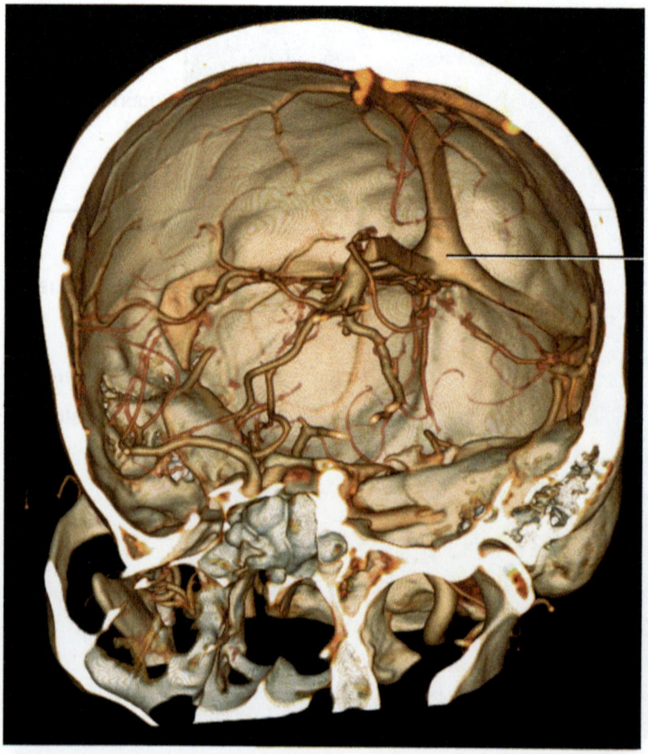

FIG. 7.4 3D CTA noting the torcular Herophili. (Courtesy Dr. Joel Curé.)

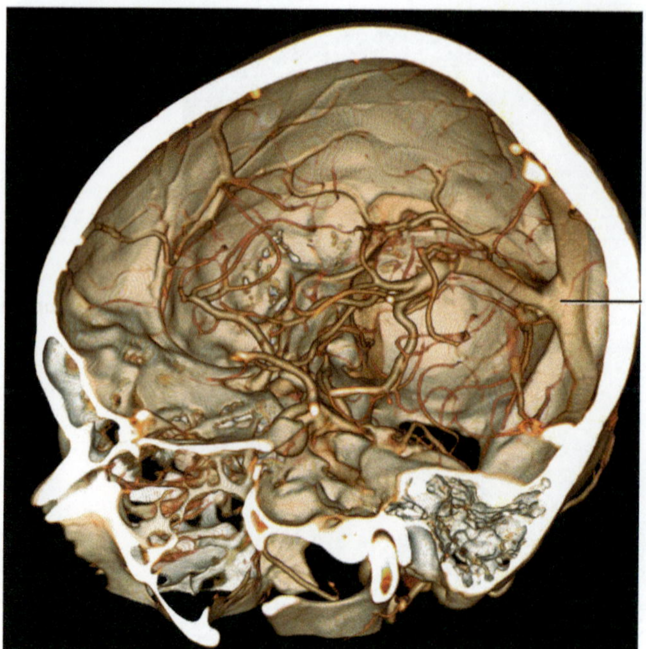

FIG. 7.5 3D CTA noting the torcular Herophili. (Courtesy Dr. Joel Curé.)

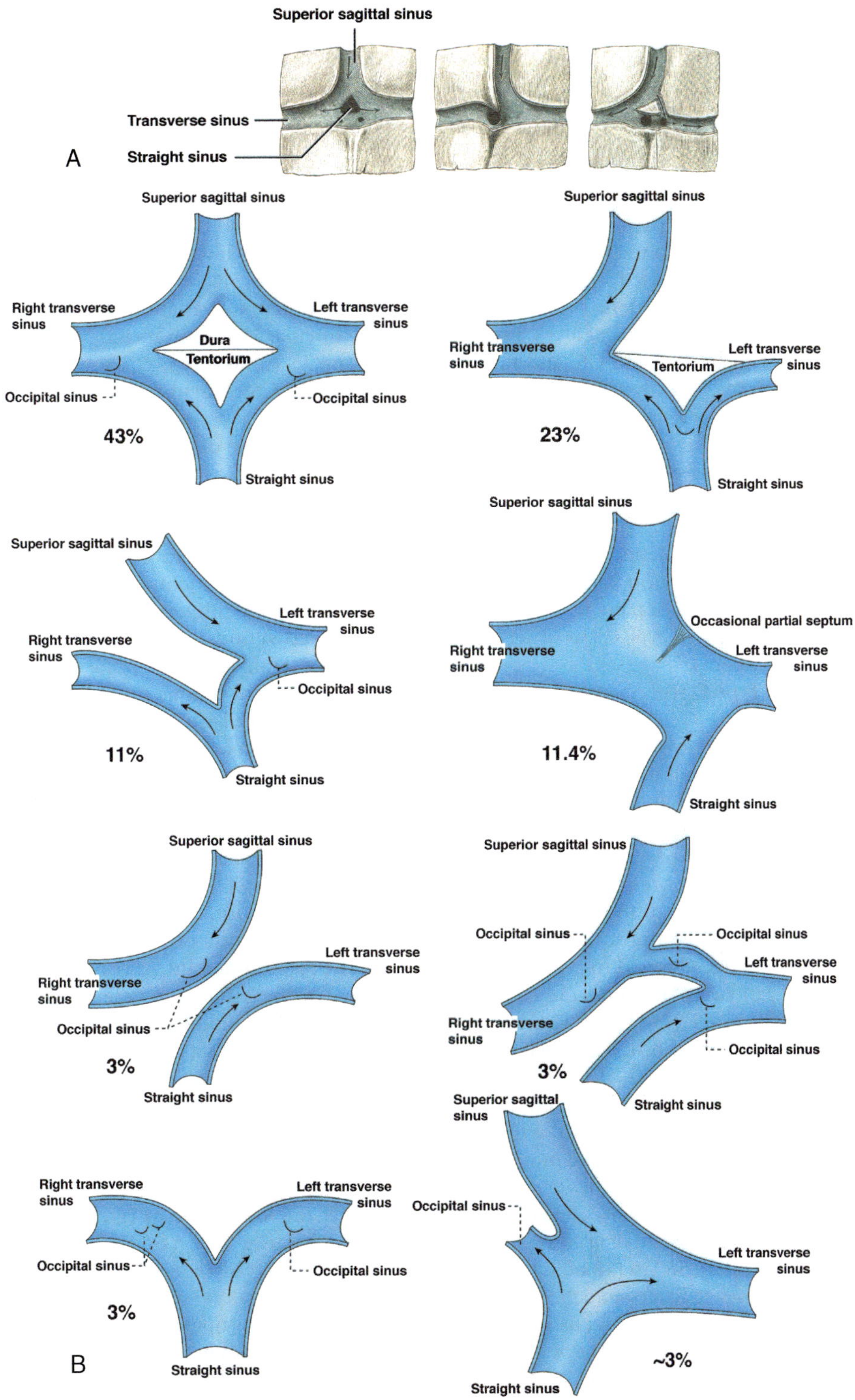

FIG. 7.6 **(A)** Variants of the composition of the torcular Herophili. After Testut; **(B)** Variations of the torcular Herophili distilled from various sources by Lang J. 1991. Clinical Anatomy of the Posterior Cranial Fossa and its Foramina. New York: Thieme.

6. Type 6—the TS was defective.
   a. Type 6a, a defective left TS, was observed in 0.4% (2 of 549) of patients.
   b. Type 6b, a defective right TS, was observed in 0.9% (5 of 249) of patients.
7. Type 7–The StS branches into bilateral TSs, and the SSS drains into the StS and the left TS. Type 7 was observed in 0.2% (1 of 549) patients.
8. Type 8–The SSS branches into the bilateral TSs, and the StS into the SSS and the left TS. Type 8 was observed in 0.4% (2 of 549) of patients.
9. Type 9–The SSS branches into the right TS and OS, the StS drains into the left TS and OS, and the SSS communicates with the StS only via the small anastomotic veins. Type 9 was observed in 0.4% (2 of 549) of patients.

The communication between the right and left TSs was classified into four types, as follows:

1. Type A–wide communication. Type A was observed in 88.1% (484 of 549) of patients.
2. Type B–narrow communication. Type B was observed in 10.2% (56 of 549) of patients.
3. Type C–no communication. Type C was observed in 0.4% (2 of 59) of patients.
4. Type D–Single TS. Type D was observed in 1.3% (7 of 549) of patients.

In Kobayashi et al.'s[9] study, the type 1 variation was observed most commonly. This variant corresponds with the historical definition of the torcular Herophili. In fact, drainage of the SSS is usually unequal, with complete or predominant drainage into the right TS three times more common than that into the left. On the other hand, the StS drains into the left transverse sinus three times as often as the right.[1] In one study, the SSS drained into the right TS in 51.6% (16 of 31) of cases, and into the center of the torcular Herophili in 45.2% (14) of specimens.[2] The study also showed that the right TS was dominant (i.e., >1.5 times the diameter of the left TS) in 35.5% (11) of cases. Comparatively, the left TS was dominant in only 3.2% (1 of 31) of cases, while the right and left TSs were symmetrical in the majority of cases (58.1% or 18 of 31 cases).[2]

The StS also varies in its point of drainage into the torcular Herophili. Park et al.[2] stated that it drained via the center of the torcular Herophili in 58.1% (18 of 31) of cases, while in 35.5% (11) of cases, it drained into the left TS.

Results from Ishizaka[3] also were consistent with those above. In his study, the torcular Herophili represented the intersection of the SSS, the StS, and the two TSs, and this arrangement was present in 29% of 52 cadaver specimens.

From the results above, Type 2a was the second variation observed most commonly, in which the StS branches into bilateral TSs and the SSS drain into the right TS.

A few rare variants also are mentioned here. Type 7 was observed in only one person among those examined. In Type 7, the StS branches into bilateral TSs, and the SSS drains into the StS and the left TS. The other rare variants, which were observed in only two patients each, were Types 5b, 6a, 8, and 9.

Some other rare variations that occur in the region of the torcular Herophili include double StSs draining into one TS (unlike Type 7 above, which drains into two TSs), the SSS dividing into three channels with two TSs on one side, one originating from a tentorial vein, and drainage of a tentorial vein into the torcular Herophili.[16]

Most studies that have examined the variability of the sinuses in the region of the torcular Herophili have involved cadaver dissections and observations of the sinus structure. Several studies also have used imaging techniques to explore the same. Singh et al.[17] used venous sinus impressions on the internal surface of the occipital bone to infer the arrangement of the dural venous sinuses in the region of the torcular Herophili. In their study, 160 dried skulls were examined macroscopically. In 41% (66 of 160) of the cases, the right dominant type was observed most frequently. In this type, the SSS drained into the right TS. The left dominant type was observed least often and was seen in 10% or 16 cases. The bifurcated type (seen in 14% or 22 cases) and the confluence type (seen in 35% or 56 specimens) made up the remainder of the observations. In the confluence type, the SSS drained into a common pool of venous sinuses. In the bifurcated type, the SSS divided and drained into the bilateral TSs.

It is believed that the level of communication between the two TSs in the vicinity of the torcular Herophili determines, to some extent, the risk of cerebral edema following obstruction of the transverse or sigmoid sinus during surgery. A variant that has a free or wide communication between the two TSs is thought to confer the lowest risk of cerebral edema.[3] As mentioned previously, Type A or the "wide communicating" type, was observed in 88.1% of subjects. Sixty-three percent of Ishizaka's specimens contained channels that possessed an open and unobstructed communication. Comparatively, 83.8% (26 of 31) of specimens Park et al.[2] examined contained sinuses that communicated freely. No communication was observed in 0.4% of Koboyashi's[9] specimens, compared to 23% of

Ishizaka's. Kobayashi et al. also observed a single TS in 1.3% of specimens.

In San Ruíz's dissertation (2006), corrosion casts of the venous systems of the skull base and the craniocervical junction of adult specimens were used to study their macroscopic and radiologic anatomy. A rare variation at the torcular Herophili was observed in one of his 12 specimens, in which an occipital emissary vein was observed to join it. This is an uncommon finding in an adult.

Variations in Partially Communicating Confluence of Sinuses

Kaplan et al.[13] studied 215 specimens of dura obtained at autopsy, and inspected the differences in the torcular Herophili sinuses' architecture. The specimens were categorized depending on their structural characteristics. In most of the specimens, there was free, unobstructed communication between the SSS, StS, OS, and the two TSs. In this section, however, we exclude the types that communicate freely to focus on their variations that demonstrated some level of obstruction.

In 10% (21 of 215) of their specimens, the caudal SSS divided into two channels of widely varying diameters in the vicinity of the torcular Herophili. In eight of these 21, the smaller channel was on the right, while it was on the left in the remaining 13. In all 21 specimens, the smaller channel seemed to have a valve-like structure at its rostral end. A thin wall (laminar chorda) was found between these two channels, the flexibility of which suggests that distension of the larger channel may occlude the smaller channel effectively. Further, distal obstruction of the outflow on the side ipsilateral to the larger channel may lead to signs and symptoms reflective of a bilateral occlusion, because the smaller outlet may become compressed eventually, which may have some bearing on procedures or accidents in which one of the jugular veins is sacrificed.

In 20% (41 of 215) of these partially communicating specimens, the lumen of one of the TSs was narrowed by thickening of the wall of the sinus just lateral to the torcular Herophili. In 29 of these 41 specimens, the thickening was found in the left TS, and was in the right TS in the remaining 12. In the majority of specimens, the StS joined the smaller TS distal to the partial obstruction. This thickening, also referred to as a mesh, was circumferential in nature, but usually was maximal on the dorsal aspect. This likely is the embryological remnant of the venous plexus from which the sinuses developed. Baló[11] mentioned these meshes, and suggested that their expansion and contraction may control venous flow in this region. However, no evidence has confirmed his postulations.

Some specimens exhibited an obvious obstruction to flow, in which it was permitted only through multiple openings smaller than the original lumen. This variation was present in 10% (21 of 215) of specimens. In some cases, valve-like structures were present where the larger openings were found. In 15 of these 21 cases, the partial obstruction was on the left, and was on the right in the remaining 6. In 17 of these cases, the StS joined the TS on the right or left, and joined the large OS in the remaining 4. Obstruction of flow at the level of the jugular vein on the side communicating freely is expected to lead to severe stasis in the superior cerebral veins.

In 5% (10 of 215) of cases, 1 of the TSs was maldeveloped. Three of these 10 occurred on the left, and 7 on the right. The SSS continued into the TS contralateral to the atretic side. In 3 of the 10 specimens, the StS joined a larger OS. Atresia of 1 of the TSs can be associated with abnormalities of other venous sinuses. In 1 of the 10 cases, there was accompanying atresia of the rostral 9 cm of the SSS.

Rare Variants

Craniopagus is an extremely rare form of conjoined twins. In some cases, the twins may share leptomeningeal and central nervous system tissue. In one case of craniopagus, two initially separate SSSs joined into one common SSS as they approached the torcular Herophili, and two separate StSs drained into this common SSS.[18–21] A single torcular Herophili existed, despite the presence of two well-developed brains, thereby compounding surgical separation further. This solitary torcular Herophili was the point of intersection of a common SSS (into which two StSs drained), an OS, and two TSs.

Vein of Galen malformations lead to dilatation of the dural venous sinuses (Figs. 7.9 and 7.10). One unusual variant is a more superiorly located accessory torcular Herophili as we have previously termed such (Figs. 7.7 and 7.8). The torcular Herophili can be malformed with bilateral splitting of the distal SSS (Fig. 7.11), the basal vein of Rosenthal can drain into the torcular Herophili (Fig. 7.12) and the torcular Herophili can take on a circular configuration (Fig. 7.13).

IMAGING

Several imaging modalities have outlined the structure of the torcular Herophili successfully. This section reviews the imaging techniques used to obtain information on the macroscopic structure of the torcular Herophili, and by extension, the pathology in this region. Imaging types used in prenatal, post-natal to adulthood, and post-mortem cases are discussed.

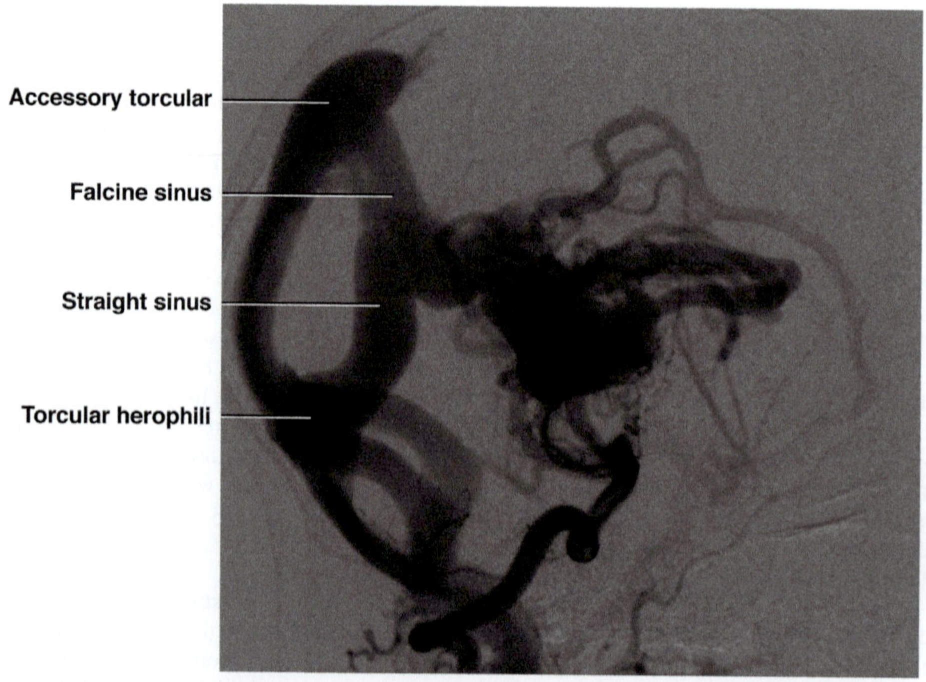

FIG. 7.7 Vein of Galen malformation noting enlarged straight and persistent falcine sinuses. Also not the so-called accessory torcular at the junction between the falcine sinus and superior sagittal sinus. The torcular Herophili is easily seen.

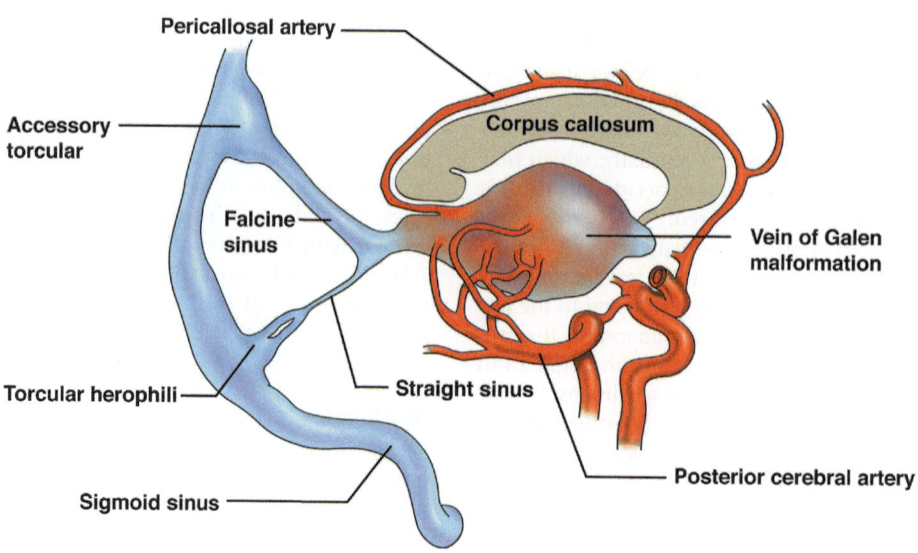

FIG. 7.8 Schematic drawing of Fig. 7.7.

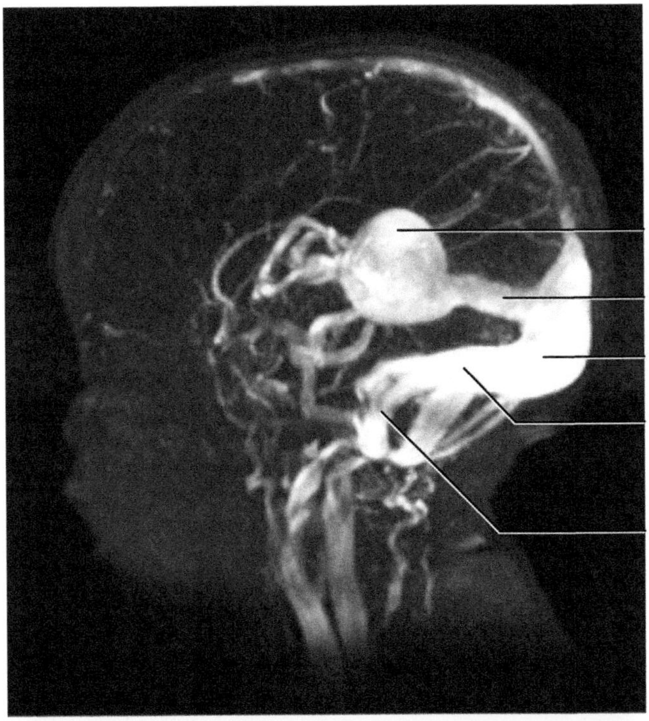

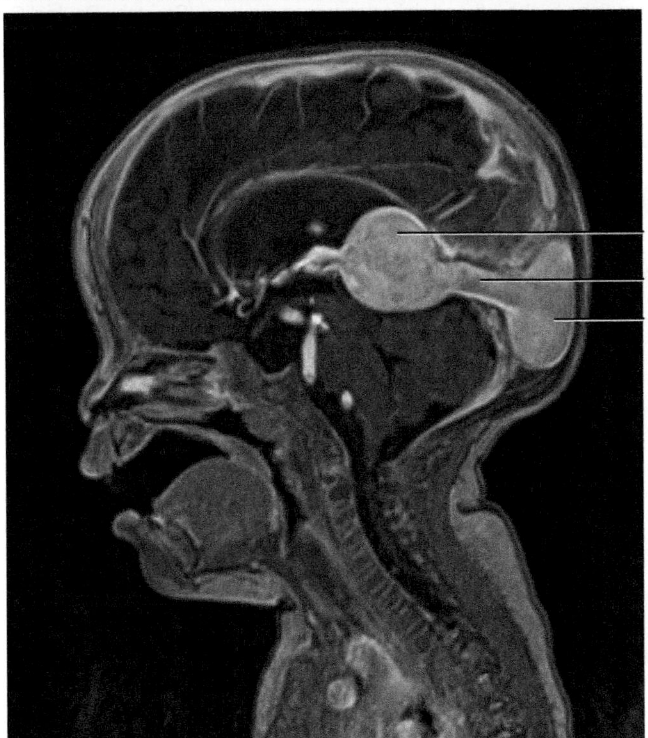

FIGS. 7.9 AND 7.10 Vein of Galen malformations with hugely dilated torcular Herophili.

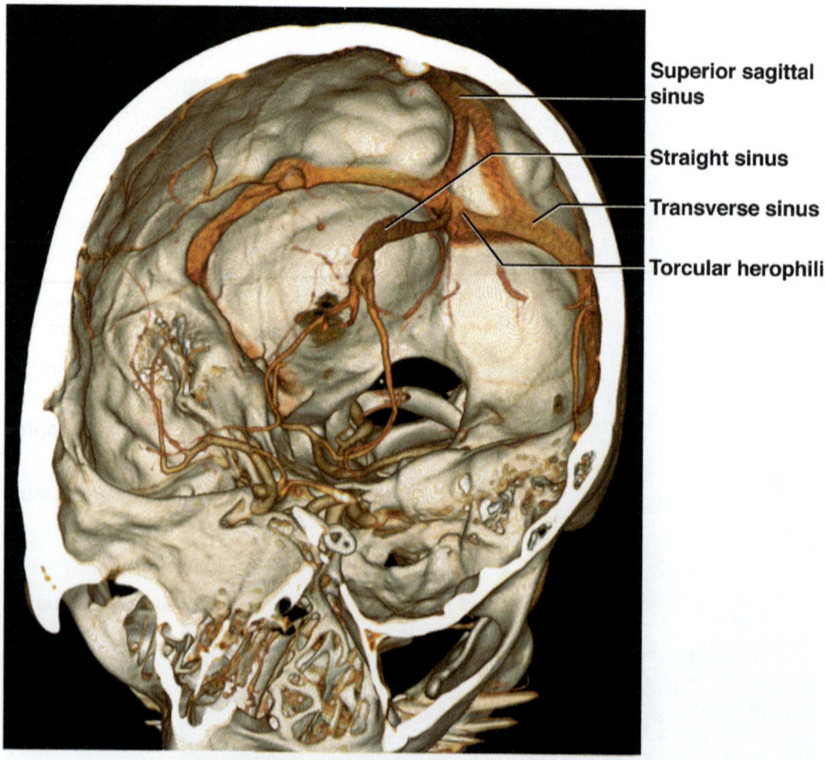

FIG. 7.11 3D CTA noting the torcular Herophili in a case of a high splitting of the superior sagittal sinus with more or less equal contributions to the left and right transverse sinuses. (Courtesy Dr. Joel Curé.)

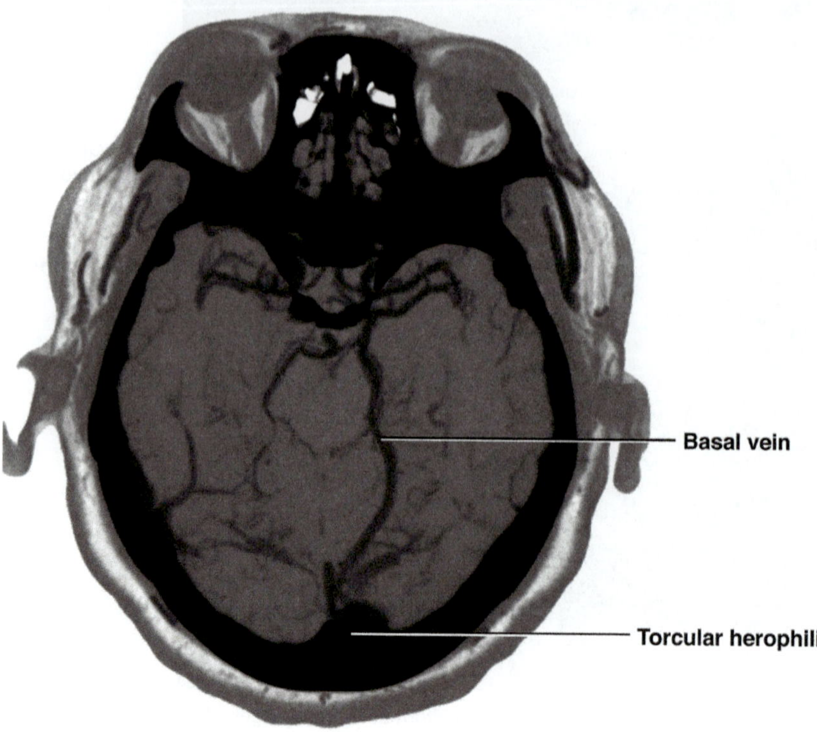

FIG. 7.12 An interesting case demonstrating the basal vein of Rosenthal draining directly into the torcular Herophili. (Courtesy Dr. Joel Curé.)

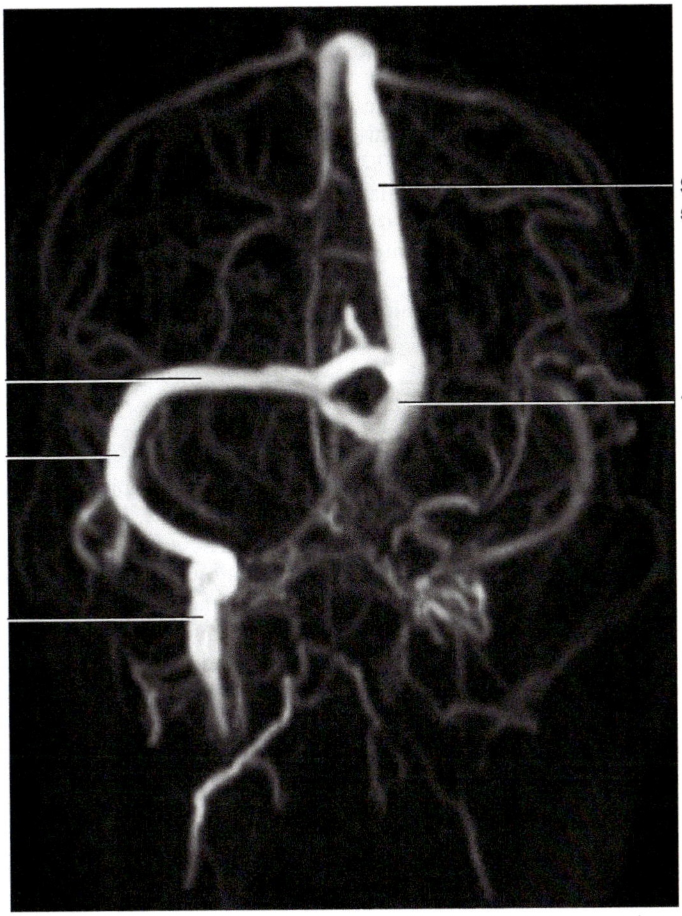

FIG. 7.13 MRV noting an unusual configuration of the torcular Herlophili with the transverse sinus splitting into two parts thus forming a circular configuration at the torcular.

Conventional Angiography

Conventional angiography has long served as the gold standard to visualize vascular structures. However, it is falling out of favor now as less invasive procedures, such as magnetic resonance imaging (MRI) and computed tomography (CT), have gained in popularity.

Angiography of the venous sinuses is accomplished by catheterizing the internal carotid artery and, less commonly, the femoral artery. In neonates, the umbilical vein may be used as the vessel of entry.[22] Images can be optimized using photographic or digital subtraction techniques. Venous sinuses usually opacify in the anteroposterior direction.

As with all imaging modalities, users must be aware of the limitations of conventional angiography. Because venous sinuses drain from different sources, filling defects may be seen as contrast drains into some regions of the sinuses before others. Intraluminal arachnoid granulations or cavernous nodules, septations or fenestrations, or duplication of sinuses also may produce apparent filling defects. Aplasia and thrombosis of venous structures also are virtually impossible to distinguish from each other.[1,23–25] Arteries and veins may be difficult to distinguish from each other in cases where they overlap as well, and small vessels may be difficult to delineate if they are very close to the bone.[26]

Magnetic Resonance Imaging (MRI)

MRI, magnetic resonance angiography (MRA), and magnetic resonance venography (MRV) continue to be noninvasive means to visualize internal structures. The choice of machine settings and interpretation of results, however, depend highly on trained personnel.

On routine MRI, dural venous sinuses show signal voids. In some cases, flow-related artifactual enhancement may be seen in some planes with patent sinuses. On the other hand, depending on the repetition time, sinus thrombosis may be overlooked when the luminal clot consists largely of constituents that produce T2 shortening, such as deoxyhemoglobin and intracellular methemoglobin. These are a few examples where the untrained eye may misinterpret images. One also must be aware of false-positive filling defects secondary to arachnoid granulations or cavernous nodules, luminal septa, or fenestrations.

MRV permits contrast-enhanced imaging of the venous system. Techniques such as time-of-flight (TOF) and phase contrast help obtain optimal images of the sinus structures. Both of these techniques can potentially yield 3-D images, which can be rotated for scrutiny in various views. However, 3-D images are more time consuming, and 2-D images usually are sufficient to answer diagnostic questions. Numerous examples of magnetic resonance use in visualizing the torcular Herophili are available.[1,9,24,25,27–29]

One should note that the lower spatial resolution of 3-D TOF MRV may lead to poor disclosure of small veins.[26] Previous demonstrations revealed that it may depict incorrectly that one of the TSs is absent. In such cases, a 2-D TOF should follow for confirmation.[30]

Computed Tomography

Computed tomography (CT) scans provide a rapid, non-invasive method of intracranial imaging. Because of their increasing availability today, access is no longer an issue, and their use in accident and emergency departments has been established well.

Because of advancements in MRI technology, the use of CT scans and CT angiograms to visualize dural venous sinuses in nonemergent cases is less common. However, they still have some value in emergent cases.[31]

Similar to conventional angiograms, it can be difficult to distinguish between arteries and veins that overlap on CT angiograms. Further, small vessels that are close to bone may not be outlined easily.

Sonography (Prenatal)

Sonography is the investigative modality of choice in pregnant patients, as it is noninvasive and quite safe. Schwartz et al.[32] highlighted a case of thrombosis in the region of the torcular Herophili that was diagnosed in a fetus[32] without the need for a confirmatory MRI, which is the norm.[33,34] The mass was visualized first on a routine growth scan at 34+ weeks, and 2-D and 3-D neurosonography was able to diagnose the lesion accurately in the third trimester. The pathological findings corroborated well with the sonogram findings.

This case serves to show that improvements in ultrasound technology mean that they now cannot be ruled out completely as an option to visualize venous sinuses, particularly prenatally and in infants. Segal and Rosenberg[10] established this fact when they performed sonograms on 12 infants aged 2 days to 7 months, and visualized the torcular Herophili in all cases. Its size varied and the shape was triangular or elongated. It appeared anechoic and was located inferior to the occipital lobes, posterior to the cerebellum, and just inside the cranial vault.[10]

INTERVENTIONAL RADIOLOGY

The torcular Herophili is of great importance to cerebral blood flow because of its location and complexity. These two characteristics make therapeutic interventions in this region challenging, and at times, the combined efforts of endovascular and neurosurgical techniques may be required.[35]

The endovascular procedures that form the framework of the field of interventional radiology have particular importance in sinus thrombosis and arteriovenous malformations. In the case of dural arteriovenous fistulas in the region of the torcular Herophili, transarterial embolization may be used to decrease the blood flow into the malformation. This involves inserting a catheter into the entry of the systemic arterial system, advancing it into the region of the torcular Herophili, and releasing the embolization material into the arterial lumen. Examples of such materials include polyvinyl alcohol foam particles or *N*-butyl-cyanoacrylate.[22,25,35]

Transvenous embolization is a close relative of the transarterial coiling used to manage intracranial aneurysms. In transvenous coiling, diseased areas are packed tightly with microcoils. These platinum-based wires may be detachable coils, interlocking detachable coils, or short, fibred coils. If the transvenous approach is not possible, then access to the area can be gained via a small craniectomy or burr hole. Once this is accomplished, the sinus is packed with larger fibered occlusion coils.[22,25,35,36]

PATHOLOGY

Disease entities in the vicinity of the torcular Herophili have the potential to lead to life-threatening dural venous hypertension and cerebral edema. This fact stems from the role the torcular Herophili plays as a common point in the drainage of dural venous sinuses.

Thrombosis at the Confluence of Sinuses

Torcular Herophili thrombosis can be diagnosed in all age groups, from fetuses to adults.[29,31–34] In many cases, the underlying cause of the thrombosis formation in this region is unknown. However, one must be careful to rule out congenital hypercoagulable disorders (such as deficiencies of protein C, protein S, and antithrombin III, as well as factor V Leiden mutation), tumors, and other pathologies that may predispose one to abnormalities in the Virchow triad (such as postinvasive neurosurgical procedures and arteriovenous fistulas).[29,31,34]

Clinical manifestations, which include hemianopsia, vary and may depend on the degree of blockage, as well as the period of time the blockage took to form.[29] Anitcoagulation is the mainstay of therapy, although if diagnosed prenatally, spontaneous recanalization of the structure is a possibility.[33,34]

Dural Arteriovenous Fistulas

Arteriovenous fistulas are abnormal, unregulated connections between arteries and veins, and often are only part of a more complex pathological process .[37] Typically, dural arteriovenous fistulas (DAVF) lie between the dura and represent connections between middle meningeal arteries and venous sinuses, meningeal veins, or cortical veins.[38] They can occur at or near the torcular Herophili,[22,25,35,36,39] and usually are acquired, but also may be congenital, albeit this is rare.[22] When congenital, they may be referred to as arteriovenous malformations and may lead to thrombosis formation. Dural arteriovenous malformations located at the torcular Herophili actually have a poorer prognosis.[34]

Signs and symptoms that may be seen in a child with a congenital DAVF include cranial bruits, cardiac failure, dilated scalp veins, macrocephaly and hydrocephaly, delayed neurological development, seizures, and focal neurological deficits. In the case of neonates, a transumbilical approach usually is the ideal portal of entry for transarterial and transvenous embolization.[22] In adults, the clinical manifestations vary widely and depend on the specific characteristics of the DAVF, such as size, location, and venous territory.[35,40–42]

Other Less Common Pathologies

Hemangiopericytomas are tumors that are composed of rounded or spindle-shaped cells proliferating around endothelial-lined capillaries that are derived from the pericytes of Zimmerman. Hemangiopericytomas can occur anywhere in the central nervous system. When present, they are found often along dural surfaces and at the midline near venous sinuses.[27,43] Their occurrence within the sinuses is very uncommon and only a few cases have been described at the torcular Herophili. Signs and symptoms include blurred vision, headaches, and papilledema.[25,27]

Other uncommon to rare pathologies that may involve the torcular Herophili include Masson's vegetant intravascular hemangioendothelioma, malignant neoplasms, and meningoencephaloceles.[24,28,44]

SURGERY

As with surgical procedures anywhere in the body, an understanding of the anatomy in the region obviously is necessary. The torcular Herophili penetrates to the occipital bone and is approximately at the midline. Therefore, an occipital or suboccipital craniotomy is performed to gain surgical access to the torcular Herophili.

Surgery at the torcular Herophili can be particularly complex because disruption of drainage here can lead to venous sinus congestion that is not limited to one particular sinus distribution. This has the potential to progress rapidly to clinically evident intracranial hypertension.

Open surgical procedures in the vicinity of the torcular Herophili may serve as an alternative, or an adjunct, to endovascular procedures for dural arteriovenous fistulas.[35] A previous publication outlined the resection of the TS and torcular Herophili as an effective way to manage multiple dural venous fistulas.[39] In some cases, access to the region of the torcular Herophili was necessary for tumor resection.[24,27]

Postoperatively, a subdural monitor may be used to monitor intracranial pressure because thrombosis of the major venous sinuses may follow invasive intervention.[24]

REFERENCES

1. Curé JK, Tassel PV, Smith MT. Normal and variant anatomy of the dural venous sinuses. *Semin Ultrasound CT MR*. 1994;15:499–519.
2. Park HK, Bae HG, Choi SK, et al. Morphological study of sinus flow in the confluence of sinuses. *Clin Anat*. 2008;21:294–300.
3. Ishizaka H. Anatomical study of the torcular Herophili. *Neurol Med -Chir*. 1985;25:873.
4. Shao Y, Sun JL, Yang Y, Cui QK, Zhang QL. Endoscopic and microscopic anatomy of the superior sagittal sinus and torcular Herophili. *J Clin Neurosci*. 2009;16:421–424.
5. Tubbs RS, Salter G, Oakes WJ. Superficial surgical landmarks for the transverse sinus and torcular Herophili. *J Neurosurg*. 2000;93:279–281.

6. Tubbs RS, Salter G, Oakes WJ. Landmarks for the transverse sinus and torcular Herophili-response. *J Neurosurg*. 2001;94:687.
7. Streeter GL. The development of the venous sinuses of the dura mater in the human embryo. *Am J Anat*. 1915;18:145–178.
8. Butler H. The development of certain human dural venous sinuses. *J Anat*. 1957;91:510.
9. Kobayashi K, Matsui O, Suzuki M, Ueda F. Anatomical study of the confluence of the sinuses with contrast-enhanced magnetic resonance venography. *Neuroradiology*. 2006;48:307–311.
10. Segal SR, Rosenberg HK. Sonographic appearance of the torcular Herophili. *AJNR Am J Neuroradiol*. 1985;6:919–922.
11. Baló J. The dural venous sinuses. *Anat Rec*. 1950;106:319–325.
12. Browder J, Browder A, Kaplan HA. The venous sinuses of the cerebral dura mater: I. Anatomical structures within the superior sagittal sinus. *Arch Neurol*. 1972;26:175–180.
13. Kaplan HA, Browder J, Knightly JJ, Rush BF, Browder A. Variations of the cerebral dural sinuses at the torcular Herophili: importance in radical neck dissection. *Am J Surg*. 1972;124:456–461.
14. Tokiguchi S, Ando K, Tsuchiya T, Ito J. Fat in the dural sinus. *Neuroradiology*. 1986;28:267–270.
15. Tokiguchi S. Investigation of fat in the dural sinus. *Nippon Igaku Hoshasen Gakkai Zasshi*. 1991;51:871–882.
16. Bisaria KK. Anatomic variations of venous sinuses in the region of the torcular Herophili. *J Neurosurg*. 1985;62:90–95.
17. Singh M, Nagashima M, Inoue Y. Anatomical variations of occipital bone impressions for dural venous sinuses around the torcular Herophili, with special reference to the consideration of clinical significance. *Surg Radiol Anat*. 2004;26:480–487.
18. Lasjaunias P, Kwok R, Goh P, Yeong KY, Lim W, Chng SM. A developmental theory of the superior sagittal sinus(es) in craniopagus twins. *Childs Nerv Syst*. 2004;20:526–537.
19. Goh KYC. Surgeon's reply. *Singap Med J*. 2005;46:2.
20. Khan ZH. Separated but oceans apart and fathoms deep: the conjoined twins' legacy. *Singap Med J*. 2005;46:1.
21. Khan ZH, Hamidi S, Miri SM. Craniopagus, Laleh and Ladan twins, sagittal sinus. *Turk Neurosurg*. 2006;17:27–32.
22. Komiyama M, Nishikawa M, Kitano S, et al. Transumbilical embolization of a congenital dural arteriovenous fistula at the torcular Herophili in a neonate: case report. *J Neurosurg*. 1999;90:964–969.
23. Huang YP, Okudera T, Ohta T, Robbins A. Anatomic variations of the dural venous sinuses. In: Kapp JP, Schmidek HH, eds. *The Cerebral Venous System and its Disorders*. Orlando, FL: Grune and Stratton; 1984:109–168.
24. Wen DY, Hardten DR, Wirtschafter JD, Sung JH, Haines SJ. Elevated intracranial pressure from cerebral venous obstruction by Masson's vegetant intravascular hemangioendothelioma: case report. *J Neurosurg*. 1991;75:787–790.
25. Kurisu K, Motegi H, Osanai T, Kobayashi H, Terasaka S, Houkin K. Regression of dural arteriovenous fistulae after venous flow reconstructive surgery in a case with hemangiopericytoma at the confluence of sinuses. *Case Rep Neurol*. 2014;6:207–212.
26. San Millán Ruíz D. *Venous Systems of the Skull Base and Craniocervical Junction. Macroscopic and Radiological Anatomy and Clinical Implications*. PhD Diss., University of Geneva; 2006.
27. Collignon FP, Cohen-Gadol AA, Piepgras DG. Hemangiopericytoma of the confluence of sinuses and the transverse sinuses: case report. *J Neurosurg*. 2003;99:1085–1088.
28. Carvalho CH, Acioly MA, Will B, Tatagiba M. Magnetic resonance angiography of a complex occipital meningoencephalocele involving the confluence of sinuses. Case illustration. *J Neurosurg Pediatr*. 2008;1:261.
29. Meguro T, Sasaki T, Haruma J, et al. Transient homonymous hemianopsia due to thrombosis of the confluence of sinuses after occipital transtentorial removal of pineal region tumor. *Noshinkeigeka*. 2010;38:927–931.
30. Carriero A, Magarelli N, Samuele F, Palumbo L, Bocola V, Iezzi A. The torcular Herophili: the diagnostic pitfalls in TOF 3D magnetic resonance angiography. *Radiol Med*. 1994;87:441–446.
31. De-Giorgio F, Peschillo S, Vetrugno G, d'Aloja E, Spagnolo AG, Miscusi M. Cerebral venous sinus thrombosis due to spontaneous, progressive, and retrograde jugular vein thrombosis causing sudden death in a young woman. *Forensic Sci Med Pathol*. 2015;11:88–91.
32. Schwartz N, Monteagudo A, Bornstein E, Timor-Tritsch II, Zagzag D, Kudla M. Thrombosis of an ectatic torcular Herophili: anatomic localization using fetal neurosonography. *J Ultrasound Med*. 2008;27:989–991.
33. Grigoriadis S, Cohen JE, Gomori JM. Prenatal thrombosis of torcular Herophili with spontaneous resolution and normal outcome. *J Neuroimaging*. 2008;18:177–179.
34. Spampinato MV, Hardin V, Davis M, Chang E, Rumboldt Z. Thrombosed fetal dural sinus malformation diagnosed with magnetic resonance imaging. *Obstet Gynecol*. 2008;111:569–572.
35. Goto K, Sidipratomo P, Ogata N, Inoue T, Matsuno H. Combining endovascular and neurosurgical treatments of high-risk dural arteriovenous fistulas in the lateral sinus and the confluence of the sinuses. *J Neurosurg*. 1999;90:289–299.
36. Gupta R, Miyachi S, Matsubara N, et al. A unique type of dural arteriovenous fistula at confluence of sinuses treated with endovascular embolization: a case report. *Neurointervention*. 2013;8:34–40.
37. Lasjaunias P, Berenstein A. *Arteriovenous Fistulas (AVFs). Surgical Neuroangiography*. Berlin, Heidelberg: Springer-Verlag; 1987:175–233.
38. Yako R, Masuo O, Kubo K, Nishimura Y, Nakao N. A case of dural arteriovenous fistula draining to the diploic vein presenting with intracerebral hemorrhage. *J Neurosurg*. 2004;101:832–835.

39. Fiumara E, Tumbiolo S, Bellomonte ML, Savatteri P, Finazzo F, La Gattuta F. Resection of the transverse sinuses and confluence of sinuses for treatment of multiple dural arteriovenous fistulas: case report. *J Neurosurg*. 2004;100:348–352.
40. Houser OW, Baker Jr HL, Rhoton Jr AL, Okazaki H. Intracranial dural arteriovenous malformations 1. *Radiology*. 1972;105:55–64.
41. Lasjaunias P, Chiu M, Brugge KT, Tolia A, Hurth M, Bernstein M. Neurological manifestations of intracranial dural arteriovenous malformations. *J Neurosurg*. 1986;64:724–730.
42. Viñuela F, Fox AJ, Pelz DM, Drake CG. Unusual clinical manifestations of dural arteriovenous malformations. *J Neurosurg*. 1986;64:554–558.
43. Nunnery EW, Kahn LB, Reddick RL, Lipper S. Hemangiopericytoma: a light microscopic and ultrastructural study. *Cancer*. 1981;47:906–914.
44. Link MJ, Cohen PL, Breneman JC, Tew Jr JM. Malignant squamous degeneration of a cerebellopontine angle epidermoid tumor: case report. *J Neurosurg*. 2002;97:1237–1243.

FURTHER READING

1. Sharifi M, Kunicki J, Krajewski P, Ciszek B. Endoscopic anatomy of the chordae Willisii in the superior sagittal sinus. *J Neurosurg*. 2004;101:832–835.

CHAPTER 8

The Tentorial Sinuses

ALIREZA SHOAKAZEMI • R. SHANE TUBBS

ANATOMY

The tentorial sinuses (Figs. 8.1 and 8.2) are often encountered with neurosurgical approaches[1,2] and should not be confused with the prenatal tentorial sinus (tentorial vein of Markowski; inferior cerebral vein of Streeter). Gibbs and Gibbs first described the presence of these postnatal sinuses, primarily fed by the superior cerebellar veins and drained into the transverse sinuses.[3,4]

Drainage of the tentorium cerebelli is dependent on two groups of vessels: the dural sinuses of the tentorium cerebelli and the afferent tentorial veins.[5] In contrast to other intracranial sinuses, the intratentorial dural sinuses are not held open and tend to collapse.[5] These sinuses show variable thickness and appear as a separation of the two leaflets of the tentorium with some arachnoid granulations, mainly at entry point into transverse sinuses.[5]

The complexity and versatility of these venous structures mandates a reliable and reproducible method of classification. A reliable method of classification can assist a neurosurgeon to plan a safe surgical corridor and to prevent potential morbidities associated with sacrifice or inadvertent injury of this category of venous sinuses. Tentorial sinuses are grossly categorized into two constant, paired, bilateral but mostly asymmetric venous channels.[2,5,6] The medial group is formed by the coalescence of the veins from the superior surface of the cerebellum (Fig. 8.3), and the lateral group is commonly formed by the convergence of veins arising from the basal and lateral surface of the temporal and occipital lobes.[2] The medial group of intratentorial sinuses arises between 15–25 mm from the midline and 10–25 mm from the transverse sinus.[5] The lateral tentorial sinus (LTS), in most cases, arises at a point on the tentorium 30–40 mm from the midline, 2–10 mm from the transverse sinus, and 10 mm from petrous ridge.[5]

Both groups of intratentorial sinuses normally carry venous blood from the supratentorial and infratentorial compartments, and they also substantially contribute to the venous drainage of the floor of the middle cranial fossa.[5] On the other hand, in certain circumstances, these sinuses act as a potential connection between the supratentorial and infratentorial sinuses.

LTS. This group of sinuses arises within the lateral part of the tentorium cerebelli, and after pursuing a lateral course, it drains into the terminal segment of the transverse sinus and transverse-sigmoid junction on each side.[2,6,7] The basal and lateral occipital and temporal venous system contributes significantly in the formation of the LTS on each side.[6]

Configuration of the LTS has been classified into three categories based on neuroradiologic and cadaveric study findings: type I: venous candelabra configuration, type II: multiple independent veins, and type III: venous lakes within the tentorium, the most common type of sinuses.[6,8] Rhoton et al. classified venous branches of LTS into eight groups: (1) anterior temporal vein, (2) anterior temporobasal vein, (3) middle temporobasal vein, (4) posterior temporobasal vein, (5) occipitobasal vein, (6) posterior temporal vein, (7) vein of Labbé, and (8) middle temporal vein.[2,6,7]

Medial tentorial sinus (MTS). This group normally courses medially and empties into the straight sinus and transverse sinus confluence.[2] This category is mainly responsible for the drainage of the superior cerebellar surface.[6]

In a cadaveric study, Matsushima et al. described four types of tentorial venous sinuses.[1] In this study, the draining pattern was used as the classification criteria.

- Group I (tentorial sinuses draining the cerebral hemispheres): In this group, several cerebral veins converged at the superior surface of the tentorium to form bridging veins. They were commonly present near the transverse sinuses. In this study, the vein of Labbé was included in this category.[1]
- Group II (tentorial sinuses draining the cerebellum): In this category, bridging veins from the cerebellar tentorial surface formed the tentorial sinuses. This group of sinuses drained into the torcular or the dural sinuses nearby.[1]
- Group III: This group formed near the tentorial edge of the straight sinus. They were frequently small with no bridging veins.

Anatomy, Imaging and Surgery of the Intracranial Dural Venous Sinuses. https://doi.org/10.1016/B978-0-323-65377-0.00008-8

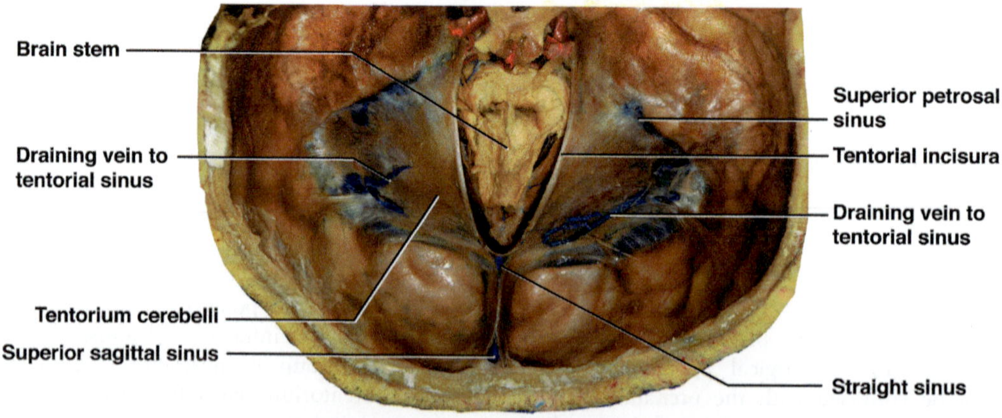

FIG. 8.1 Cadaveric example of the tentorial sinuses. The supratentorial brain has been removed.

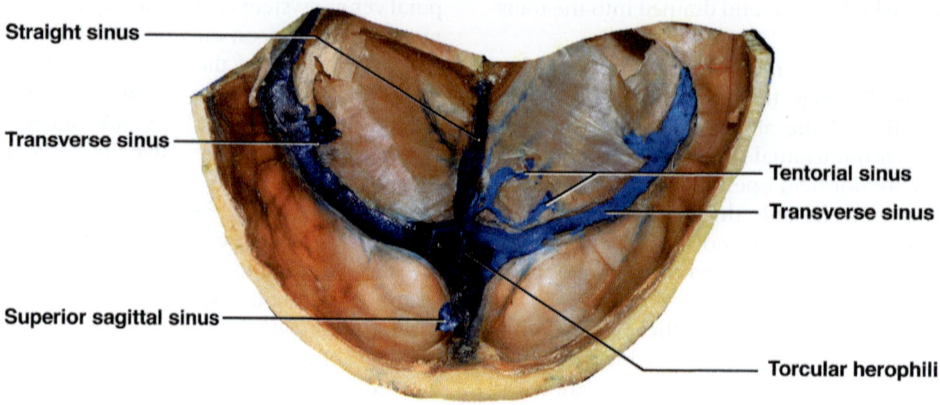

FIG. 8.2 Cadaveric example of the tentorial sinuses. This right-sided tentorial sinus is seen draining into the straight sinus.

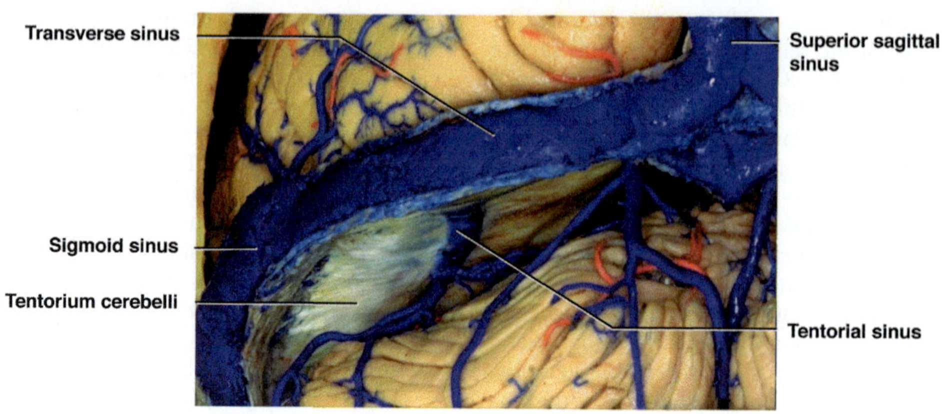

FIG. 8.3 Posterior view of the supracerebellar region noting superior cerebellar veins draining superiorly into the tentorial sinus on the left side. (Courtesy Dr. Albert Rhoton.)

- Group IV: This group was a rare subtype found in cadaveric studies. The basal vein of Rosenthal terminated as a bridging vein to the tentorial free edge forming a tentorial sinus.

The presence of venous sinuses in the tentorium cerebelli is reported in about 86% of cases in some cadaveric studies.[4] Special attention to detect the presence of these sinuses in imaging is of paramount importance.

TENTORIAL BRIDGING VEINS

This group of bridging veins is a part of the superficial group of cerebral veins that are involved with the draining of the lateral surface of the temporal lobe and the basal surface of the temporal and occipital lobes into the tentorial sinuses, transverse sinuses, or superior petrosal sinuses at the tentorial margin.[2] This group of bridging veins, except for the vein of Labbé, which normally drains into the transverse sinus, converges on the preoccipital notch to drain into the LTS. For ease of classification, a group of veins that empty into the LTS can be subdivided into two groups. The lateral branches include the anterior temporal vein, middle temporal vein, posterior temporal vein, and vein of Labbé.[6] The medial branches are composed of the anterior temporobasal vein, middle temporobasal vein, posterior temporobasal vein, and occipitobasal veins.[6] There have been some controversies with regard to the predominant type of LTS. Miabi et al. found type III to be the most common type, whereas Guppy et al. found type II to be the most common in a cadaveric study.[6,8]

EMBRYOLOGY

Padget explained the formation and development of the intracranial venous channels.[9] She highlighted that the venous development is frequently accompanied by the reversal of flow direction and that posteroinferior and middle cerebral veins drain a part of the neopallium into the transverse sinuses behind the sigmoid sinus.[9] Butler et al. reported the results of a human embryonic study depicting cranial venous anatomy.[10] During the embryonic phase, the posterior tentorial fold runs along the superior border of the otic capsule and then sweeps onto the posterior surface of the otic capsule.

PATHOLOGY

The tentorial sinuses can be the main venous drainage pathway in conditions, such as vein of Galen aneurysms and holoprosencephaly, in which the posterior dural venous sinuses are absent are compromised.[6] In these conditions, interventional radiology or surgical manipulation of this group of vessels should be considered more carefully. This group of sinuses can be affected with other pathologies that normally affect other sinuses, such as tumors and vascular anomalies.

IMAGING

Understanding the location and different types of tentorial sinuses facilitates an easier detection of these sinuses on different imaging modalities. Although an LTS is commonly detectable by catheter angiogram or magnetic resonance imaging (MRI) (Figs. 8.4–8.6), it is commonly misinterpreted as a cortical vein close to the vein of Labbé.[6] Miabi et al. investigated the accuracy of the conventional T1-weighted, spin-echo, contrast-enhanced MR imaging to visualize the LTS and found this method to be reliable for detecting this category of sinuses.[6]

Although in the majority of cases, the previously mentioned LTS and MTS anatomic classifications are reflected in imaging findings, case reports of a tentorial sinus draining the telencephalic and diencephalic tributaries of the basal vein has been reported in the literature.[11] Braun et al. on a neuroradiologic study found that the LTSs are taking up the contrast via the superficial veins of the temporal and occipital lobes (anterior circulation angiography), whereas the MTSs are more obvious during vertebral angiography studies.[5]

In radiologic studies, two types of venous formations can be found: an inverted cone and a rectilinear formation.[5]

Choosing the appropriate imaging modality, interpreting the resultant data, and determining the architecture of the sinuses in anticipation of performing a surgery, which can potentially involve manipulation or sacrifice of these sinuses, can prevent potential morbidities accompanied by the chosen surgical approach.

SURGERY

Certain neurosurgical approaches involve manipulation or sectioning of the tentorial sinuses or adjacent venous structures.[1] Special attention to the presence, location, and anatomic configuration of the tentorial sinuses is crucial to prevent devastating intraoperative bleeding and potential postoperative complications associated with damage to these sinuses.[4] For ease of classification, surgical approaches can be categorized according to the part of the TS that can potentially be affected.

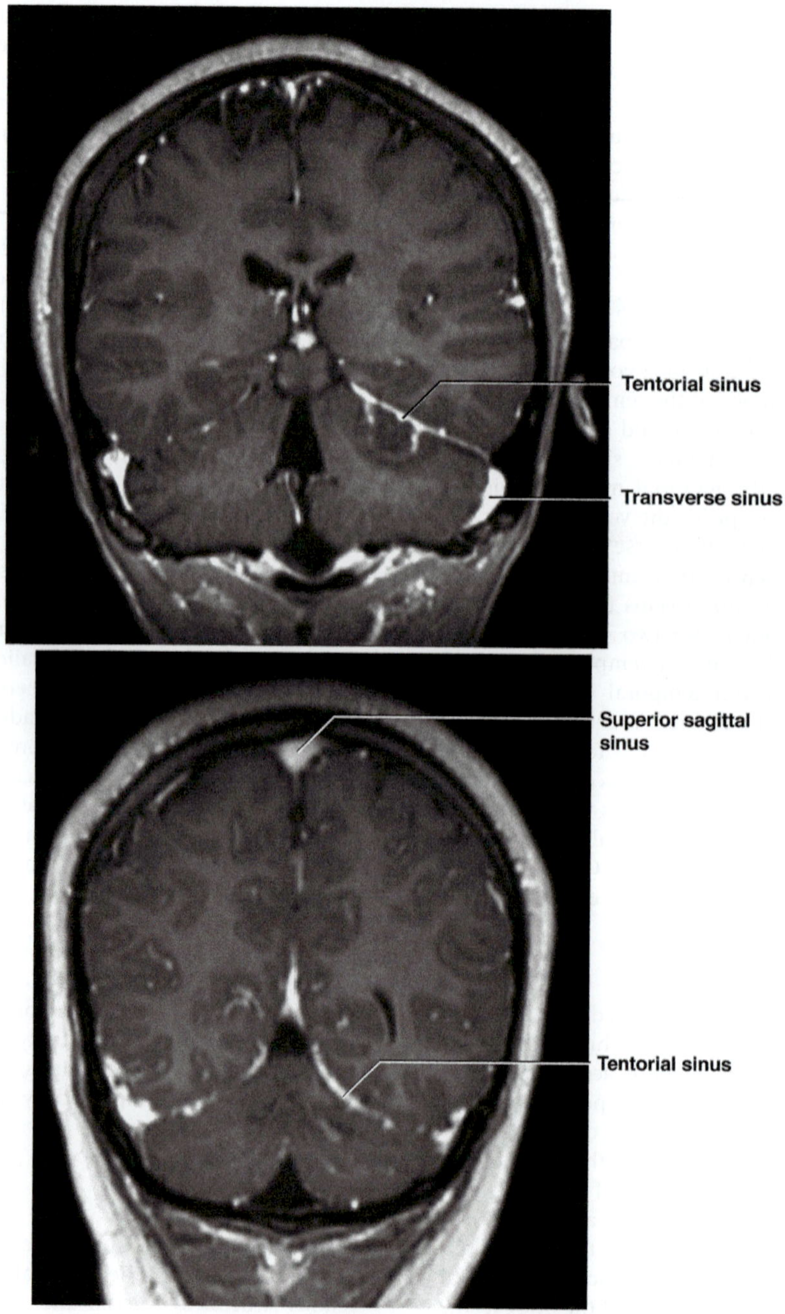

FIGS. 8.4–8.6 Coronal MRIs illustrating the tentorial sinuses.

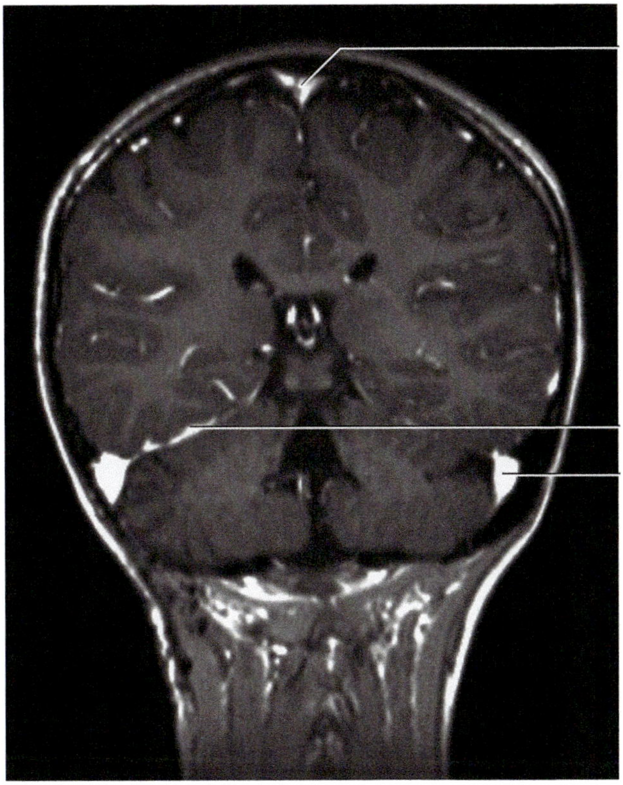

FIGS. 8.4–8.6, cont'd

1. **Surgical approaches that can affect the LTS.** Certain surgical approaches that involve manipulation of the posterior temporal lobe area can have a deleterious effect on the LTS venous structures with possible resultant venous infarction.[6] Collaboration between a neurosurgeon and neuroradiologist before a middle cranial fossa approach, which can potentially involve retraction and damage to the LTS, is of paramount importance. To define the LTS type, termination of the vein of Labbé and venous drainage dominance and presence of sphenoparietal sinus should be considered before embarking a surgical approach.[6] To define the type of LTS can be helpful to modify a surgical approach accordingly. Other approaches in which the LTS can be affected are the transoccipital transtentorial, infratentorial supracerebellar, and subtemporal transtentorial approaches.[1] Some authors recommended avoiding dividing the tentorium cerebelli in patients displaying type I or III LTS.[6] The possibility of a tentorial sinus acting as a collateral circulation should be considered when sacrifice of the sinus is considered.[4]
2. **Surgical approaches that can affect the MTS.** A supracerebellar infratentorial approach can potentially affect the venous structures of the bridging veins, which empty into the MTSs. Similar approaches to tentorial meningiomas often manipulate the MTS-related bridging veins.

REFERENCES

1. Matsushima T, Suzuki SO, Fukui M, Rhoton AL, de Oliveira E, Ono M. Microsurgical anatomy of the tentorial sinuses. *J Neurosurg*. 1989;71(6):923–928.
2. Rhoton AL. *Rhoton's Cranial Anatomy and Surgical Approaches*. LWW; 2007.
3. Gibbs EL, Gibbs FA. The cross section areas of the vessels that form the torcular and the manner in which flow is distributed to the right and to the left lateral sinus. *Anat Rec*. 1934;59(4):419–426.
4. Muthukumar N, Palaniappan P. Tentorial venous sinuses: an anatomic study. *Neurosurgery*. 1998;42(2):363–371.

5. Braun JP, et al. Anatomical and neuroradiological study of the veins of the tentorium and the floor of the middle cranial fossa, and their drainage to dural sinuses. *J Neuroradiol*. 1978;5(2):113–132.
6. Miabi Z, et al. Delineation of lateral tentorial sinus with contrast-enhanced MR imaging and its surgical implications. *AJNR Am J Neuroradiol*. 2004;25(7):1181–1188.
7. Oka K, et al. Microsurgical anatomy of the superficial veins of the cerebrum. *Neurosurgery*. 1985;17(5):711–748.
8. Guppy KH, et al. Venous drainage of the inferolateral temporal lobe in relationship to transtemporal/transtentorial approaches to the cranial base. *Neurosurgery*. 1997;41(3):615–619; discussion 619–20.
9. Padget DH. The cranial venous system in man in reference to development, adult configuration, and relation to the arteries. *Am J Anat*. 1956;98(3):307–355.
10. Butler H. The development of certain human dural venous sinuses. *J Anat*. 1957;91(4):510–526.
11. Terbrugge K, Lasjaunias P. Tentorial sinus. Radiologic and anatomic features of a case. *Surg Radiol Anat*. 1988;10(3):243–246.

CHAPTER 9

Falcine Venous Plexus

R. SHANE TUBBS

The falx cerebri is an intracranial midline partition composed of the meningeal layer of dura mater. This structure has a superior attached portion and an inferior free part housing the superior and inferior sagittal sinuses, respectively. The extant medical literature has scant statements regarding other potential veins within the falx cerebri. Crosby[1] had stated that the inferior sagittal sinus "begins in about the middle of the border of the falx with the convergence of the falcial plexus of veins." The superior sagittal sinus may communicate with the inferior sagittal sinus through a venous channel in the falx cerebri[2] (Figs. 9.1 and 9.2). Rhoton[2] had stated that this connection may rarely be so large that the superior sagittal sinus drains primarily into the inferior sagittal and straight sinuses. This latter configuration, not to be confused with a falcine venous plexus, most likely represents a persistent falcine sinus (to be discussed later). Kaplan et al.[3] had stated that freely anastomosing small plexiform channels may be present throughout the falx cerebri.

Tubbs et al.[4] found that these vascular channels ranged in size from 0.5 mm to 1.1 cm (mean 0.6 mm). All of these vessels communicated with the inferior sagittal sinus. Typing of these vessels was as follows: type I falcine veins had no communication with the superior sagittal sinus, type II falcine veins had limited communication with the superior sagittal sinus, and type III falcine veins had significant communication with the superior sagittal sinus. No draining veins were found that communicated with these identified veins within the falx cerebri. In total, 17 of 27 specimens (63%) had communication with the superior sagittal sinus (types II and III). Further subdivision revealed 10 type I (37%), 7 type II (26%), and 10 type III (37%) falcine venous plexuses. Generally, most falcine veins in the falx cerebri were found in its posterior one-third and within this posterior one-third, in the inferior two-thirds.

An important distinction should be made between the rare persistent fetal falcine sinus and the falcine venous plexus. The falcine sinus is a normal in utero venous structure located in the falx cerebri that normally involutes before birth.[5] This sinus develops from mesenchyme in the mesencephalic flexure, the same area that gives rise to the straight sinus. When the straight sinus is absent or rudimentary, the falcine sinus may be recanalized.[6,7] It is extremely rare to find a persistent falcine sinus without associated anomalies (Figs. 9.3 and 9.4). Associated anomalies include bifid cranium, vein of Galen malformation, agenesis of the corpus callosum, Apert syndrome, osteogenesis imperfecta, Chiari II malformation, occipital encephalocele, absent tentorium cerebelli, parietal cephaloceles, and bilateral giant parietal foramina.[6,8–10]

Streeter[11] defined the sagittal plexus (in the 20-mm embryo) as a mesh of anastomotic loops from which the superior sagittal and straight sinuses develop. Similarly, the inferior sagittal sinus is thought to develop from the ventral aspect of the sagittal plexus with the disappearance of the smaller channels of this plexus.[11] However, in its posterior one-third, more than one channel of the sagittal plexus might contribute to the development of the superior sagittal sinus. Residual vessels of previous stages dwindle and disappear with the progression of normal development. The superior sagittal sinus in the 50-mm embryo is plexiform in its caudal part.[12]

This sinus within the falx cerebri may receive a bridging vein.[13] Tubbs et al.[4] identified a relatively "safe area" where the falcine venous plexus was not as concentrated. This area was in most specimens (types I and II) in the anterior two-thirds of the falx cerebri between the superior and inferior sagittal sinuses. Surgical ramifications of these findings center mainly around approaches for lesions near the falx. Both transtentorial approaches and posterior transcallosal routes come into close contact with the posterior one-third of the falx. Large meningiomas may involve this region and caution must be taken in dissection around or removal of this specific area. Occasionally, surgical windows in the falx cerebri are opened to allow access to the opposite hemisphere, to assist in complete tumor removal, or to rotate as a flap around a bleeding superior sagittal sinus. Therefore, the potential for bleeding from the venous plexus of the falx cerebri should be considered.

Anatomy, Imaging and Surgery of the Intracranial Dural Venous Sinuses. https://doi.org/10.1016/B978-0-323-65377-0.00009-X

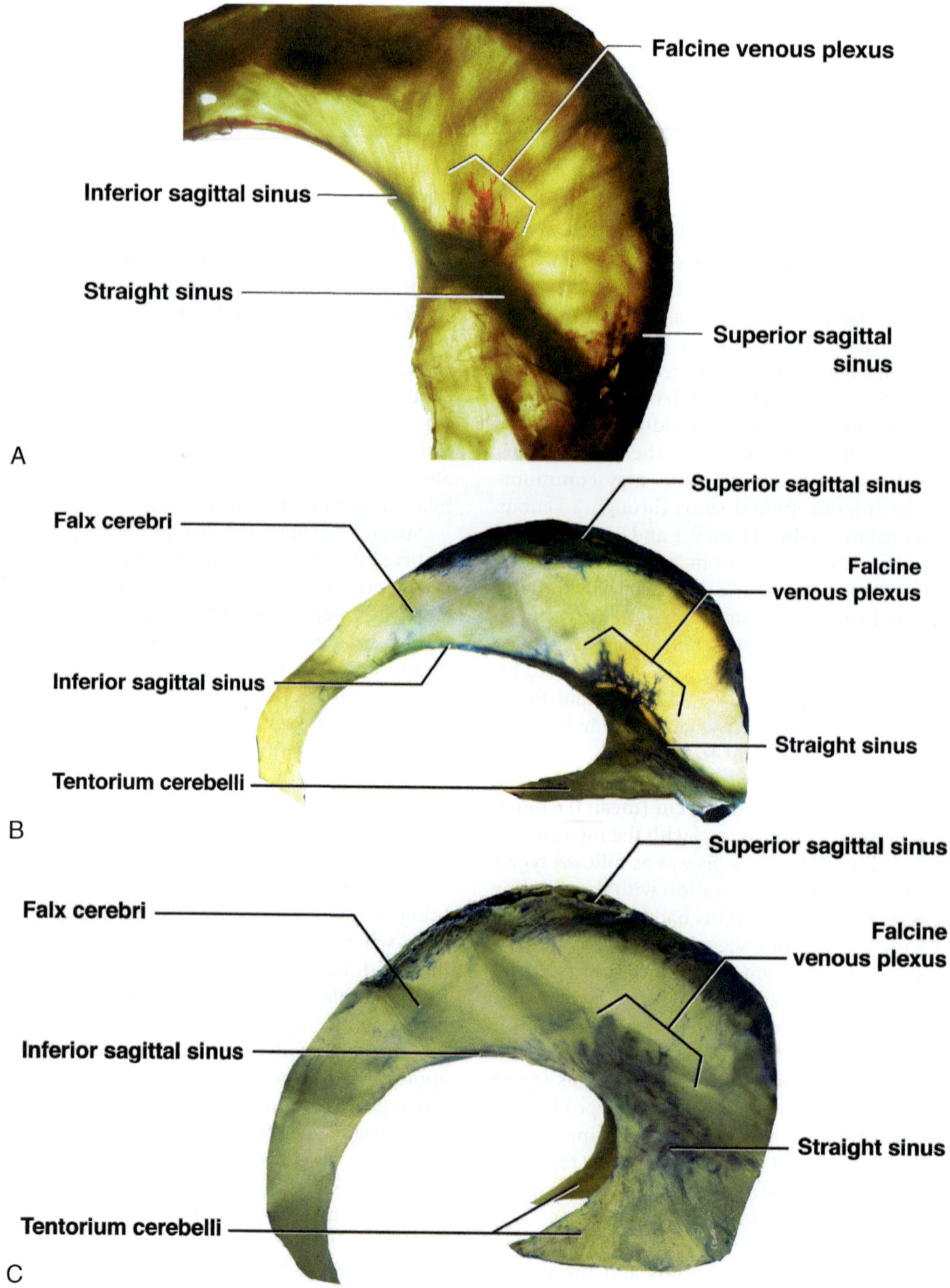

FIG. 9.1 **(A–C)**; Cadaveric examples of falcine venous plexuses.

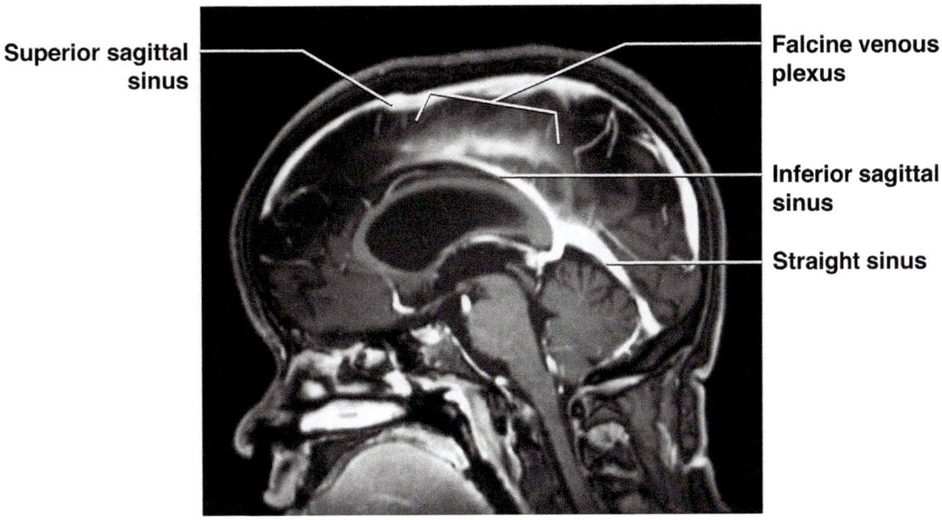

FIG. 9.2 T1-weighted midsagittal MRI after contrast administration. Note the falcine venous plexus.

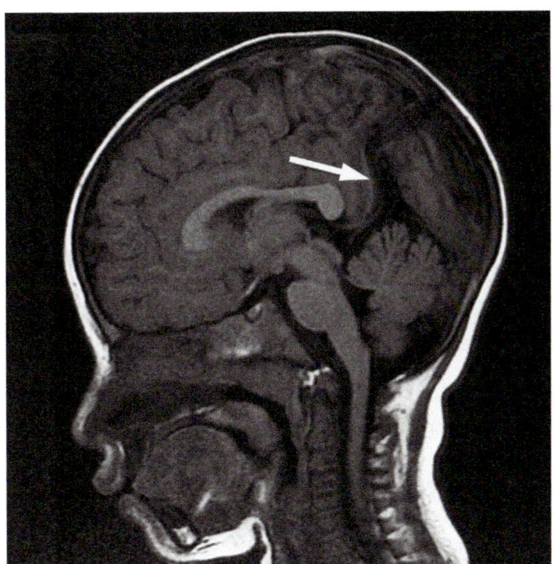

FIG. 9.3 T1-weighted midsagittal MRI noting a persistent falcine venous sinus (*arrow*) in a patient with a parietal cephalocele.

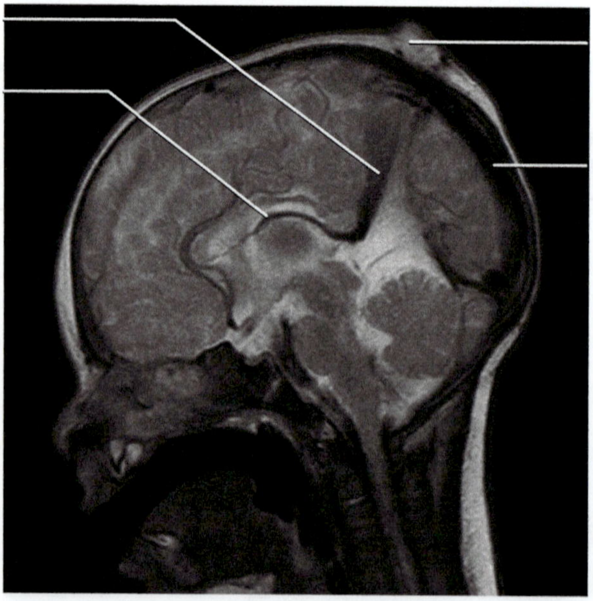

FIG. 9.4 T2-weighted midsagittal MRI of patient seen in Fig. 9.3. Note the parietal cephalocele.

REFERENCES

1. Crosby EC. *Correlative Anatomy of the Nervous System*. New York: The Macmillan Company; 1962:568.
2. Rhoton AL. *Rhoton Cranial Anatomy and Surgical Approaches*. Schaumburg: The congress of neurological surgeons; 2003.
3. Kaplan HA, Browder J, Krieger AJ. Venous channels within the intracranial dural partitions. *Neuroradiology*. 1975;115:641–645.
4. Tubbs RS, Loukas M, Louis Jr RG, et al. Anatomy of the falcine venous plexus. *J Neurosurg*. 2007;107:155–157.
5. Manoj KS, Krishnamoorthy T, Thomas B, Kapilamoorthy TR. An incidental persistent falcine sinus with dominant straight sinus and hypoplastic distal superior sagittal sinus. *Pediatr Radiol*. 2006;36:65–67.
6. Kesava PP. Recanalization of the falcine sinus after venous sinus thrombosis. *AJNR Am J Neuroradiol*. 1996;17:1646–1648.
7. Strub WM, Leach JL, Tomsick TA. Persistent falcine sinus in an adult: demonstration by MR venography. *AJNR Am J Neuroradiol*. 2005;26:750–751.
8. Bartels RH, Merx JL, van Overbeeke JJ. Falcine sinus and occipital encephalocele: a magnetic resonance venography study. *J Neurosurg*. 1998;89:738–741.
9. Reddy AT, Hedlund GL, Percy AK. Enlarged parietal foramina association with cerebral venous and cortical anomalies. *Neurology*. 2000;54:1175–1178.
10. Sener RN. Association of persistent falcine sinus with different clinicoradiologic conditions: MR imaging and MR angiography. *Comput Med Imaging Graph*. 2000;24:343–348.
11. Streeter GL. The development of the venous sinuses of the dura mater in the human embryo. *Am J Anat*. 1915;18:145–178.
12. Browder J, Kaplan HA. *Cerebral Dural Sinuses and Their Tributaries*. Springfield: Charles C. Thomas; 1976:29.
13. Yaşargil MG. *Personnel Communication*; 2006.

CHAPTER 10

The Straight Sinus

MATTHEW PROTAS • R. SHANE TUBBS

EMBRYOLOGY

It was originally believed that the straight sinus developed as an outgrowth from the torcular Herophili, which was derived from the dilated caudal end of the embryonic superior sagittal sinus.[1] This hypothesis, however, has been refuted. Since then, Washington[2] described the proper development of the straight sinus. In the 20-mm embryo, one can start to see the straight sinus as it begins to differentiate from the ventral part of the deep sagittal plexus over the third ventricle. This differentiation then anastomoses with the caudal end of the sagittal plexus. At 50 mm, spontaneous migration causes the movement of the developing straight sinuses as well as the superior sagittal sinus to move more caudally. As development proceeds and the plexus develops more caudally, selection occurs of favorable loops of the plexus. As this proceeds, it causes reorganization and fusion into the tentorial plexus which completes the development of the straight sinus and formation of the torcular Herophili.[2]

Anatomy

The straight sinus travels posteriorly and inferiorly beneath the splenium of the corpus callosum toward the internal occipital protuberance between the areas where the falx cerebri meets the midline of the tentorium cerebelli[3,4] (Figs. 10.1–10.6). The length of the straight sinus ranges between 4 and 7 cm, and its width at the terminal point ranges between 2 and 5 mm.[5] In 108 cadavers studied by Hasegawa et al.[6] the length of the straight sinus was 51±5.2. In a cross-sectional view, the straight sinus appears triangular[7] (Fig. 10.4). The

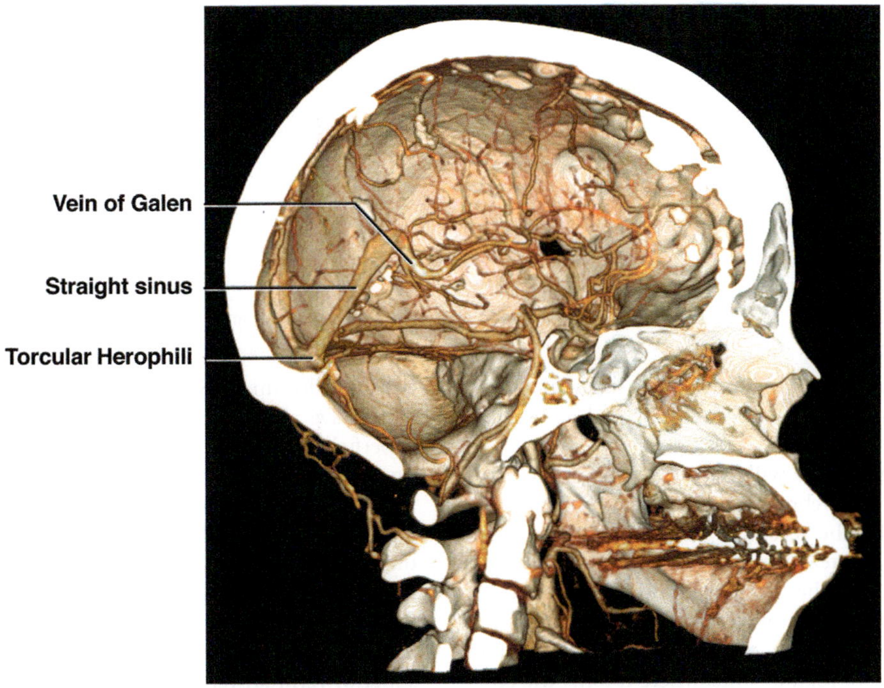

FIG. 10.1 3D CTA noting the straight sinus, medial view. (Courtesy Dr. Joel Curé.)

Anatomy, Imaging and Surgery of the Intracranial Dural Venous Sinuses. https://doi.org/10.1016/B978-0-323-65377-0.00010-6

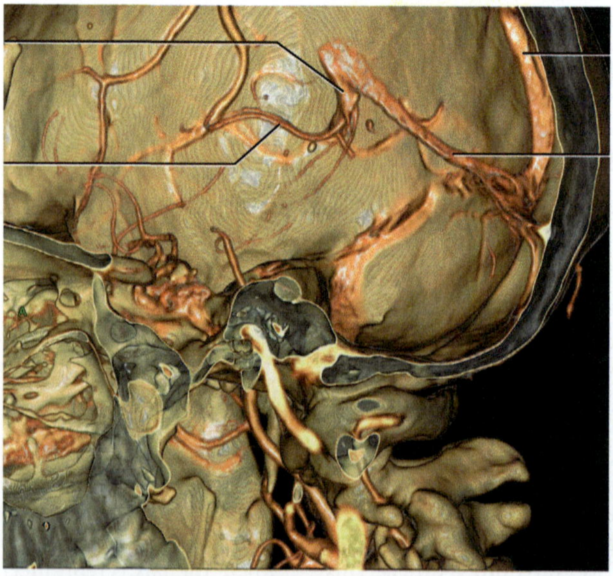

FIG. 10.2 3D CTA noting the straight sinus, lateral view. (Courtesy Dr. Joel Curé.)

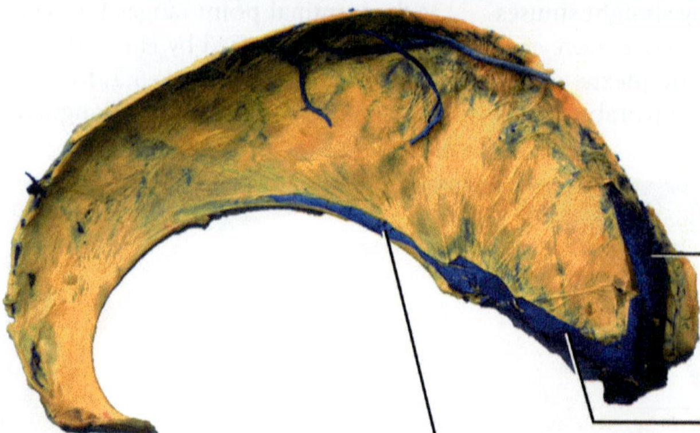

FIG. 10.3 Cadaveric example of the straight sinus.

slope of the straight sinus varies with age with a normal adult tentorial angle between 27 and 52°degrees (mean = 40).[8]

The straight sinus will receive its major drainage from the great cerebral vein of Galen, which passes caudally under the splenium of the corpus callosum to join it.[9] The great cerebral vein of Galen joins the straight sinus at the anterior tentorial edge of the straight sinus at the level of the quadrigeminal plate[10] (Figs. 10.7–10.8). Major venous drainage also comes from the inferior sagittal sinus where it joins the anterior end after it has received its tributaries from the corpus callosum.[9,11] Small contributions to the straight sinus have also been noted to come from the medial superficial cerebral veins of the occipital region, which drain centrally into the straight sinus.[9] Although little is known about the posterior meningeal venous drainage because of its multiple variations, it has been proposed that it would logically contribute to drainage into the straight sinus as well as the tocular Herophili.[9] The straight sinus receives a significant amount of venous drainage from the cerebellum (Figs. 10.9–10.11). The superior vermian veins of the cerebellum passes anteriorly and medially to join the straight sinus.[9,12] Arterial

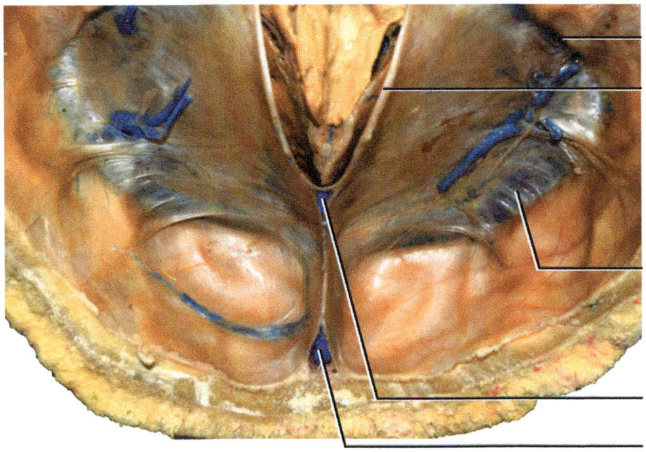

FIG. 10.4 Superior view of the junction of the falx cerebri with the tentorium cerebelli. Note the straight sinus and superior sagittal sinus.

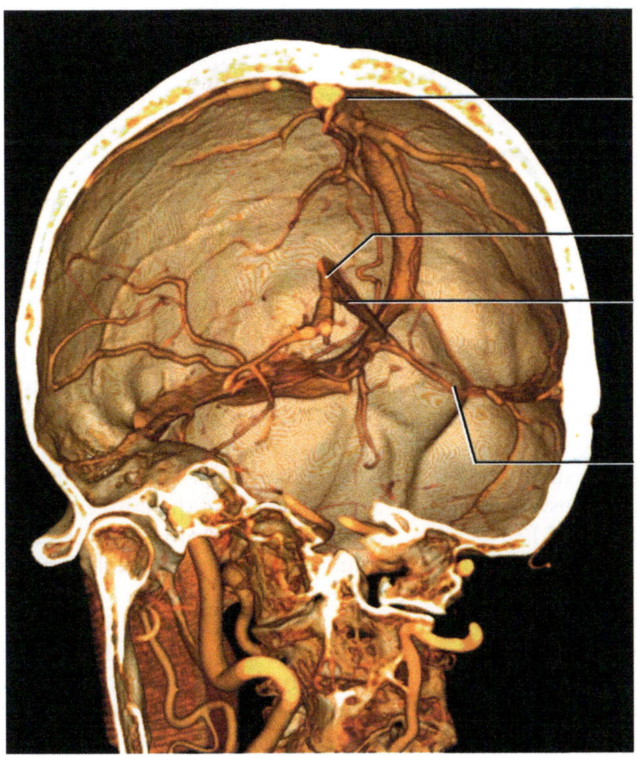

FIG. 10.5 3D CTA noting the straight sinus, anterior view. (Courtesy Dr. Joel Curé.)

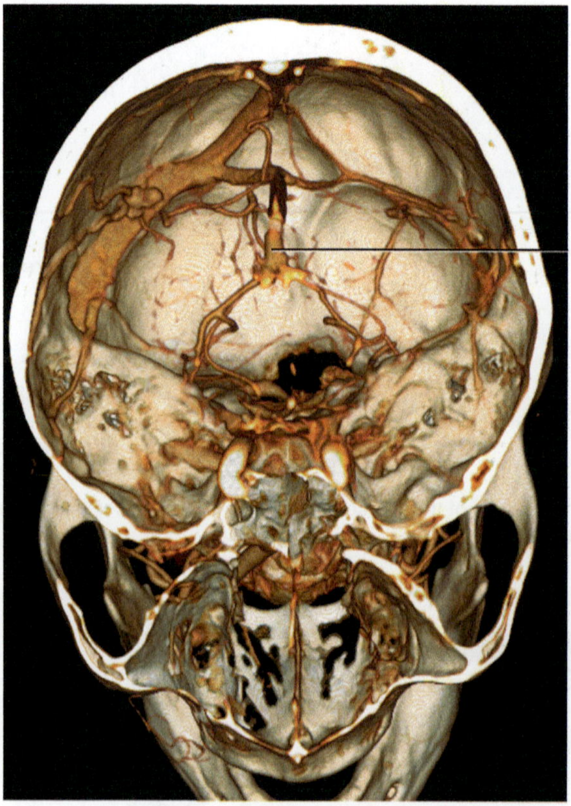

FIG. 10.6 3D CTA noting the straight sinus, superior view. (Courtesy Dr. Joel Curé.)

connections from as far as the posterior pericallosal, posterior cerebral artery, and collicular arteries have all been shown to supply the walls of straight sinus.[13]

Variations

Although most often described as draining posteriorly toward the torcular Herophili (Fig. 10.14), or commonly draining into the left transverse sinus and the superior sagittal sinus into the right transverse sinus, this arrangement can be reversed (Fig. 10.15).

The straight sinus may be doubled or tripled.[14] When duplicated in a median position, one straight sinus is superior and the other inferior. The superior straight sinus represents a continuation of the inferior sagittal sinus and the inferior of the great cerebral vein. When duplicated, the two straight sinuses may drain into either the same or contralateral transverse sinuses. In paramedian position, both sinuses lie on either side of the midline. In most instances, the left represents a continuation of the great cerebral vein and the right, the continuation of the inferior sagittal sinus. Each paramedian straight sinus drains into the ipsilateral transverse sinus.[5,14–16] Saxena et al.[14] examined the straight sinus in 43 cadavers and found that 13.85% were doubled with 9.3% in the median position and 4.65% in the paramedian position. In 56 human cadavers, Magden[15] found the straight sinus in 26.7% of cadavers to be doubled, being either median in position (one superior to the other) (17.8%) or paramedian (both lying on one side of the midline at the junction of the falx cerebri with the tentorium cerebelli) (8.9%). In two cases (3.5%), the straight sinus was tripled, being either median in position or paramedian.

A triple straight sinus is rare, and when present, the sinuses are also described as median or paramedian. In both positions, a middle straight sinus is also found in addition to the superior and inferior or right and left straight sinus, which drain in either transverse sinuses.[15] Partial duplication of the straight sinus may also be found. It usually includes the anterior part of the sinus extending to the junction with the vein of Galen. Duplication of posterior and middle parts and partial tripling has also been observed.[16]

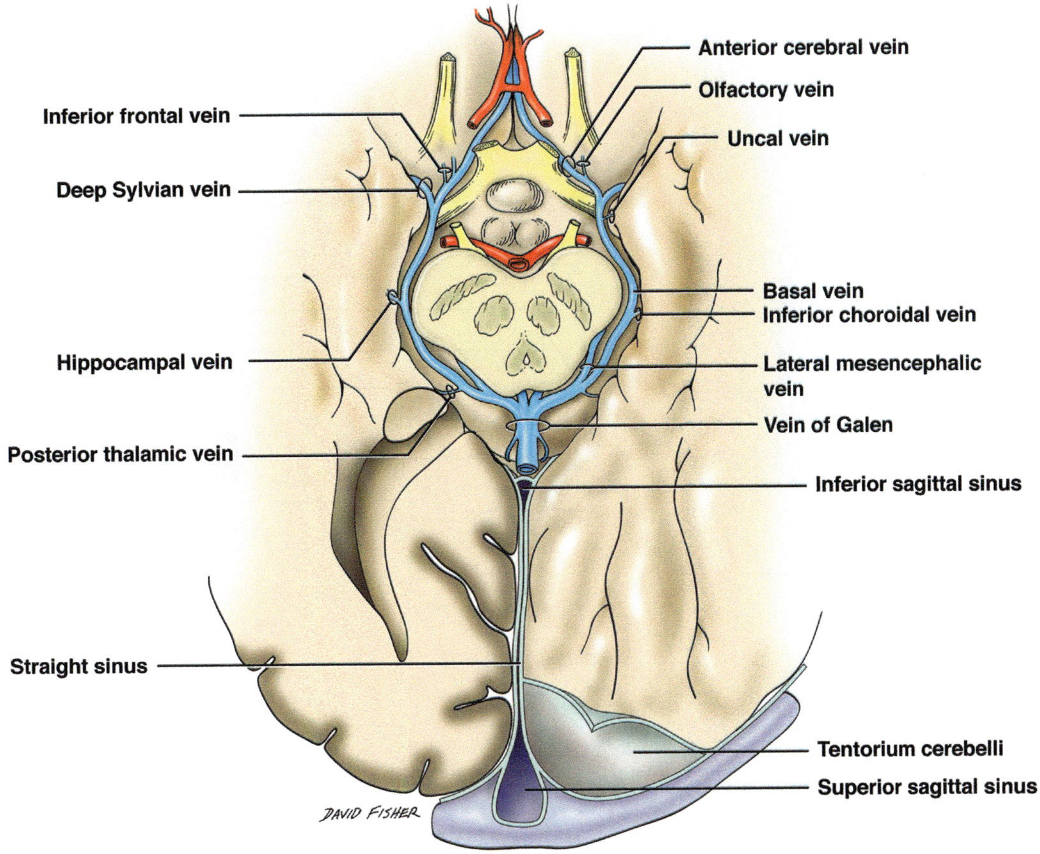

FIG. 10.7 Schematic drawing of the tributaries into the basal vein and its fusing with the internal cerebral veins to form the vein of Galen.

The straight sinus can also be completely or partially absent. Van den Bergh et al.[17] described a case of congenital absence of the straight sinus in a patient with Aarskog syndrome (X-linked recessive syndrome). Knott[18] also described one instance in which the sinus was completely absent. However, Hsu and Chalopka[19] reported a case of a 16-year-old male with a midline-persistent falcine sinus (connecting the vein of Galen and the posterior one-third of the superior sagittal sinus) with the absence of only the proximal end of the straight sinus. The distal end of the straight sinus drained the cortical veins of the occipital lobe and the superior cerebellum. Kim and Lee[20] reported two cases of persistent falcine sinus with the complete absence of the straight sinus in a 60-year-old woman and an 11-year-old girl. Ryu[21] examined the computed tomography angiogram of 586 patients and found that 12 patients had a falcine sinus with one associated with a dysplastic tentorium. Three patients had an absent straight sinus, eight patients had a rudimentary straight sinus, and four patients had a normal sinus. In a case study by Desai et al.,[22] absence of the straight sinus and great vein of Galen was reported in one patient. This led to the internal vertebral veins and the basal veins of Rosenthal to drain into a large frontal interhemispheric falcine vein. In a rare case examined by Chen et al.,[23] arachnoid granulations were found in the straight sinus of a 71-year-old female. A similar case was reported by MRI of arachnoid granulations of the straight sinus in a 19-year-old man who presented with dizziness.[24]

In cases of absent inferior sagittal sinus, the straight sinus is formed by the continuation of the great cerebral vein. It may also communicate with the occipital sinus, the cavernous sinus through tentorial veins, or with the right transverse sinus.[5,16]

Hasegawa et al.[6] examined the anatomic variations of the straight sinus and found that the angle of the straight sinus to the nasion-tuberculum sellae line was

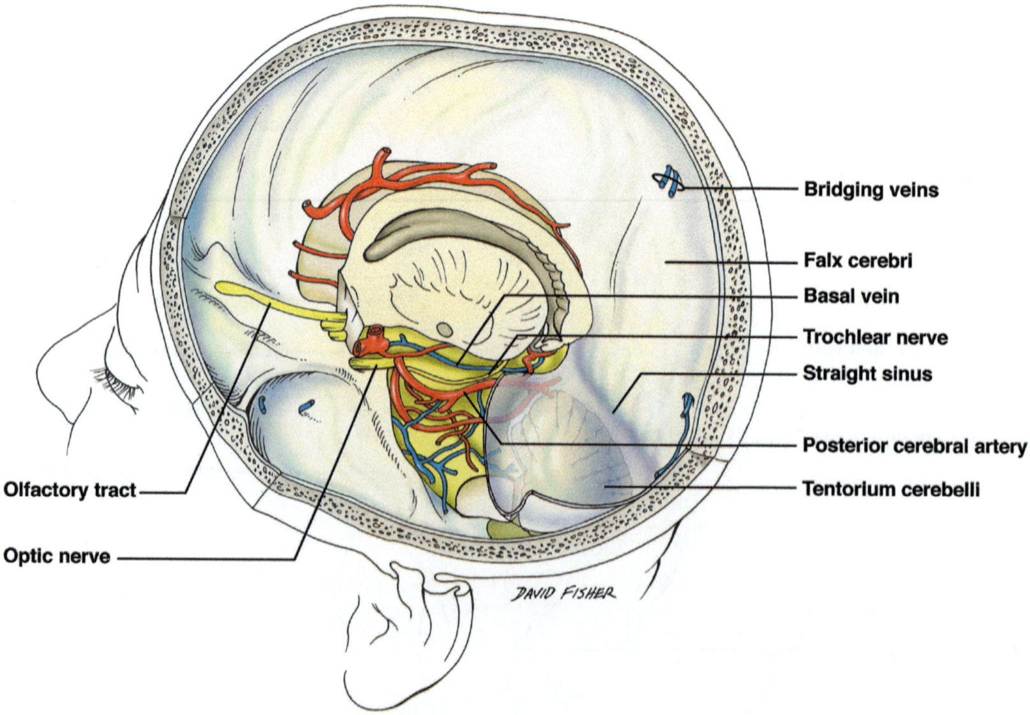

FIG. 10.8 Schematic drawing of the lateral cranium noting the intradural position of the straight sinus. (Courtesy Dr. Joel Curé.)

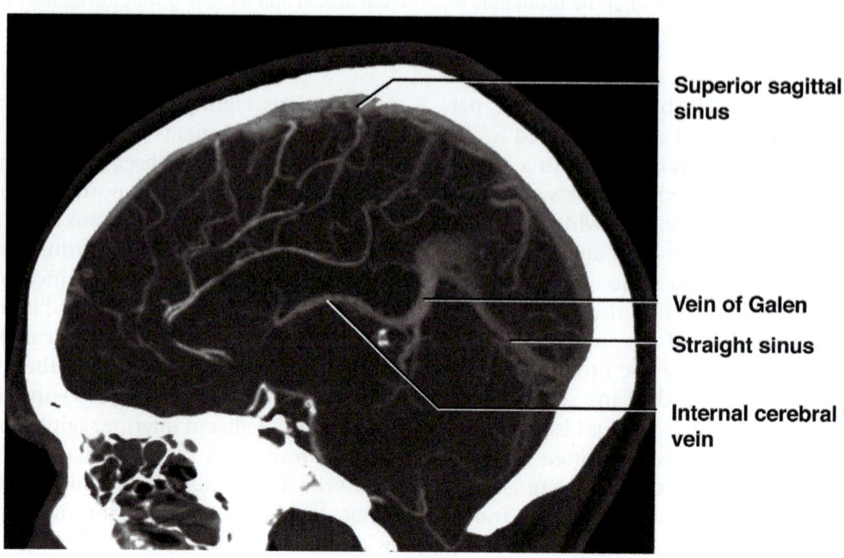

FIG. 10.9 Arteriogram illustrating the straight sinus.

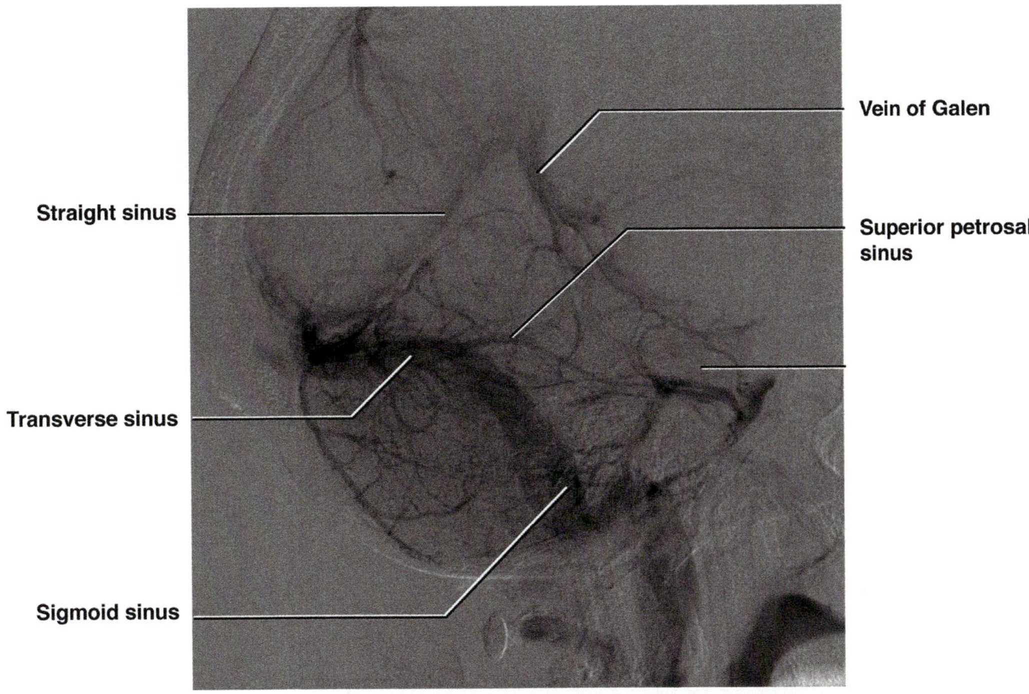

FIG. 10.10 Magnetic Resonance Venogram (MRV) of the straight sinus.

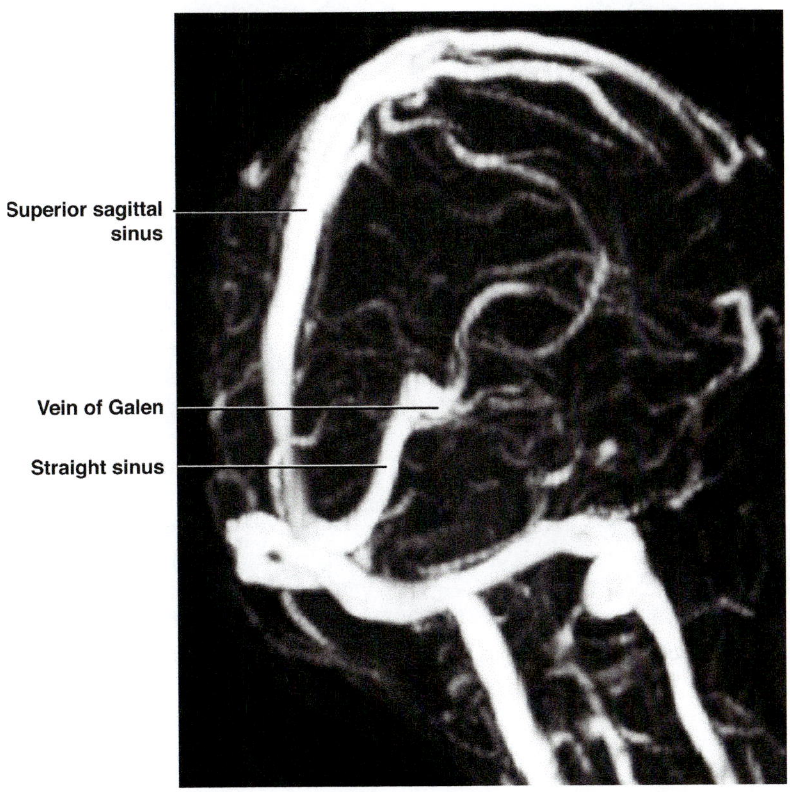

FIG. 10.11 3D CTA illustrating the straight sinus. (Courtesy Dr. Joel Curé.)

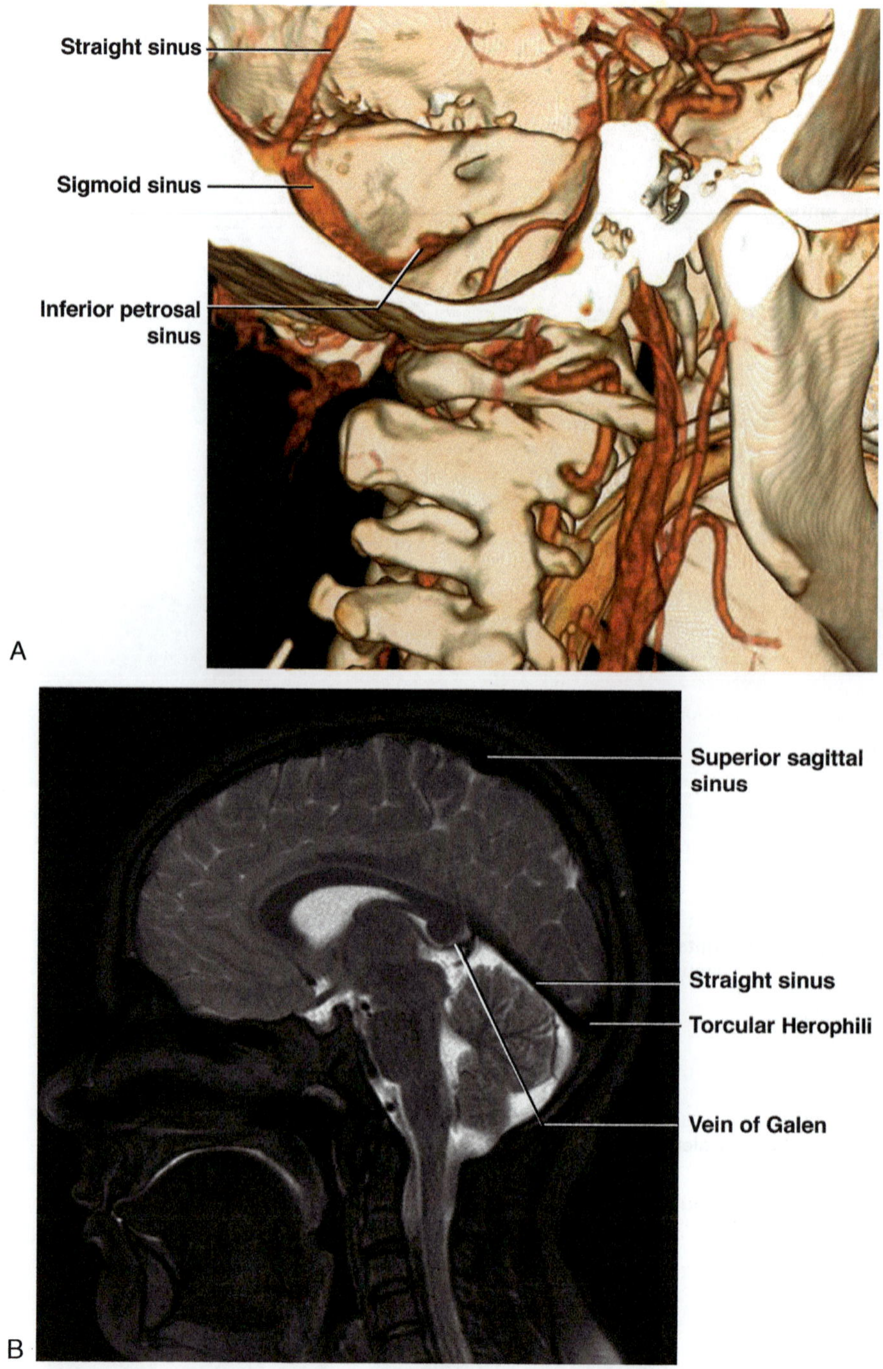

FIG. 10.12 **(A)**. CTA noting the straight sinus and **(B)**. Sagittal T2-weighted MRI illustrating the straight sinus.

51 ± 6.7 degrees (Figs. 10.12–10.13); the angle to the tuberculum sellae-inion line was 44 ± 5.0 degrees and the angle the nasion-inion line was 47 ± 5.0 degrees. The straight sinus coursed posteriorly at 1.4 ± 4.5 degrees to the bregma-inion line. The straight sinus was placed into three groups based on the relationship with the corpus callosum. They included the following:

- Type 1 (63%): the extended line of the slope of the straight sinus is tangential to the upper aspect of the splenium of the corpus callosum.
- Type 2 (26%) (high-angle type): The extended line was far above the tangent line.
- Type 3 (11%) (low-angle type): The extended line was far below the tangent line.

Multiple variations are noted in the caudal end of the straight sinus as it joins the torcular Herophili. Rare variations have even shown the inferior vermian veins to drain into the straight sinus.[25]

PATHOLOGY

Atretic Parietal Encephalocele

Atretic parietal encephaloceles cause a failure of the straight venous sinus to move more caudally leading to a retention of its early embryonic vertical positioning and is typically associated with a persistent falcine sinus.[17,26] In patients with parietal cephaloceles, the straight sinus has been shown to ascended along the interhemispheric region and anastomosed with the superior sagittal sinus. This pathology is also associated with an upward tenting of the tentorium cerebelli in three of four cases reported by Rosa et al. (2014).[27] One case report of a patient who presented with atretic parietal cephalocele had an embryonic bifid caudal superior sagittal sinus because of the vertical positioning of the straight sinus, which could best appreciated by an axial or coronal T2-weighted MRI.[28]

Sinus Thrombosis, Stenosis, and Dural Arteriovenous Fistulas

In a study examining infarctions related to cerebral venous sinus thrombosis, patients with venous sinus thrombosis of the straight sinus are more at risk for an infarction or hemorrhage (67.8% n = 28).[29] Five cases have also been reported of intracranial dural arteriovenous fistulas leading to sinus thrombosis in a study by Pierot et al.[30] Reversible parkinsonism is also of pathologic concern of patients with cortical

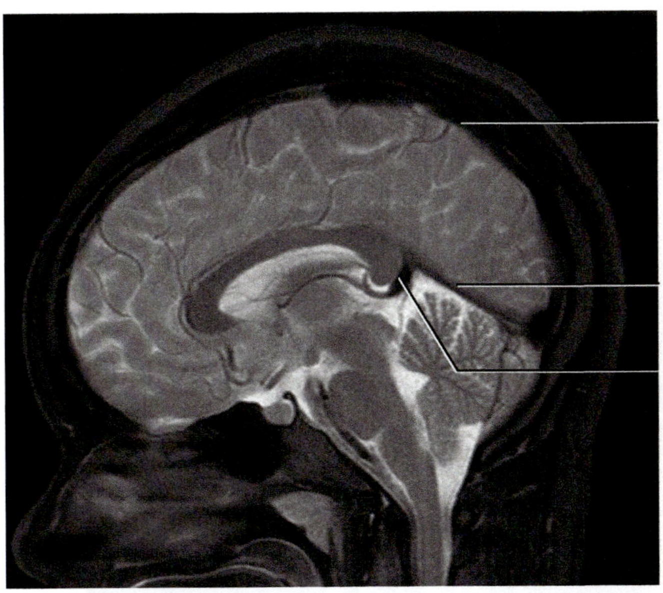

FIG. 10.13 Sagittal T2-weighted MRI noting the straight sinus. (Courtesy Dr. Joel Curé.)

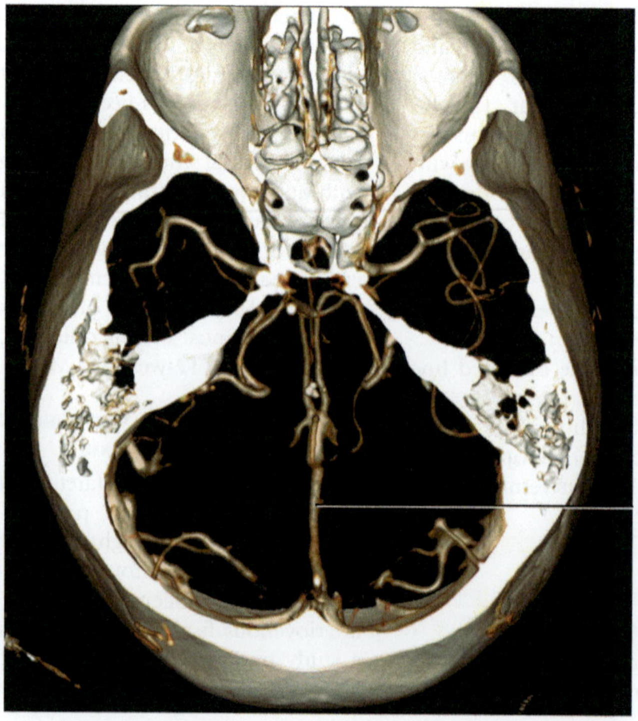

FIG. 10.14 CTA noting the straight sinus.

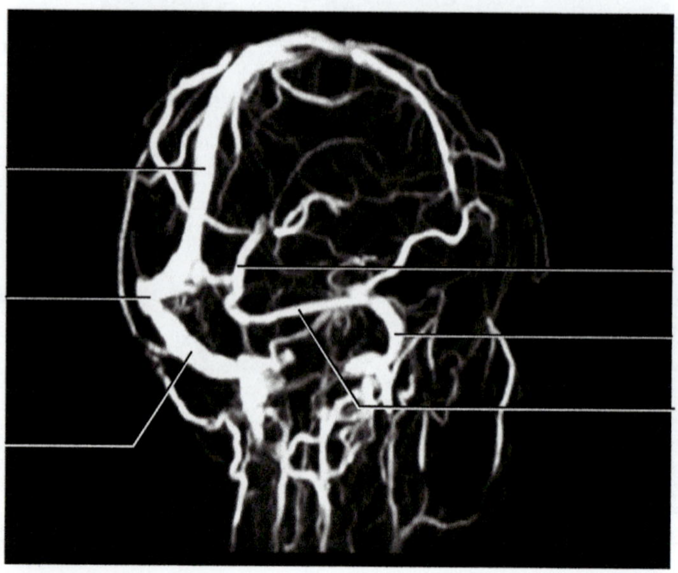

FIG. 10.15 MRV illustrating the straight sinus draining directly into the transverse sinus instead of the confluence.

venous thrombosis of the straight sinus.[30] Parkinsonism has also been attributed to increased straight sinus pressure caused by a dural arteriovenous fistula of the transverse sinus, which presented in a 52-year-old woman.[31] Parkinsonism is reversible if the fistula can be treated with embolization.[32] In a case study of a 59-year-old man, dural arteriovenous fistulas as a result of an occluded straight sinus led to retrograde blood flow causing edema of the globus pallidus causing parkinsonism.[33] Another dural arteriovenous fistula involving the straight sinus in one rare case report involving a 64-year-old man caused idiopathic hypertrophic cranial pachymeningitis.[33] Another case study of a 60-year-old man described a stenosis at the junction of the great vein of Galen and straight sinus being a probable cause of perimesencephalic nonaneurysmal hemorrhage.[34]

OTHER REPORTED PATHOLOGIES

1. Brain herniations into arachnoid granulations of the straight sinus, although extremely rare, have been reported in 1 out of 68 patients.[35]
2. Cranium bifidum with malformation of the straight sinus is rare but has been reported.[36,37] Inoue et al.[33] reported six cases of cranium bifidum causing an anomalous upward course of the straight sinus. Laak and Petridis[37] reported a similar finding in one case of a 4-month-old with crinium bifidum. The straight sinus was also positioned abnormally high and an elongated great vein of Galen.[37]
3. Pineal tumors are likely to cause anatomic variations of the straight sinus. In five cases of pineal tumors, two straight sinuses were in a normal location, whereas three presented as a high-angle or low-angle variation.[6]

Surgical

Localization of the straight sinus is best shown through lateral angiography.[7] When using straight frontal projection, the sinus will appear superimposed on other midline structures making areas such as the upper and anterior parts of the straight sinus difficult to differentiate.[7] To best show the straight sinus through angiography at this angle, the patient's head should be rotated 5–10 degress.[7] In an analysis of a team of neurologist's agreement on the localization of dural sinus thrombosis in the straight sinus of 40 separate patients through MRI, they had moderate to excellent agreement on location among the team (κ range: 0.59–0.92), which compared with the other sinuses is good, but not as accurate as the rest.[38] In a study of eight patients with dural arteriovenous fistulae of the straight sinus, a supracerebellar-infratentorial approach was the preferred method.[39] It has also been proposed that a noninvasive measurement of the elastance and reserve capacity of the craniovertebral contents can be measured via the straight sinus through the occipital window during a body tilt test.[40] When performing intercranial surgery, it is very important to take into consideration patients with dural arteriovenous fistulas of the straight sinus. A cerebellar arteriovenous malformation in a 58-year-old female blocked the straight sinus leading to the occipital sinus providing the only drainage for it and the superior sagittal sinus.[41]

REFERENCES

1. Bailey FR, Miller AM. *Text-book of Embryology*. New York: W. Wood and Co; 1911.
2. Washington CI o. *Contributions to Embryology*. Carnegie Institution of Washington; 1918.
3. Drake RL, Vogl W, Tibbitts AWMM, Illustrations by Richard, Richardson P. *Gray's Anatomy for Students*. Philadelphia: Elsevier/Churchill Livingstone; 2005:795.
4. Harrigan MR, Deveikis JP. *Handbook of Cerebrovascular Disease and Neurointerventional Technique*. Humana Press; 2012.
5. Saxena RC, Beg MA, Das AC. The straight sinus. *J Neurosurg*. 1974;41:724–727.
6. Hasegawa M, Yamashita J, Yamashima T. Anatomical variations of the straight sinus on magnetic resonance imaging in the infratentorial supracerebellar approach to pineal region tumors. *Surg Neurol*. 1991;36:354–359.
7. Newton TH, Potts DG. *Radiology of the Skull and Brain*. Mosby; 1974.
8. Wolpert SM. Dural sinus configuration: measure of congenital disease. *Radiology*. 1969;92(7):1511–1516. https://doi.org/10.1148/92.7.1511.
9. Jinkins JR. *Atlas of Neuroradiologic Embryology, Anatomy, and Variants*. Philadelphia, PA: Lippincott Williams & Wilkins; 2000.
10. Le Gros Clark W. On the pacchionian bodies. *J Anat*. 1920;55:40–48.
11. Naidich TP, Castillo M, Cha S, Smirniotopoulos JG. *Imaging of the Brain: Expert Radiology Series*. Elsevier Health Sciences; 2012.
12. Conn PM. *Neuroscience in Medicine*. Humana Press; 2008.
13. Velut S. Embryology of the cerebral veins. *Neurochirurgie*. 1987;33(4):258–263.
14. Saxena RC, Beg MA, Das AC. Double straight sinus- report of six cases. *J Neurosurg*. 1973;39:540–542.
15. Magden AO. Triple straight sinus--report of 2 cases. *Anat Anzeiger*. 1991;173(1):17–22.
16. Browder J, Kaplan HA, Krieger AJ. Anatomical features of the straight sinus and its tributaries. *J Neurosurg*. 1976;44(1):55–61.

17. Van den Bergh P, Fryns JP, Wilms G, Piot R, Dralands G, Van den Bergh R. Anomalous cerebral venous drainage in Aarskog syndrome. *Clin Genet.* 1984;25:288–294.
18. Knott JF. On the cerebral sinuses and their variations. *J Anat Physiol.* 1881;16:27–42.
19. Hsu S, Chaloupka JC. Atretic parietal cephalocele associated with sinus pericranii: embryological consideration. *Brain Dev.* 2012;34:325–328.
20. Kim MS, Lee GH. Two Cases with persistent falcine sinus as congenital variation. *J Korean Neurosurg Soc.* 2010;48: 82–84.
21. Ryu CW. Persistent falcine sinus: is it really rare? *AJNR Am J Neuroradiol.* 2009;31:367–369.
22. Desai K, Bhayani R, Nadkarni T, Limaye U, Goel A. Developmental deep venous system Anomaly associated with congenital malformation of the brain. *Pediatr Neurosurg.* 2002;36:37–39.
23. Chen SS, Shao KN, Chiang JH, et al. Arachnoid granulations--computerized tomography and magnetic resonance imaging features: a case report. *Zhonghua Yixue Zazhi.* 1999;62(1):46–50.
24. Shin J, Lee KH, Lee JM, Kwon US, Choi GC, Suh CD. An arachnoid granulation in the straight sinus. *Neuroradiology.* 2000;42(10):746–748. https://doi.org/10.1007/s002340000381.
25. Lasjaunias P, Berenstein A, Brugge KT. *Clinical Vascular Anatomy and Variations. Surgical Neuroangiography.* Springer Berlin Heidelberg; 2001.
26. Rumboldt Z. *Brain Imaging with MRI and CT: An Image Pattern Approach.* Cambridge University Press; 2012.
27. Perez da Rosa S, Millward CP, Bhatti MI, Healey A, Burn SC, Sinha A. MRI findings of intracranial anomalies associated with cephalocele—a case series. *Child's Nerv Syst.* 2014;30(5):891–895.
28. Murakami N, Morioka T, Kawamura N, Suzuki SO, Kira R. Venous anomaly analogous to vertical embryonic positioning of the straight sinus associated with atretic cephalocele at the suboccipital region. *Childs Nerv Syst.* 2016.
29. Zhou G, Li M, Zhu Y, Zhao J, Lu H. Cerebral venous sinus thrombosis involving the straight sinus may result in infarction and/or hemorrhage. *Eur Neurol.* 2016;75(5-6): 257–262.
30. Pierot L, Chiras J, Duyckaerts C, Jason M, Martin N. Intracranial dural arteriovenous fistulas and sinus thrombosis. Report of five cases. *J Neuroradiol.* 1993;20(1):9–18.
31. Hattori T, Takeuchi T, Kabeya R, Ando K, Tosaki F. Transverse-sigmoid sinus dural arteriovenous fistula presenting with parkinsonism. *Neurol Med -Chir.* 2013;53(4):224–227.
32. Shahar T, Gadoth A, Nossek E, Giladi N, Ram Z, Maimon S. Reversible freezing of gait caused by dural arteriovenous fistula and congestion of the globus pallidus. *Mov Disord.* 2012;27(13):1690–1693.
33. Hamada J, Yoshinaga Y, Korogi Y, Ushio Y. Idiopathic hypertrophic cranial pachymeningitis associated with a dural arteriovenous fistula involving the straight sinus: case report. *Neurosurgery.* 2000;47(5):1230–1233.
34. Shad A, Rourke TJ, Hamidian Jahromi A, Green AL. Straight sinus stenosis as a proposed cause of perimesencephalic non-aneurysmal haemorrhage. *J Clin Neurosci.* 2008;15(7):839–841.
35. Malekzadehlashkariani S, Wanke I, Rüfenacht DA, San Millán D. Brain herniations into arachnoid granulations: about 68 cases in 38 patients and review of the literature. *Neuroradiology.* 2016;58(5):443–457.
36. Inoue Y, Hakuba A, Fujitani K, et al. Occult cranium bifidum. Radiological and surgical findings. *Neuroradiology.* 1983;25(4):217–223.
37. van Laak D, Petridis AK. A case of occult cranium bifidum combined with abnormal high position of the straight sinus. *Clin Anat.* 2010;23(8):877–878.
38. Ferro JM, Morgado C, Sousa R, Canhao P. Interobserver agreement in the magnetic resonance location of cerebral vein and dural sinus thrombosis. *Eur J Neurol.* 2007;14(3):353–356.
39. Lawton MT, Sanchez-Mejia RO, Pham D, Tan J, Halbach VV. Tentorial dural arteriovenous fistulae: operative strategies and microsurgical results for six types. *Neurosurgery.* 2008;62(3 suppl 1):110–124; discussion 124–115.
40. Shakhnovich AR, Shakhnovich VA, Galushkina AA. Noninvasive assessment of the elastance and reserve capacity of the craniovertebral contents via flow velocity measurements in the straight sinus by TCD during body tilting test. *J Neuroimaging.* 1999;9(3):141–149.
41. Hamnett N, Ogungbo B, Nasher H, Javadpour M. Anomalous cerebral venous sinus drainage. *Br J Neurosurg.* 2010;24(4):497–498.

CHAPTER 11

The Inferior Petrosal Sinus

SELEIPIRI AKOBO • SHENELL BERNARD • ANDRE GRANGER • R. SHANE TUBBS

The inferior petrosal sinus (IPS) (Figs. 11.1–11.4) occupies an important position at the skull base and must be considered with surgical approaches to this area. Moreover, more recent, minimally invasive intravascular procedures necessitate sampling blood from this sinus. Therefore, detailed knowledge of its anatomy and variations is important in clinical practice.

EMBRYOLOGY

The IPS is an important paired cerebral venous channel at the skull's base. It drains the cavernous sinus and receives inflow from the auditory structures and drains into the sigmoid sinus and the superior jugular bulb on each side.[1]

In 1915, Streeter observed and documented the development of dural venous sinuses in human embryos ranging from a crown-rump length (CRL) of 4–80 mm. In the early stages of development of the cerebral venous system, the vena capitis medialis, or the medial head vein, can be seen lying medial to the emerging cranial nerve roots and otic vesicle.[2,3]

As the fetuses grow to a 5–10-mm CRL, the medial head disappears and is replaced by the vena capitis lateralis or the lateral head vein,[1,3] which is located lateral to the otic vesicle, medial to the trigeminal nerve, and lateral to the facial and vestibular nerves.[2] It is connected to the precardinal vein, which is the precursor of the internal jugular vein (IJV).[1]

In a fetus's 14–18-mm CRL, a venous channel parallel to the lateral head vein connecting these plexuses develops.[2] This channel provides the basis for the cerebral venous structures that are rostral to the jugular bulb.[2]

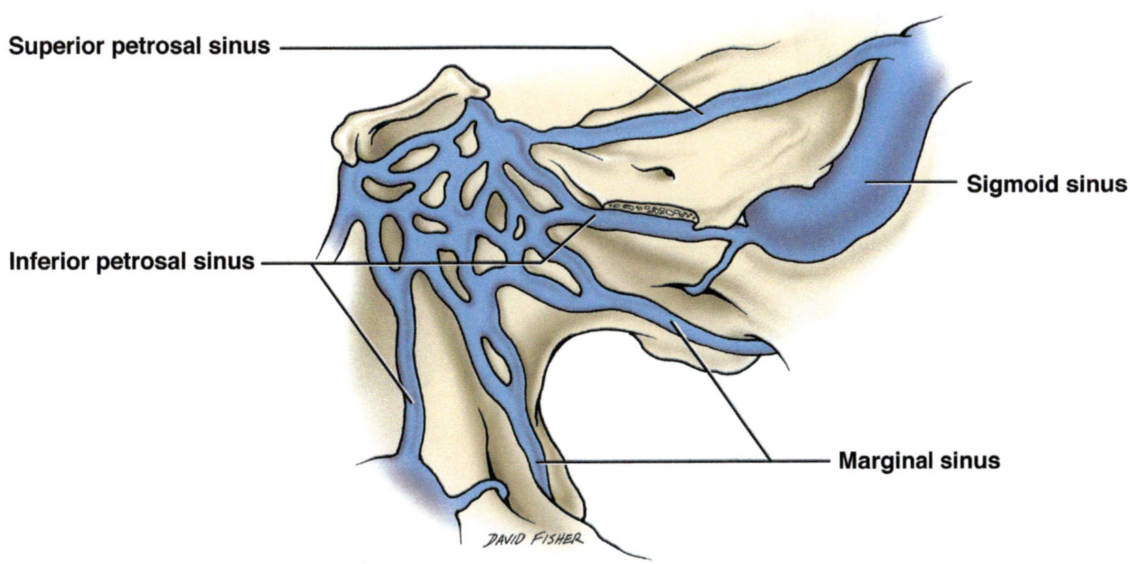

FIG. 11.1 Schematic drawing of the major venous sinuses of the floor of the posterior cranial fossa illustrating the inferior petrosal sinus.

Anatomy, Imaging and Surgery of the Intracranial Dural Venous Sinuses. https://doi.org/10.1016/B978-0-323-65377-0.00011-8

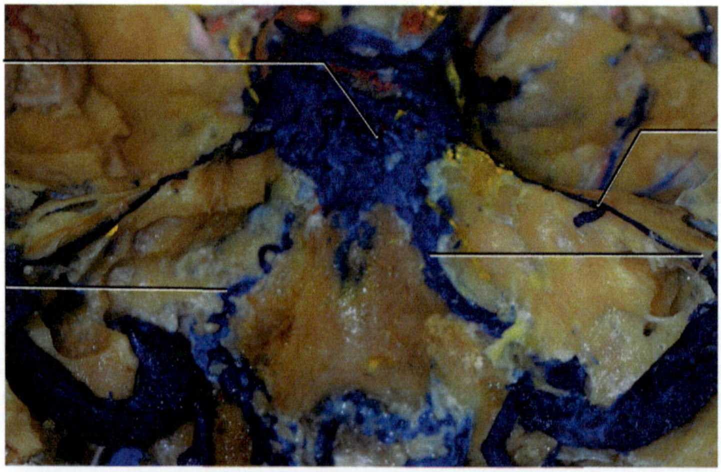

FIG. 11.2 Latex-injected cadaveric specimen illustrating the inferior petrosal sinus on the right side and with removal of the left inferior petrosal sinus, the inferior petrooccipital vein.

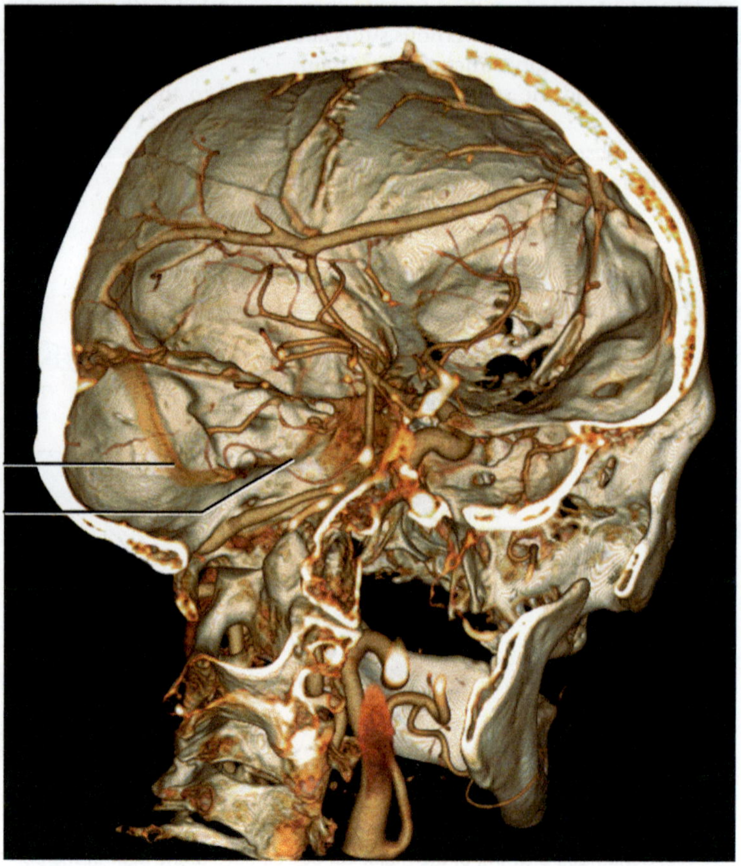

FIG. 11.3 3D CTA illustrating the inferior petrosal sinus. (Courtesy Dr. Joel Curé.)

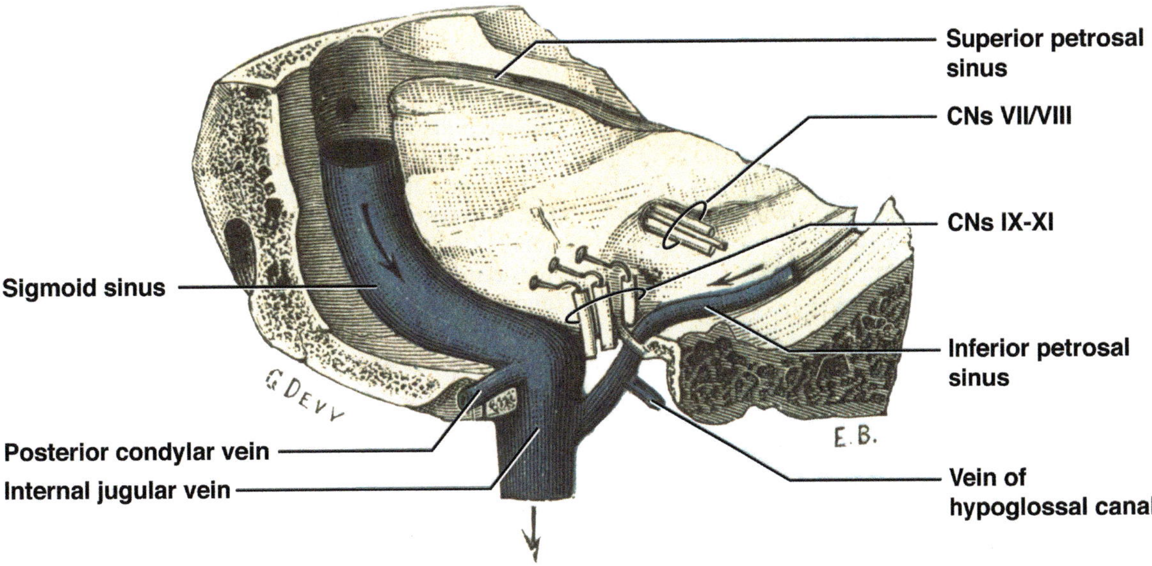

FIG. 11.4 Drawing of the relationship of the inferior petrosal sinus at its confluence with the internal jugular vein, which is below the skull in this case, that is, outside the jugular foramen (After Testut).

In 24–40-mm CRL fetuses, the anterior component of the lateral head vein persists as the cavernous sinus whereas its posterior component disappears. The IPS can be seen forming as a new channel that is medial to the otic vesicle connecting the cavernous sinus to the jugular bulb vesicle vein.[2]

In fetuses, the junction of the IPS with the IJV is entirely extracranial. In adults, however, the junction occurs at the anterior surface of the jugular bulb.[2,3]

The remnant of the head sinus after it forms the sigmoid sinus, the preotic sinus, and proximal ventral myelencephalic vein contributes to the formation of the IPS. This occurs at the level of CN VI in continuity with the emerging cavernous sinus draining the orbit.[4]

ANATOMY

The cerebral venous system can be divided into superficial and deep systems. The deep system consists of the lateral sinus, straight sinus, and sigmoid sinus along with draining deeper cortical veins. The superficial system comprises sagittal sinuses and cortical veins, which drain superficial surfaces of both cerebral hemispheres.[5] Both of these systems mostly drain into IJVs[5] via the IPS.

The IPS can drain intra- or extracranially (Fig. 11.5). Intracranial drainage has been reported in roughly 20% of cases. It rests in the lower parts of the foramen and has no relationship with the jugular foramen in about 7% of people.[6] It originates from the side of the cavernous sinus projecting between the sphenoid and temporal bones.[7]

Along its course, it receives venous drainage from the internal auditory vein, medulla oblongata, pons, and inferior cerebellar surface.[1,2] It is the major drainage of the cavernous sinus, with numerous branches communicating with the anterior condylar vein (ACV), lateral condylar vein (LCV), basilar plexus, and the vertebral venous plexus (VVP).[8] The size of the IPS increases as it progresses through its path, bending enough to leave its imprints on both the temporal and sphenoid bones and entering into both the cavernous sinus and the jugular vein, where they collect the contents of the lateral sinuses.[7] The size ranges in diameter from 2.85 mm in its lower part to about 7–10 mm through its many channels.[6]

The IPS is housed in the petrooccipital suture or groove and runs from the cavernous sinus to the IJV, close to the basilar artery.[7,9] It is posterior and superior to the internal carotid artery and carries blood to the IJV.[10] The IPS enters the jugular foramen between CN's IX and X, while draining the basilar venous plexus.[11] It also lies between the petrous apices and the clivus along the path of the petrooccipital fissure[12].

VARIATIONS

Osborn (1999) stated that it is common for the IPS to display quite a number of variations in its appearance,

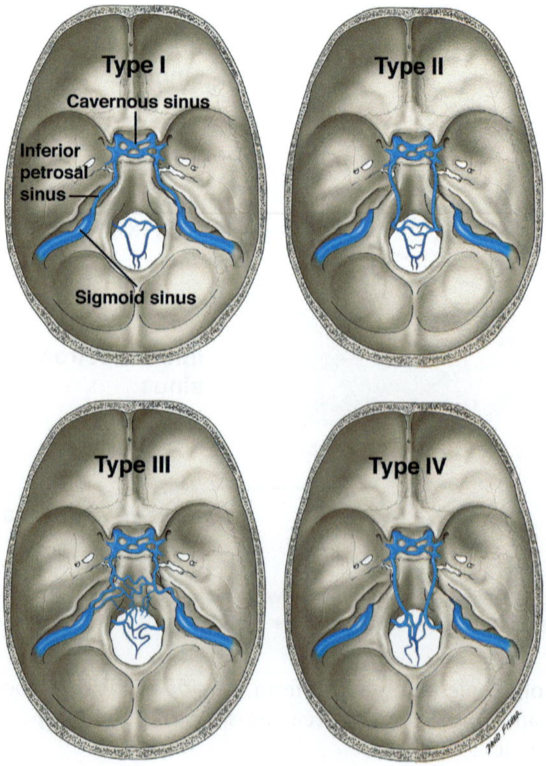

FIG. 11.5 Four types of morphology reported for the inferior petrosal sinus.

ranging in size, anastomoses, and relationship to the nerves that surround it as they enter the jugular foramen (Osborn, 1999).[13] Variations of this sinus depend on the level of dominance of anastomosing landmarks associated with the sinus. Any one of these may be more dominant, but in the majority of people, these anastomotic channels/landmarks are symmetric. However, 1.0% of people do not have an IPS that connects with the IJV.[14] Despite the variance in the anatomy of the anastomoses between the IPS, the IJV, and the venous plexuses at the base of the skull, it is still almost always possible to catheterize the IPS.

VARIATIONS IN THE LEVEL OF TERMINATION

The normal anatomy of the IPS is discussed in the section of this chapter titled Anatomy. In brief, the IPS forms a connection with the posteroinferior portion of the cavernous sinus. It then follows an approximately posterolateral course along the petrous ridge to drain into the IJV at the jugular bulb.

Gailloud et al.[15] described a variant of the IPS with respect to its point of termination. In the cadaver of an 85-year-old male, the IPS was noted to have its point of drainage into the IJV approximately 4.0 cm below the jugular bulb, which is its normal point of termination. This was generally the same bilaterally in this patient, with minor differences. Among these differences were the exact distance below the jugular bulb that the IPS joined the IJV, the number and size of the tributaries between the IJV and this extended version of the IPS, and finally the thickness of the connective tissue separating these two vessels.

To have an idea of the prevalence of this variant, Gailloud et al.[15] observed 100 consecutive routine neuroradiologic angiographies. This low-terminating version of the IPS was observed in four of these cases (the drainage pattern in the other 96 cases was not mentioned). Benndorf and Campi[16] reported two similar cases in patients undergoing endovascular management of cavernous sinus lesions.

In the 27 cases evaluated by Rubenstein et al.,[17] three different locations of the junction of the IPS and the IJV were identified. In four cases, the junction was located within the jugular foramen. In eight cases, it was found in the extracranial opening of the jugular foramen. Its location was below the skull base in the remaining 15 cases.

The work of Knott[18] was carried out on 22 sinuses. Here, the level of termination of the IPS was near the lower margin of the jugular foramen in eight sinuses. In nine sinuses, it was slightly above the jugular foramen, and in five sinuses, it was slightly below the jugular foramen.

The level of the IPS-IJV junction was classified into six main types by Mitsuhashi et al.[19] based on a study of 3D rotational venograms of 83 venous sinus sides in 63 patients. In type A (seen in one side), the IPS drained directly into the superior part of the jugular bulb. In type B (seen in 29 sides), the point of drainage of the IPS was at the level of the extracranial opening of the hypoglossal canal. The types where the IPS drained into the lower extracranial IJV were classified as type C (seen in 31 sides). Type C was subclassified into type C1, where the IPS had a single communication with the IJV and type C2 where another upper venous route existed. In type D (seen in five sides), the IPS adopted a plexiform architecture, and multiple connections between the IPS and the IJV existed around the jugular foramen. In type E (seen on three sides), the IPS drained directly into the VVP without communicating with the IJV. The IPS was absent in type F (seen in 14 sides). Types D and E correspond, respectively, to types III and IV as mentioned by Shiu et al.[20] (Fig. 11.6).

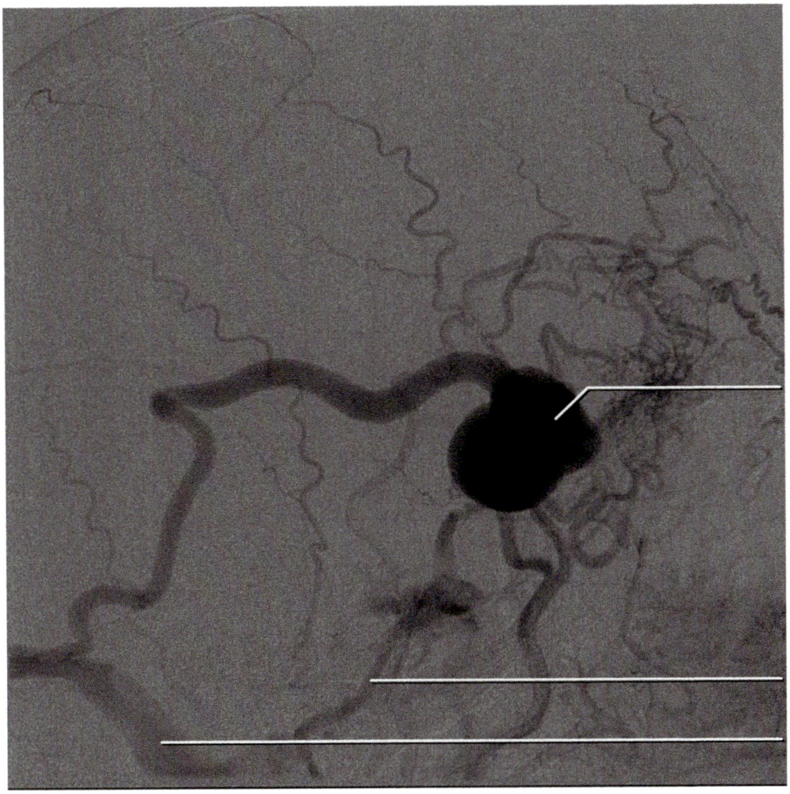

FIG. 11.6 Angiogram of a patient with an arteriovenous fistula (AV fistula) in which the inferior petrosal sinus is well seen.

If one were to also consider the patterns of anastomosis between the IPS and the sigmoid sinus, ACV, LCV, and the VVP, then several further subdivisions of the six categories named by Mitsuhashi et al. can be obtained.[8] Type A can be divided into A1, where the IPS drains directly into the jugular bulb, and type A2 where the IPS connects with the sigmoid sinus and the jugular bulb via two branches. Type B was subdivided into two categories: B1 where the IPS drained into the IJV at the hypoglossal canal, and B2 where it also had a communication with the sigmoid sinus. To type C, the subtype C3 was added in which one branch of the IPS drained into IJV at a lower extracranial level either alone or with a higher branch draining into the IJV or jugular bulb. Also present in C3 was a communicating branch with the sigmoid sinus. Type D was divided into two subtypes: D1 in which the plexiform IPS drained into the IJV near the jugular foramen, and D2 that was plexiform and possessed a communicating branch with the sigmoid sinus.

Variation in Inferior Petrosal Sinus-Internal Jugular Vein Communication

In 1968, Shiu et al. wrote on their experience with cavernous angiography. From the venography of 53 patients, they commented on the variations of the IPS. They found four distinct patterns (Fig. 11.6) of drainage into the IJV as follows:

1. Type I (45% of patients): It is the *textbook* version where the IPS drains directly in to the IJV.
2. Type II (24% of patients): In these cases, the IPS drained into a communicating vein that united the internal jugular bulb with the deep cervical plexus.
3. Type III (24% of patients): In type III variants, the IPS exists essentially as a plexus of veins. The cavernous sinus drains into various locations via this plexus.
4. Type IV (7% of patients): The IPS, in these cases, is well formed. However, instead of draining into the superior jugular bulb, it drains into the deep cervical plexus of veins.

The results obtained by Miller et al.[14] had slightly different results. Type II, as defined above, was the most common type. The prevalence of type IV in their study was only 1 in 133 subjects in their series.

Miller et al.[14] mentioned an observed architecture described as a variant of type II and type III and termed as an incomplete type IV. The anatomy of this type is characterized by a normal-sized IPS, as it leaves the cavernous sinus. The channel, however, is very small from the IJV to the point where the IPS anastomoses with the VVP. The IPS may otherwise exhibit type II or type III anatomy. This incomplete type IV was found in 2.6% of the 268 evaluated IPSs.

With regard to the clinical significance of these variants, type I and type II permit sufficient filling of the cavernous sinus and orbital veins during venography. In type III, although a venous plexus now replaces the IPS, when the contrast is injected at the IPS, the cavernous sinus is usually outlined. In type IV, investigation of the cavernous sinus via the IPS is not possible.

VARIATIONS IN THE INFERIOR PETROSAL SINUS COURSE

The course of the IPS at the entrance to the jugular foramen relative to the location of the glossopharyngeal nerve may be variable. Rubinstein et al.[17] investigated these variations using 25 specimens, in which in 22, the IPS passed as inferior to the horizontal portion of the glossopharyngeal nerve at its entrance into the jugular foramen. In the remaining three specimens, the IPS passed anterior and medial or medial to the descending portion of the glossopharyngeal nerve.

Variations of the course within the jugular foramen was also examined in 20 specimens by Rubinstein et al.,[17] where they noted that the IPS took a route between glossopharyngeal and vagus/accessory nerves in 16 cases. In four of the cases, IPS passed medial to all three cranial nerves.

Imaging

The cerebral venous system can be imaged in numerous ways, traditionally via digital subtraction angiography (DSA).[21] DSA has remained the most definitive diagnostic tool, or reference standard, in the investigation of intracranial venous disease.[22]

MAGNETIC RESONANCE IMAGING

Magnetic resonance imaging (MRI) is a constantly developing imaging modality that offers a variety of solutions for imaging of the intracranial venous system.[21] It can be used to study the IPS by demonstrating its morphology and route of the intracranial IPS.[8] With the recent advances in MR angiography, it is possible to visualize the dural venous sinuses without the use of invasive techniques or ionizing radiation.[22] MR angiography that uses either time-of-flight or motion-induced phase shifts has been reported to be comparable with high-resolution CT in the diagnosing of dural sinus thrombosis.[22]

In venous sinus thrombosis using MR venography, the images show a lack of flow and enhancement[23] of the petrosal sinus. The intensity of venous thrombosis varies with time and the state of the thrombosis within the sinuses on planar imaging.[23] In T1- and T2-weighted images, the signal intensity of the blood products can make it difficult to appreciate the thrombus on conventional planar imaging.[23] As the thrombus ages and there is recanalization of the sinus, MR venography will demonstrate a filling defect[23] within the petrosal sinus. This filling defect may be evident for many years.[23]

MULTIPLANAR RECONSTRUCTION AND CURVE MULTIPLANAR RECONSTRUCTION

These modalities can accurately image the parallel relationship between the IPS and the IJV, along with its confluence and 3D structural features, making it possible to measure the diameter of the IPS in different segments.[24] Although the MRI can be used to image the dural venous system, its parameters and low space resolution can result in an unclear image of a normal IPS.[24]

Zhang et al. (2009)[25] using volume-enhanced scanning with a slice thickness of 0.0625 mm demonstrated the IPS in transverse planes and clearly showed the beginning, vertical segment, horizontal segment, going-out segment, and extracranial segment of the IPS, especially its anastomosis with the ACV, LCV, and VVP and its confluence with the IJV (Zhang, 2009).

COMPUTER TOMOGRAPHIC CEREBRAL VENOGRAPHY

High-resolution computer tomographic cerebral venography (CTV) is comparable with magnetic resonance angiographic techniques in diagnosing dural sinus thrombosis.[23] The advantages of using this imaging modality include its widespread availability and its more rapid image acquisition that reduces the negative effects of patient motion-related artifacts.[23] It also avoids the contraindications that may prevent or limit MR imaging in patients.[23] However, CTV requires the use of iodinated contrast material and exposure to ionizing radiation.[23]

Surgery

Clinically, the IPS is an important route for the embolizing treatment of cavernous sinus dural arteriovenous fistula (Fig. 11.6), along with the embolization of the IPS, the ACV, LCV, and other anastomoses before resection of tumors in the area of the jugular foramen.[24]

The benefits of using this surgical approach are numerous from significantly reducing bleeding and postoperative complications to diagnosing and the differential diagnoses of pituitary microadenoma, as well as for the localization of tumors for resection via sphenoidal sinus with its therapeutic efficacy of about 90%.[24]

Interventional Radiology

The role of the IPS in the diagnosis of Cushing's syndrome is well established. Cushing's syndrome involves excess cortisol production frequently secondary to an altered hypothalamic-pituitary-adrenal axis. Diagnostic tests and procedures that aid in establishing the presence of hypercortisolemia include urinary-free cortisol, late-night salivary cortisol, and the low dexamethasone suppression test. After confirmation of high cortisol, the exact cause should then be sought. Tests important in this stage of the workup include ACTH measurement, a high-dose dexamethasone suppression test, and corticotropin-releasing hormone stimulation test. Pituitary MRI, IPS sampling, and identification of ectopic ACTH-producing tumors are also critical steps in definitively identifying the cause of Cushing's syndrome.[26]

Arnaldi et al.[26] recommend bilateral inferior petrosal sinus sampling (BIPSS) in patients with ACTH-dependent Cushing's syndrome whose workup has been nonconfirmatory after clinical, biochemical, or radiologic studies. BIPSS is considered highly accurate. Its specificity and sensitivity were found to be 96% and 100%, respectively, according to a metaanalysis review of 21 studies.[27]

After the patient is positioned, cleaned, and draped, both femoral veins are used as access points. Catheters are advanced into the bilateral IJVs with the aid of a wire. Microcatheters are then introduced over the wire and directed medially toward the orifice of the IPS. Hand injection of the contrast is then used to highlight the anatomy of the venous structures. Samples are taken before and after corticotropin-releasing hormone administration. One must also note that variations of the IPS-IJV junction may affect the ability to obtain accurate results, or any results whatsoever, from this approach.[28]

In fact, Doppman et al.[29] reported 4 of their 501 cases (0.8%) had false-negative BIPSS in patients with surgically confirmed Cushing's disease. The presence of hypoplastic or plexiform IPS variants was stated as the cause of these results.

Deep vein thrombosis, pulmonary emboli, and brain stem vascular damage are a few of the serious, but rare, complications associated with BIPSS.[26,30] To minimize the risk of thrombosis of the IPS, heparin is usually administered via the catheter.[28]

REFERENCES

1. Mortazavi M, Denning M, Yalcin B, Shoja M, Loukas M, Tubbs RS. The intracranial bridging veins: a comprehensive review of their history, anatomy, histology, pathology, and neurosurgical implications. *Childs Nerv Syst.* 2013;29:1073–1078.
2. Mortazavi MM, Griessenauer CJ, Krishnamurthy S, Verma K, Loukas M, Tubbs RS. The inferior petrosal sinus: a comprehensive review with emphasis on clinical implications. *Childs Nerv Syst*. 2014;30:831–834.
3. Streeter. *Development of the Cerebral Dural Sinuses and Their Tributaries*; 1915.
4. Dolenc VV, Rogers L. *Cavernous Sinus: Developments and Future Perspectives*. Springer Science& Business Media; 2009:37–41.
5. Kilic T, Akakin A. Anatomy of cerebral veins and sinuses. In: Caso V, Agnelli G, Paciaroni M, eds. *Handbook on Cerebral Venous Thrombosis. Front Neurosci*. Vol. 23. Basel: Karger; 2008:4–15.
6. Lang J. *Clinical Anatomy of the Head: Neurocranium, Orbit, Craniocervical Regions*. Springer Science & Business Media; 2012:331–334.
7. Swedenborg E. *The Pituitary Gland, the Cerebellum and the Medulla Oblongata. The Brain Considered Anatomically, Physiologically and Philosophically*. Vol 2. 1887:143–147. James Speirs.
8. Zhang W, Ye Y, Chen J, et al. Study on inferior petrosal sinus and its confluence pattern with relevant veins by MSCT. *Surg Radiol Anat*. 2010a;32:563–572.
9. Stoltz E. Cerebral veins and sinuses. In: Baumgartner RW, ed. *Handbook on Neurovascular Ultrasound. Front Neurosci*. Vol. 21. Basel: Karger; 2006:182–193.
10. Dolenc VV, ed. *The Cavernous Sinus: A Multidisciplinary Approach to Vascular and Tumorous Lesions*. Springer Science Business Media; 2012:113–115.
11. Petruzzeli GJ. *Practical Head and Neck Oncology*. Plural Publishing; 2008:209–210.
12. Osborn AG, Jacobs JM. *Diagnostic Cerebral Angiography*. 2nd ed. Lippincott Williams &Wilkins; 1999:201–207.
13. Miller DL, Doppman JL. Petrosal sinus sampling: technique and rationale. *Radiology*. 1991;178:37–47.
14. Miller DL, Doppman JL, Chang R. Anatomy of the junction of the inferior petrosal sinus and the internal jugular vein. *Am J Neuroradiol*. 1993;14(5):1075–1083.

15. Gailloud P, Fasel JH, Muster M, Desarzens F, Ruefenacht DA. Termination of the inferior petrosal sinus: an anatomical variant. *Clin Anat*. 1997;10:92–96.
16. Benndorf G, Campi A. Aberrant inferior petrosal sinus: unusual transvenous approach to the cavernous sinus. *Neuroradiology*. 2002;44(2):158–163.
17. Rubinstein D, Burton B, Walker A. The anatomy of the inferior petrosal sinus, glossopharyngeal nerve, vagus nerve, and accessory nerve in the jugular foramen. *Am J Neuroradiol*. 1995;16:185–194.
18. Knott JF. On the cerebral sinuses and their variations. *J Anat Physiol*. 1881;16:27–42.
19. Mitsuhashi Y, Nishio A, Kawahara S, et al. Morphologic evaluation of the caudal end of the inferior petrosal sinus using 3D rotational venography. *Am J Neuroradiol*. 2007;28:1179–1184.
20. Shiu PC, Hanaffee WN, Wilson GH, Rand RW. Cavernous sinus venography. *Am J Roentgenol*. 1968;104(1):57–62.
21. Patel N. Venous Anatomy and imaging of the first centimeter. *Semin Ultrasound CT*. 2009;30:513–524.
22. Scott JN, Farb RI. Imaging and anatomy of the intracranial venous systems. *Neuroimag Clin N Am*. 2003;13:1–12.
23. Agid R, Shelef I, Scott JN, Farb RI. Imaging of the intracranial venous system. *Neurol*. 2008;14:12–22.
24. Zhang WG, Ye YY, Chen JH, Chen R, Kuang LQ, Li X. Imaging study of the long extracranial extension of the inferior petrosal sinus with MSCT. *Clin Anat*. 2010b;23:160–167.
25. Lv X, Jiang C, Zhang J, Li Y, Wu Z. Complications related to percutaneous transarterial embolization of intracranial dural arteriovenous fistulas in 40 patients. *AJNR Am J Neuroradiol*. 2009;30(3):462–468.
26. Arnaldi G, Angeli A, Atkinson AB, et al. Diagnosis and complications of Cushing's syndrome: a consensus statement. *J Clin Endocrinol Metab*. 2003;88(12):5593–5602.
27. Newell-Price J, Trainer P, Besser M, Grossman A. The diagnosis and differential diagnosis of Cushing's syndrome and pseudo-Cushing's states. *Endocr Rev*. 1998;19(5):647–672.
28. Deipolyi A, Karaosmanoğlu A, Habito C, et al. *The Role of Bilateral Inferior Petrosal Sinus Sampling in the Diagnostic Evaluation of Cushing Disease*; 2011.
29. Doppman JL, Chang R, Oldfield EH, Chrousos G, Stratakis CA, Nieman LK. The hypoplastic inferior petrosal sinus: a potential source of false-negative results in petrosal sampling for Cushing's disease. *J Clin Endocrinol Metab*. 1999;84(2):533–540.
30. Gandhi CD, Meyer SA, Patel AB, Johnson DM, Post KD. Neurologic complications of inferior petrosal sinus sampling. *Am J Neuroradiol*. 2008;29(4):760–765.

FURTHER READING

1. Booth GL, Redelmeier DA, Grosman H, Kovacs K, Smyth HS, Ezzat S. Improved diagnostic accuracy of inferior petrosal sinus sampling over imaging for localizing pituitary pathology in patients with Cushing's disease. *US Natl Libr Med*. 1998;83(7):2291–2295.
2. Browder J, Kaplan HA. *Cerebral Dural Sinus and Their Tributaries*. pp. 1–12.
3. Browder J, Browder A, Kaplan HA. The venous sinuses of the cerebral dura mater. Anatomical structures within the superior sagittal sinus. *Arch Neurol*. 1972;26:175–180.
4. Browder J, Browder A, Kaplan HA. Anatomical relationships of the cerebral and dural venous systems in the parasagittal area. *Anat Rec*. 1973;176:329–332.
5. Butler H. *The Development of Certain Human Dural Venous Sinuses*; 1957.
6. Gaillard F. *Inferior Petrosal Sinus Sampling*; 2015. http://radiopaedia.org/articles/inferior-petrosal-sinus-sampling.
7. Guari M. *Petrosal Sinus Sampling*; 2013. http://emedicine.medscape.com/article/2114270-overview.
8. Jinkins JR. *Atlas of Neuroradiologic Embryology, Anatomy, and Variants*. Lippincott Williams & Wilkins; 2000:374–381.
9. Koo JW, Hong SK, Kim DK, Kim JS. Superior semicircular canal dehiscence syndrome by the superior petrosal sinus. *J Neurosurg Psychiatr*. 2010;81(4):465–467.
10. Matsushima K, Carvalhal Ribas ES, Kiyosue H, Komune N, Miki K, Rhoton AL. Absence of the superior petrosal veins and sinus: surgical considerations. *Surg Neurol Int*. 2015;6:34.
11. Mitsos AP. *Endovascular Neurosurgery through Clinical Cases*. Springer; 2014:8–10.
12. Padget DH. The cranial venous system in man in reference to development, adult configuration and relation to the arteries. *Am J Anat*. 1956;98:307–355.
13. Roche PH, Fournier HD, Sameshima T, Fukushima T. The combined petrosal approach. Anatomical principles, surgical technique and indications. *US Natl Libr Med*. 2008;54(1):1–10.
14. Salamon G, Huang YP. *Radiologic Anatomy of the Brain*. Springer Science & Business Media; 2012:331–335.
15. Shibao S, Borghei-Razavi H, Orii M, Yoshida K. Anterior transpetrosal approach combined with partial posterior petrosectomy for petroclival meningiomas with posterior extension. *World Neurosurg*. 2015;84(2):574–579.
16. Simonds GR, Truwit CL. Anatomy of the cerebral vasculature. *Neuroimag Clin N Am*. 1994;4:691–706.
17. Tubbs RS, Mortazavi MM, Krishnamurthy S, Verma K, Griessenauer CJ, Cohen-Gadol AA. The relationship between the superior petrosal sinus and the porus trigeminus: an anatomical study. *J Neurosurg*. 2013;119(5):1221–1225.
18. Watanabe T, Igarashi T, Fukushima T, Yoshino A, Katayama Y. Anatomical variation of the superior petrosal vein and its management during surgery for cerebellopontine angle meningiomas. *Acta Neurochir*. 2013;155:1871–1878.
19. Yuranga W, Gaillard F. *Inferior Petrosal Sinus*; 2015. http://radiopaedia.org/articles/inferior-petrosal-sinus.

CHAPTER 12

The Superior Petrosal Sinus

SELEIPIRI AKOBO • R. SHANE TUBBS

ANATOMY

The dural venous sinuses can be categorized into two groups: (1) the posterosuperior group that includes the sagittal, transverse, sigmoid, and occipital sinus and (2) the anteroinferior group that includes the basilar plexus and cavernous and petrosal sinuses.[20] Swedenborg[30] described the superior petrosal sinus as the longer but smaller and slenderer sinuses of the base or of the sella turcica, the posterior petrous angle, and the interior basilar sinuses. This author also described the connection of this sinus with the cavernous sinus as having a shape of the letter e.

The superior petrosal sinus (Figs. 12.1–12.4) (*sinus tentoria lateralis* or *sinus petrosus basilaris*) emerges from the posterosuperior aspect of the cavernous sinus and runs caudally beneath the oculomotor and trochlear nerves[4] and along the dorsal ridge of the petrous part of the temporal bone, on which it leaves a small depressed groove, where the tentorium cerebelli is attached,[7,10] to the petrous ridge.[21–23] The superior petrosal sinus also traverses the superior aspect of the trigeminal ganglion in the roof of Meckel's cave.[4] It originates from a small cerebral vein derived from the basal surface of the hindbrain and empties into the prootic vein.[28] This long slender passage channel passes over the cochlear part of the otic capsule and empties the cavernous sinuses[12] into the transverse sinus.[28,4] This passage runs in the posterosuperior margin of the pyramid of the sphenoid bone and acts as a connector between the cavernous and sigmoid sinuses,[27] which extend to the transverse venous sinus from the cavernous sinus,[7,10] from where they receive their blood supply as well as from the many veins that enter into them from the inferior and anterior parts of the cerebrum.[30] The anterior end of the superior petrosal sinus connects to the cavernous sinus near the proximal trigeminal nerve at the anterior aspect of the posterior clinoid process.[30] Conversely, Rhoton (2012)[23] stated that the medial end of the superior petrosal sinus is affixed to the posterior end of the cavernous sinus, with its lateral ends blending in with the junction of the transverse and sigmoid sinuses. The venous receptive function of the superior petrosal sinus is vast, consisting of the veins of the pons, upper medulla oblongata, cerebellum, and the inner ear.[7,10] The superior petrosal sinus is responsible for draining the anterior portion of the cerebellum via the superior petrosal vein—one of the largest and most constant veins of the posterior fossa[16] and the vein of the lateral recess or cerebellomedullary fissure.[12] The veins also receive the contents of the circular, cavernous, and anterior occipital sinuses via little trabeculae, which are valvular and emanate from the internal wall of the sinus. They also act in concert with the inferior petrosal sinus to drain the interior of the bones of the skull.[30] In general, the veins that enter the superior petrosal sinus emerge from the cerebellum and brain stem.[23]

This sinus is usually larger posteriorly and becomes smaller near its apex.[33] It receives drainage from the cerebellum, the inferior cerebral veins, and the veins of the tympanic cavity.[33]

The superior petrosal sinus can be divided into three types: (1) medial if it empties into the cavernous sinus, (2) lateral if it empties into the transverse-sigmoid junction, and (3) if it empties into both (Matsushima et al., 2013).[16]

The relationship between the superior petrosal sinus and Meckel's cave also known as the *porus trigeminus* varies. Tubbs et al.[33] reported three types of sinus courses in relation to porus trigeminus, which was found to be inferior to, or around the opening of Meckel's cave, in more than 30% of the specimens and 68% of specimens.[33] The superior petrosal sinus traverses in a somewhat triangular form via the duplication of the dura mater over the base of the cranium. This mater is impressed upon the temporal bones as they open into the cavernous sinuses and terminate in the transverse sinus.[30]

EMBRYOLOGY

The anatomy of the dural venous sinuses has been extensively documented dating back to Streeter's account in 1915 using fetuses ranging from crown rump length of

Anatomy, Imaging and Surgery of the Intracranial Dural Venous Sinuses. https://doi.org/10.1016/B978-0-323-65377-0.00012-X

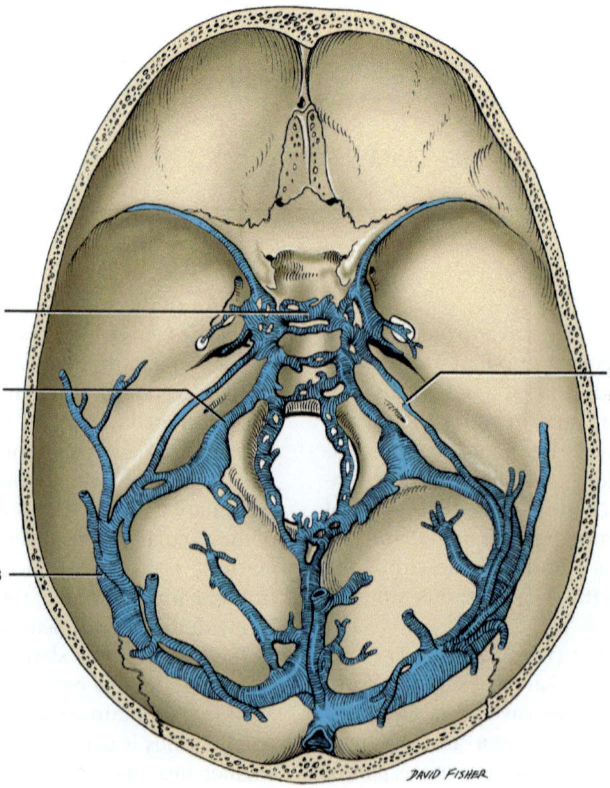

FIG. 12.1 Schematic drawing of the superior petrosal sinus and other sinuses of the skull base.

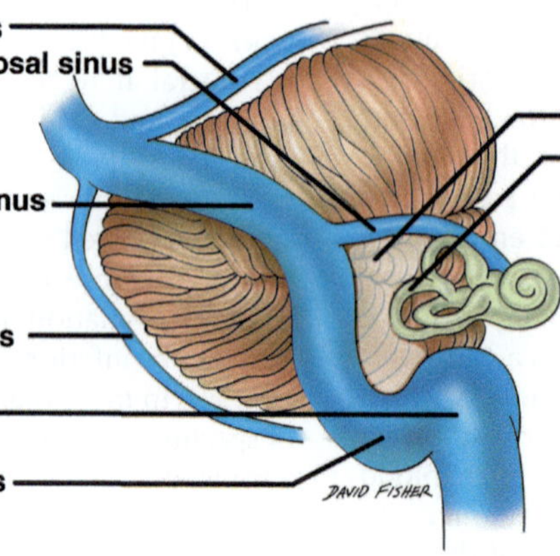

FIG. 12.2 Lateral drawing of the venous sinuses of the skull base noting the right superior petrosal sinus.

4–80 mm, to Salzer in 1985 who described the dural sinus development in rabbits, guinea pigs, pigs, cats, and humans.

The primary venous plexus of the head divides into three strata: outer, middle, and deeper. The outer plexus becomes the basis for the vascular channels of the dura mater. The deeper plexus of the head connects with the superficial plexus via intermediate channels. These intermediate channels are eventually obliterated with the development of the meninges that grow from the base of the skull and gradually extend dorsally around the neural tube to the vertex of the head.[3,4,11,28]

The anterior dural plexus gives off a capillary plexus that forms a cephalic network into the fore and

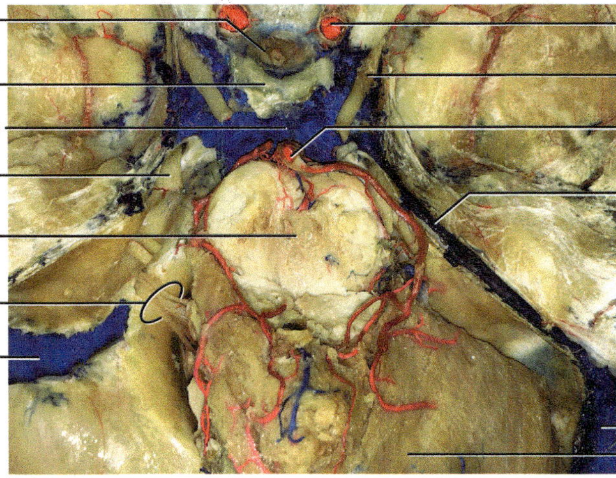

FIG. 12.3 Skull base in a latex injected cadaveric specimen noting the superior petrosal sinus on the right side.

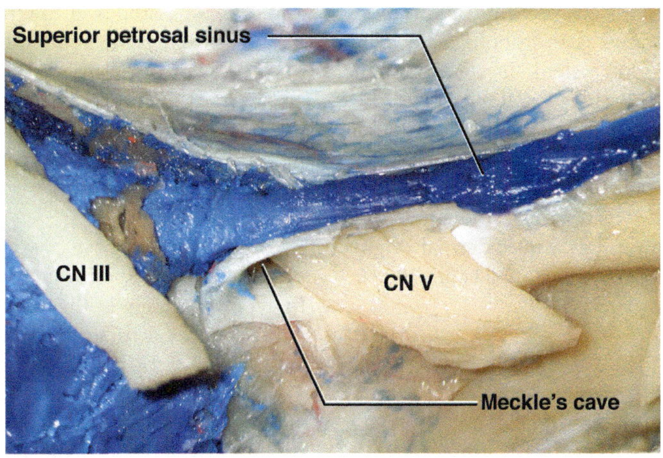

FIG. 12.4 Right skull base in a latex injected cadaveric specimen noting the superior petrosal sinus and its relationship to Meckle's cave and the trigeminal nerve.

midbrain. These networks culminate into the primary head plexus. This mesh of this venous network further divides into three strata: outer, middle, and deeper head plexuses. The outer plexus becomes the basis for the vascular channels of the dura mater. The deeper plexus of the head connects with the superficial plexus via intermediate channels. These intermediate channels are eventually obliterated with the development of the meninges that grow from the base of the skull and gradually extend dorsally around the neural tube to the vertex of the head.[4,11,28]

The development of these dural venous sinuses emanates from an amalgamation of the junction of vena capitis medialis and lateralis to a middle cerebral vein to form the superior petrosal sinus.[4] Thus, the superior petrosal sinus is the last of the major dural venous sinuses to become definitive in human development. Additionally, this sinus is new in phylogenetic development. Changes in the stem of the middle dural plexus and the middle section of the primary head vein result in the superior petrosal sinus, which lies in the cavum epipterícum close to the anterior layer of the tentorium cerebelli. At some point during the embryologic development of the superior petrosal sinus, it runs along the upper margin of the otic capsule above the trigeminal ganglion in the roof of Meckel's cave. It later joins the cavernous sinus and then rests beneath the trigeminal ganglion and between the oculomotor and trochlear nerves.[4]

When first developed, the anterior layer of the tentorial fold is reflected on the inner surface of the orbital cartilage, well anterior to the otic capsule, and the cavum epiptericum is wide in an anteroposterior direction. The third and fourth nerves and the superior petrosal sinus are close to the anterior dural fold and well in front of the otic capsule from which they are separated by the trigeminal ganglion.[4] The posterior tentorial fold runs along the superior border of the otic capsule and then sweeps onto the posterior surface of the otic capsule.

As the temporal lobe of the cerebral hemisphere expands and excavates the middle cranial fossa, it presses the anterior tentorial layer backward, together with the third and fourth nerves, the trigeminal ganglion, and the superior petrosal sinus toward the otic capsule. The cavum epiptericum is thereby reduced in size, and the line of attachment of the anterior tentorial fold is between that of the posterior layer and the superior border of the otic capsule.[5]

The superior petrosal sinus has very little association with the cavernous sinus and is morphologically part of the metencephalic venous system. Its development occurs late in the process of sinus development as the last of the main adult sinuses to form. It appears in 14- to 18-mm embryos[28,6] and rises as a result of the melding of the proximal ventral metencephalic vein into the petrous crest.[24] The petrous apex, which houses the sinus and some of its related structures, has a mesodermal origin and osseous and fatty components (Hanna et al., 2008).

VARIATIONS

The superior petrosal sinus can be completely absent or enlarged, passing into the mastoid foramen to compensate for a small or absent transverse sinus.[13,34,36] A communication between an ophthalmic vein and the superior petrosal sinus has been described.[13] Theile also noted an aberrant termination of the superior petrosal sinus into the foramen spinosum of the middle cranial fossa.[29] On rare occasions, the basal vein of Rosenthal may drain into the superior petrosal sinus.[35] The vein of Labbé may drain into the superior petrosal sinus, which can make surgical approaches at the skull base extremely difficult or impossible.[1] Seven percent of the 14 fixed cadaver heads examined by Avci et al.[1] showed the vein of Labbé draining directly into the superior petrosal vein. The superior petrosal sinus may be absent.[13,9] Matsushima et al.[16] also showed in their study of one venogram and another anatomic specimen a case where the superior petrosal vein and sinus were absent, thus necessitating that the drainage of the posterior cranial fossa be done via the vein of Galen, the lateral mesencephalic vein, and other tentorial groups of veins.

Tubbs et al.[33] observed different arrangements of the superior petrosal sinus from studying the relationship between the superior petrosal sinus and the porous trigeminus. In the 25 (50 sides) cadaver heads, 68% of the superior petrosal sinuses were superior to the opening of Meckel's cave, 18% were inferior, and 16% surrounded the opening of Meckel's cave. It was also observed that the superior petrosal sinuses that coursed inferiorly to the porous trigeminus were generally smaller than those that coursed superiorly or around the opening of Meckel's cave.[33]

Coates[5] examined 31 cadavers (63 sinuses identified) to determine the relationship of the superior petrosal sinus to the trigeminal nerve. In eight specimens, both right and left sinuses passed over the cranial surface of the trigeminal nerve root. Both right and left sinuses passed under the trigeminal nerve root in three cases. The sinus divided on both sides in three cases with some portions passing under the trigeminal root and others passing over the trigeminal nerve root.

Occasionally, the superior petrosal sinus may communicate with the superior ophthalmic veins through an aberrant vein termed the ophthalmopetrosal sinus in up to 9% of the cases, according to Knott.[2] The foramen of the ophthalmopetrosal sinus of Hyrtl is rarely seen in humans and may vary in size and be found on one or both sides.[25]

Tanoue et al. [32] have classified the proximal communication of the superior petrosal sinus into three types. In type A, which is the most common, the superior petrosal sinus runs along the lesser sphenoid wing and connects with the anterior aspect of the cavernous sinus.

In type B sinuses, the superior petrosal sinus runs along the lesser sphenoid wing and connects with the foramen ovale venous plexus or the pterygoid venous plexus, in addition to the anterior aspect of the cavernous sinus.

In type C sinuses, a hypoplastic superior petrosal sinus connects with the anterior aspect of the cavernous sinus.[32] On other occasions, the superior petrosal sinus communicates via an aberrant vein with the superior ophthalmic vein.[2] The superior petrosal sinus can be completely absent.[34]

Streeter[28] stated that the prootic vein of Markowski is one in the same as the superior petrosal sinus, although there are dissenting views.

The sphenopetrosal sinus, an infrequent tributary of the superior petrosal sinus that collects drainage for the sylvian veins, may be a variation of the superior petrosal sinus.

Matsushima et al.[16] in their work on the classification of the superior petrosal sinus and veins noted that the obliteration of the superior petrosal sinus is a variation that may have a congenital or iatrogenic cause. Iatrogenically, this can result after transpetrosal surgery. This result occurs when the superior petrosal group of veins and their tributaries are compromised, which poses an issue as these veins, most notably the veins of the cerebellopontine fissure, serve as a major drainage pathway into and from the superior petrosal sinus. This occurrence is usually seen after surgery for cerebellopontine angle meningiomas such as petroclival, tentorial, anterior petrous, and posterior petrous tumors.[35]

IMAGING

Transcranial ultrasonography: Like the sphenoparietal or cavernous sinuses, the superior sagittal sinus and the transverse sinus, the superior petrosal sinus, which is a major tributary of the cavernous sinus, can be shown by an ultrasound.[27] On transcranial Doppler sonography (TCD), the carotid siphon acts as a landmark to detect the superior petrosal sinus. The transcranial color-coded duplex sonography (TCCS) uses the same landmarks as the TCD but provides a better view of the parenchymal structures as well as the direction of flow of the vessels. The TCCS begins in the mesencephalic plane. Flow in the TCCS is directed away from the probe as opposed toward the flow in TCD.[27] In a cerebral venous thrombosis, superior petrosal sinus should not be measured in proximity to the cavernous sinus to prevent tapering of the vessel diameter because of the increased comparative flow in the cavernous sinus.[27] The flow can be reversed in the superior petrosal sinus with pressure directed at the transverse sinus. Ultrasound lacks the ability to differentiate between thrombotic occlusion or partial thrombosis and aplasia or hypoplasia,[27] and therefore, it is imperative that MRI and angiography be used to increase the sensitivity and specificity of ultrasound imaging in the diagnosis of cerebral venous thrombosis. TCD or TCCS can, however, be used for follow-ups.[27]

*Fluid-attenuated inversion recovery (FLAIR) magnetic resonance imag*ing: This is a type of diffusion-weighted imaging. This imaging modality uses a special inversion recovery sequence with long basic pulse sequences to taper the effects of fluid from images. This technique is utilized when there is a need to detect subtle changes in the brain's parenchyma from edema, infarction, hemorrhage, and other head injuries (Radiopaedia.org). In superior petrosal sinus thrombosis, FLAIR MR shows extensive hyperintensity, albeit less than apparent in acute infarction, a picture seen in vasogenic edema.

Computer tomographic cerebral venography (CTV): This high-resolution CT is comparable with magnetic resonance angiographic techniques in diagnosing dural sinus thrombosis (Agid, 2008).

The advantage of using this imaging modality includes its widespread availability and more rapid image acquisition that reduces the negative effects of patient motion-related artifacts (Agid, 2008). It also avoids the contraindications that may prevent or limit MR imaging in patients such as implants (Agid, 2008). However, CTV requires the use of iodinated contrast material and exposure to ionizing radiation (Agid, 2008), which may limit its use in patients with an allergy to contrast or contraindications from other medications.

PATHOLOGY

Diseases in the superior petrosal sinus and the structures around it vary, and their removal poses a problem as the majority of these structures are fragile and may be precarious when disturbed. Pathology may be primary tumors or lesions of the petrous apex like chondrosarcomas or may be from structures and regions close to the petrous apex such as petroclival meningiomas, trigeminal schwannomas, and chordomas (Hanna et al., 2008).

1. Superior canal dehiscence by the superior petrosal sinus: Patients with this defect are seen to have a dehiscence (separation) of the superior semicircular canal in the middle cranial floor adjacent to the superior petrosal sinus. Patients with this pathology present with hearing loss, ipsilateral tinnitus, autophony, and disequilibrium.[14] They are also found to have conductive hearing loss and decreased vestibular evoked potential on the ipsilateral side of the lesion.
2. Dural arteriovenous fistulae of the superior petrosal sinus.
3. Petrous apex meningioma.
4. Superior petrosal sinus thrombosis: Contrary to the rate at which thrombosis occurs in the transverse, sigmoid, or straight sinuses, the superior petrosal sinus rarely thromboses. This stems from the amount of collateral circulation present in the infratentorial region around the superior petrosal sinus. However, there has been a report of thrombosis of the superior petrosal sinus that presented in a cerebellar fashion, with vertigo, nausea, gait abnormalities. Tumors or arterial occlusions are absent on angiography. MRI images show a hyperintense lesion in the distribution of the SPV/superior petrosal sinus. Variants of this lesion may include a hemorrhagic component and mimic brain tumors. Anticoagulation is usually sufficient in alleviating the symptoms from this lesion, with complete spontaneous resolution within months.[15]

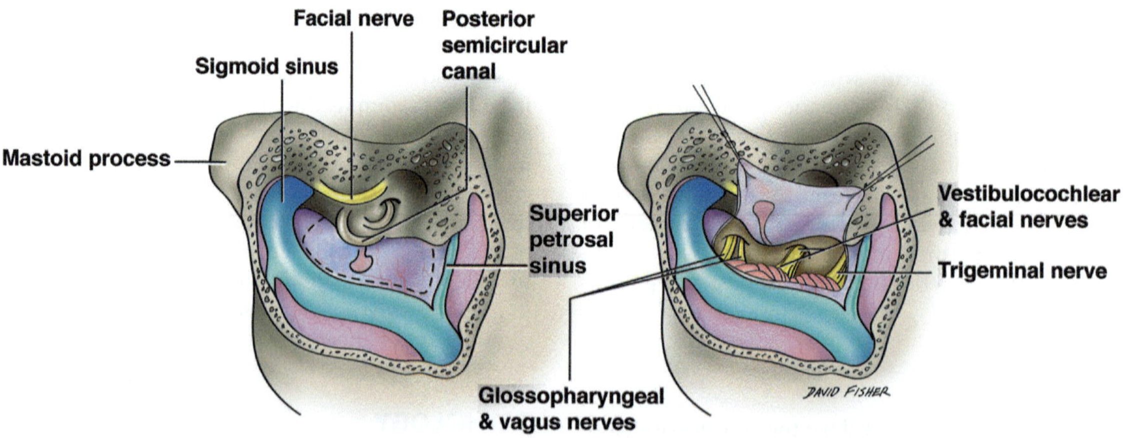

FIG. 12.5 Schematic drawings demonstrating approaches through Trautmann's triangle with the superior petrosal sinus as its superior border.

SURGERY

The superior petrosal sinus is a small, narrow venous channel located at the junction between the middle and posterior cranial fossae. It is adjacent to many important cranial structures, and its vicinity to these structures makes it a very important landmark for surgical approaches to the skull bases.[33] The superior petrosal sinus forms the superior border of Trautmann's triangle (Figs. 12.2 and 12.5) and the medial border of the Kawase's triangle used in anterior prosectomy.[33]

Surgical approaches and access to the superior petrosal sinus can be direct or indirect, depending on the location of the tumor or pathology. Most of the time, this sinus is a conduit to other sinuses that empty into it such as the cavernous and transverse sinuses. The extent to which the sinus or its critical surrounding structures may be entered depends on the kind and location of the tumor. Below are some of the approaches with which the superior petrosal sinus can be accessed.

1. *Anterior transpetrosal approach (ATPA):* This approach can be used for the removal of petroclival meningiomas.[26] The use of this approach has many advantages such as devascularization of feeder arteries from the meningohypophyseal trunk and separation of the dural attachment of the tumor.[26] ATPA allows for direct visualization of the brain stem, making the safe detachment of adhesions possible.[26] It cannot, however, be solely used when a lesion extends beyond the anterior loop of the carotid artery, along the lower clivus, or posterolaterally to the internal acoustic meatus along the petrous edge, its major limitation.[26]
2. *Retrosigmoid suboccipital approach*: This approach of surgical access to the superior petrosal sinus utilizes the third group of superior petrosal veins located superior and medial to the Meckel's cave and empties directly into the sinus. This approach allows for direct access to the superior petrosal sinus.[15,33,35] It allows for access to the cerebellopontine angle from the anterolateral aspect by the ligation and division of the superior petrosal and transverse sinuses. It is commonly used in concert with the supratentorial approach.[8]
3. Transpetrous (petrosal) approach: Involves the use of a combination of approaches to attempt to access both the middle and posterior fossae.[18] It also enables access to the petroclival area of the infratentorial fossa. A combined middle fossa-retrolabyrinthine and a middle fossa-translabyrinthine approach are usually used.[18] The proper use of this technique circumvents the usual problematic factors with safe ligation of the superior petrosal sinus and the sectioning of the tentorium. This involves the use of a combined petrosal approach with the anterior first and then the posterior as well as an extra step to preserve the superior petrosal sinus. This overall approach favors the removal of clival tumors that are laterally extended (Hanna et al., 2008)
4. *Middle fossa approach*: Attempting to plug dehiscence of the superior semicircular canal may relieve signs of dizziness, vertigo, disequilibrium, and autophony.[14] The middle fossa approach is attempted using Kawase's approach in which the temporal lobe is retracted extradurally, and the petrous apex is accessed anterior to the internal acoustic meatus to contact the upper clivus, brain stem, and the posterior cranial fossa. This approach has its downsides such as injury to cranial nerves VII, IX, the internal

carotid artery, etc., and yet has many benefits as well, such as a lower risk of injury to cranial nerves VII and VIII, thus allowing for concurrent access to middle and posterior fossae. It also reduces bleeding during the procedure from early cauterization of vessels so that seeing the entrance location allows early identification of crucial markers such as the glossopharyngeal nerve and the superior petrosal sinus.[19] Lack of precision in drilling the petrous apex can cause injury to the inferior petrosal sinus and abducens nerve. Bony removal of Kawase's triangle can provide adequate space for the suture and ligation of the superior petrosal sinus.[16]

5. Petrosal-tentorial triangular approach: This approach like all the others is used to access tumors and other pathologies of the cerebellopontine angle, as well as the petroclival region. The trigeminal nerve forms an important landmark in this approach. The edge of the tentorium cerebelli near the cerebral peduncle forms a part of the triangle with the petrosal surface of the cerebellum and the superior petrosal sinus/veins to allow for entry and access to remove whatever pathologies may exist in the region.[17,31] Utilizing this approach creates a wide window that allows access to the superior petrosal sinus and the infratentorial areas without increased bleeding that may result from the superior petrosal sinus and the veins around it. This approach also protects the fourth and fifth cranial nerves that may be affected with other approaches.[31]

One of the major risks associated with ligation of the superior petrosal sinus during surgery is the interruption of the flow of the vein of Labbé, which provides drainage to the posterior temporal and inferior parietal lobes. This interruption can be as a result of a propagated blood clot along the superior petrosal sinus or prolonged occlusion. The consequences include infarction of the temporal lobe that can result in brain herniation and eventually death.[18] Injury to the trochlear nerve is also possible with prolonged ligation of the superior petrosal sinus near the free edge of the tentorium cerebelli, resulting in unilateral hearing loss in patients.[18]

REFERENCES

1. Acvi E, Dagtekin A, Akture E, Uluc K, Baskaya MK. Microsurgical anatomy of the vein of Labbe. *Surg Radiol Anat.* 2011;33:569–573.
2. Bergman R, Thompson SA, Afifi AK, Saadeh FA. Cardiovascular system. In: Bergman R, ed. *Compendium of Human Anatomic Variation.* Baltimore-Munich: Urban & Schwarzenberg; 1988:93.
3. Browder J, Kaplan HA. *Cerebral Dural Sinus and Their Tributaries.* 1976:1–12.
4. Butler H. *The Development of Certain Human Dural Venous Sinuses.* 1957:511–523.
5. Coates AE. A note on the superior petrosal sinus and its relation to the sensory root of the trigeminal nerve. *J Anat.* 1934;68:428.
6. Dolenc VV, Rogers L. *Cavernous Sinus: Developments and Future Perspectives.* Springer Science& Business Media; 2009:37–41.
7. Jinkins JR. *Atlas of Neuroradiologic Embryology, Anatomy, and Variants.* Lippincott Williams & Wilkins; 2000:374–381.
8. Hay ID, Wass JAH, eds. *Clinical Endocrine Oncology.* 2nd ed. John Wiley& Sons; 2009:308.
9. Hyrtl J. Der sinus opththalmo-petrosus. *Wien Med Wochenschr.* 1862;12:290–291.
10. Jinkins RJ. *Venous Drainage of the Cranium. Atlas of Neuroradiologic Embryology, Anatomy and Variants.* Philadelphia: Lippincott Williams and Wilkins; 2000b.
11. Kaplan HA, Browder J, Krieger AJ. Venous channels within the intracranial dural partitions. *Radiology.* 1975;115:641–645.
12. Kilic T, Akakin A. Anatomy of cerebral veins and sinuses. In: Caso V, Agnelli G, Paciaroni M, eds. *Handbook on Cerebral Venous Thrombosis.* Front Neurosci; Vol. 23. Basel: Karger; 2008:4–15.
13. Knott JF. On the cerebral sinuses and their variations. *J Anat Physiol.* 1881;16:27–42.
14. Koo JW, Hong SK, Kim DK, Kim JS. Superior semicircular canal dehiscence syndrome by the superior petrosal sinus. *J Neurol Neurosurg Psychiat.* 2010;81(4):465–467.
15. Masuoka J, Wakamiya T, Mineta T, Takase Y, Kawashima M, Matsushima T. Thrombosis of the superior petrosal vein mimicking brain tumor- case report. *Neurol Med -Chir.* 2009;49:359–361.
16. Matsushima K, Ribas ESC, Kiyosue H, Komune N, Miki K, Rhoton AL. Absence of the superior petrosal veins and sinus: surgical considerations. *Surg Neurol Int.* 2015;6:34.
17. Monroy-Sosa A, Mendoza-Falcon G, Macias-Duvignau MA, et al. Neurosurgical importance of the superior petrosal venous complex. *Neurocirugia.* 2013;24(2):70–77.
18. Nadol JB, Mckena MJ. *Transtemporal and Transpetrous Approach to the Cranial Base. Surgery of the Ear and Temporal Bone.* Lippincott Williams & Wilkins; 2005:146–149.
19. Oghalai JS, Driscoll CLW. *Middle Fossa Appraoches. Atlas of the Neurotologic and Lateral Skull Base Surgery.* Springer; 2015:19–23.
20. Patel N. Venous Anatomy and imaging of the first centimeter. *Sem Ultrasound CT.* 2009;30:513–524.
21. Rhoton AL. The cerebral veins [suppl]. *Neurosurgery.* 2002;51:159–205.
22. Rhoton ALJ. The sellar region. *Neurosurgery.* 2002;51:1–374.
23. Rhoton A. Rhoton's cranial anatomy and surgical approaches. In: Rhoton A, ed. *Schaumburg: Congress of Neurological Surgeons.* 2003.
24. Salamon G, Huang YP. *Radiologic Anatomy of the Brain.* Springer Science & Business Media; 2012:331–335.

25. Shapiro R, Robinson F. The foramina of the middle cranial fossa: a phylogenetic, anatomic and pathologic study. *Am J Roentgenol Radium Ther Nucl Med*. 1967;101:779–794.
26. Shibao S, Borghei-Razavi H, Orii M, Yoshida K. Anterior transpetrosal approach combined with partial posterior petrosectomy for petroclival meningiomas with posterior extension. *World Neurosurg*. 2015;84(2):574–579.
27. Stoltz E. Cerebral veins and sinuses. In: Baumgartner RW, ed. *Handbook on Neurovascular Ultrasound*. Front Neurosci; Vol. 21. Basel: Karger; 2006:182–193.
28. Streeter. *Development of the Cerebral Dural Sinuses and Their Tributaries*. 1915.
29. Streit H. Ueber otologisch wichtige anormalien der hirnsinus, uber accessorische sinus und bedeutendere venenverbindungen. *Arch f Ohneuheilk*. 1903;58(85):161.
30. Swedenborg E. The Pituitary gland, the cerebellum and the medulla oblongata. *The Brain Considered Anatomically, Physiologically and Philosophically*. Vol. 2. James Speirs; 1887:490–498.
31. Tandon NT, Ramamurthi R. 3rd ed. *Textbook of Neurosurgery*. Vol. 1. 2012:1996–1998.
32. Tanoue S, Kiyosue H, Okahara M, et al. Para-cavernous sinus venous structures: anatomic variations and pathologic conditions evaluated on fat-suppressed 3D fast gradient-echo MR images. *AJNR Am J Neuroradiol*. 2006;27:1083–1089.
33. Tubbs RS, Mortazavi MM, Krishnamurthy S, Verma K, Griessenauer CJ, Cohen-Gadol AA. The relationship between the superior petrosal sinus and the porus trigeminus: an anatomical study. *J Neurosurg*. 2013;119(5): 1221–1225.
34. Waltner J. Anatomic variations of the lateral and sigmoid sinuses. *Arch Otolaryngol Head Neck Surg*. 1944;39:307–312.
35. Watanabe A, Nagaseki Y, Ohkubo S, et al. Anatomical variations of the ten triangles around the cavernous sinus. *Clin Anat*. 2003;16:9–14.
36. Williams HL. Apparent unilateral absence of sigmoid sinus noted at operation. *Arch Otolaryngol*. 1930;12: 339–341.

FURTHER READING

1. Agid R, Shelef I, Scott JN, Farb RI. Imaging of the intracranial venous system. *Neurol*. 2008;14:12–22.
2. Campero A, Abarca-Olivas J, et al. Presigmoid approach. *3D Neuroanatomy Approaches*. 2013;3(3):1–10.
3. Di Muzio B, Niknejad MT, et al. *Fluid Attenuation Inversion Recovery*. Retrieved from: http://radiopaedia.org/articles/fluid-attenuation-inversion-recovery on 09/23/15.
4. Dolenc VV. *The Cavernous Sinus: A Multidisciplinary Approach to Vascular and Tumorous Lesions*. Springer Science Business Media; 2012:113–115.
5. Gray H. *Anatomy of the Human Body*. Philadelphia: Lea & Febiger, 1918; 2000. Bartleby.com. www.bartleby.com/107/.
6. Hafez A, Nader R, Al-Mefty O. Preservation of the superior petrosal sinus during the petrosal approach- Technical note. *J Neurosurg*. 2011;114:1294–1298.
7. Harris F, Rhoton Jr A. Anatomy of the cavernous: a microsurgical study. *J Neurosurg*. 1976;45:169–180.
8. Hanna EY, Demonte F, eds. *Comprehensive Management of Skull Base Tumors*. CRC Press; 2008:277–279; 371–375.
9. Lookabaugh S, Kelly HR, et al. Radiologic classification of superior canal dehiscence: implications for surgical repair. *Otol Neurotol*. 2015;36(1):118–125.
10. Matsushima T, Suzuki SO, et al. Microsurgical anatomy of the tentorial sinuses. *J Neurosurg*. 1989;71:923–928.
11. Matsushima K, Matsushima T, et al. Classification of the superior petrosal veins and sinus based on drainage pattern. *Neurosurgery*. 2014;10(suppl 2):357–367.
12. Matsushima T. *Microsurgical Anatomy and Surgery of the Posterior Cranial Fossa: Surgical Approaches and Procedures Based on Anatomical Study*. Springer; 2015:269–275.
13. Mitsos AP. *Endovascular Neurosurgery through Clinical Cases*. Springer; 2014:8–10.
14. Ng PP, Halbach VV, Quinn R, Balousek P, et al. Endovascular treatment for dura arteriovenous Fistulae of the superior petrosal sinus. *Neurosurgery*. 2003;53:25–33.
15. Osborn AG, Jacobs JM. *Diagnostic Cerebral Angiography*. 2nd ed. Lippincott Williams &Wilkins; 1999:201–207.
16. Padget DH. The cranial venous system in man in reference to development, adult configuration and relation to the arteries. *Am J Anat*. 1956;98:307–355.
17. Petruzzeli GJ. *Practical Head and Neck Oncology*. Plural Publishing; 2008:209–210.
18. Rubinstein D, Burton B, Walker A. The anatomy of the inferior petrosal sinus, glossopharyngeal nerve, vagus nerve, and accessory nerve in the jugular foramen. *Am J Neuroradiol*. 1995;16:185–194.
19. Scott JN, Farb RI. Imaging and anatomy of the intracranial venous systems. *Neuroimaging Clin*. 2003;13:1–12.
20. Simonds GR, Truwit CL. Anatomy of the cerebral vasculature. *Neuroimag Clin North Am*. 1994;4(4):691–706.
21. Smith AT, Williams XY, Lang C. The superior petrosal sinus. *Clin Anat*. 2015;20:23–34.
22. Tanoue S, Kiyosue H, et al. Venous structures at the craniocervical junction: anatomical variations evaluated by multidetector row CT. *Br J Radiol*. 2010;83:831–840.
23. Theile. Beiträge zur angiologie und osteologie des menschen. Zeitschr f rat Med Neue Folge V und VI.
24. Watanabe T, Igarashi T, Fukushima T, Yoshino A, Katayama Y. Anatomical variation of the superior petrosal vein and its management during surgery for cerebellopontine angle meningiomas. *Acta Neurochir*. 2013;155:1871–1878.

CHAPTER 13

The Basilar Plexus

CHIRAG PATEL • R. SHANE TUBBS

Dural venous sinuses surround the brain while receiving contributions from the brain itself, the meninges, diploë, as well as the veins outside the skull via the emissary channels. The anterior inferior group of sinuses includes the cavernous sinuses, superior petrosal sinus and the basilar plexus. The majority of the blood through these channels flows posteriorly through the sigmoid sinuses into the internal jugular veins or directly into the cavernous sinus, the veins of the orbit and the vertebral venous plexus.[1,2]

ANATOMY

The basilar venous plexus (Figs. 13.1 and 13.2) also known as the posterior clinoid sinus, anterior occipital sinus, plexus basilaris of Virchow, sinus of Littré, *sinus transversus*, and *sinus fossae basilaris*, is scarcely mentioned in the literature; however, when it has appeared, it is associated with several different names: sinus basilaris, sinus fossae basilaris, sinus basilaris anterior, sinus occipitalis anterior, or the sinus occipitalis transversus.[3]Schaeffer[4] considered the basilar plexus as being "serially homologous with the longitudinal vertebral venous sinuses on the posterior surfaces of the bodies of the vertebrae."

Overall, the basilar venous plexus consists of interconnecting channels that join both the inferior petrosal sinuses and the internal vertebral venous plexus.[3,5] The communicating channels lie between the dural sheets above the dorsum sellae of the sphenoid bone and the bony skull base. With the largest and most constant connection being between the cavernous sinus and the pars basilaris of the sphenoid bone. Lower portions of the plexus connect with both the inferior petrosal sinuses and with the anterior internal vertebral venous plexus.[6] Posteriorly, the sinus communicates with the sinus intercavernosus and at times with the superior petrosal and cavernous sinuses anteriorly.[2] In a study by Tubbs et al.,[7] using 20 latex-injected cadavers, they found the plexus in all specimens and that it was always plexiform and very variable in nature. This structure was dorsal to the clivus superiorly and dorsal to the tectorial membrane inferiorly. The diameter of the channels forming the basilar plexus ranged from 0.5 to 1.6 mm (mean 1.1 mm). The basilar venous plexus more or less covered the entire dorsal aspect of the clivus. The thickness of this venous sinus was approximately 1 mm in all specimens. Communication was always found between the basilar plexus and the inferior petrosal sinuses, which were the main outflow of this system of veins. In fact, these two venous structures were more or less contiguous across the midline at multiple levels. In seven specimens (35%), the basilar plexus communicated with veins draining into the hypoglossal canal. The basilar plexus communicated with the marginal sinus in 12 specimens (60%).[7] We found visible connections between the internal vertebral plexus and the basilar plexus in two specimens. No specimen was found to have connections with veins of the anterior brain stem although some historical anatomists have mentioned this. We found that no direct connections between the basilar plexus and occipital sinus were observed. The concentration of venous channels in the basilar plexus decreased, as this structure descended inferior to a plane between the left and right jugular tubercles.

If the marginal sinus is enlarged, it may also communicate anteriorly with the basilar plexus[7] or as San MillánRuíz et al.[8] reported, with the anterior condylar vein (venous plexus of the hypoglossal nerve) in approximately one-fourth of the studied sides. The basilar plexus may also indirectly communicate with the pterygoid plexus and facial veins through the cavernous sinus and superior ophthalmic vein, respectively, or with the suboccipital cavernous sinus.[9] Hollinshead and Rosse[10] and Wackenheim and Braun[11] have written that this venous sinus may also receive small veins from the brain stem or cerebellum. Additionally, Takahashi et al.[12] reported a dural arteriovenous fistula that venography revealed communication between the right transverse pontine vein and the basilar plexus. There may also be transosseous (transclival) connections between the basilar plexus and the inferior side of the clivus via the basilar canal when present.[13] Lang[14] in his textbook

Anatomy, Imaging and Surgery of the Intracranial Dural Venous Sinuses. https://doi.org/10.1016/B978-0-323-65377-0.00013-1

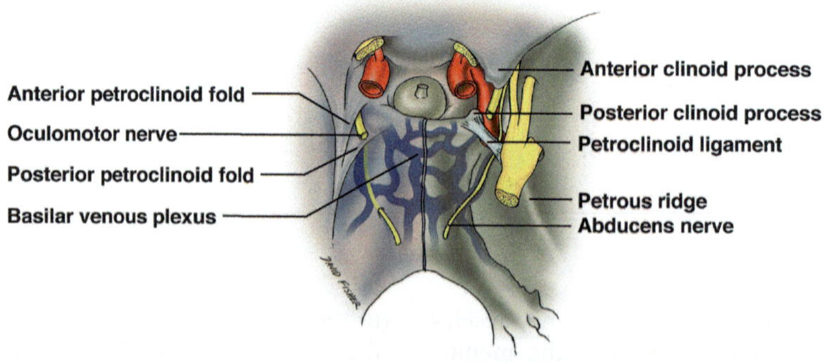

FIG. 13.1 Schematic drawing of the basilar venous plexus and related cranial nerves. Note the proximity of Dorello's canal to this plexus and its communication with the cavernous sinus anteriorly.

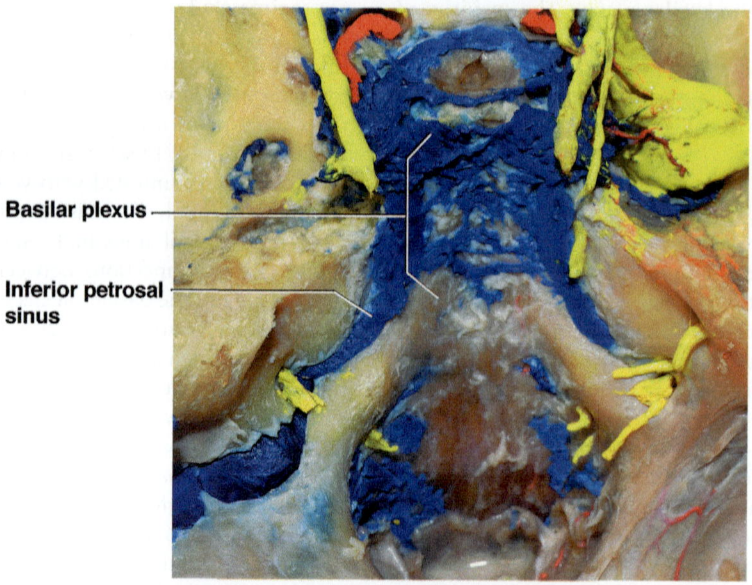

FIG. 13.2 Cadaveric dissection of the basilar plexus after blue latex injection into the left and right internal jugular veins. The regional cranial nerves are colored yellow for clarity.

regarding the anatomy of the posterior cranial fossa, also described communications of the basilar plexus with the venous network of the hypoglossal canal, condylar emissary veins, and rarely (~2%), transclival veins to the inferior aspect of the skull base.

Although uncommonly mentioned in the literature, the basilar plexus has become quite important because of its communication with the vertebral venous plexus of Batson. Venous tributaries from the pons and medulla oblongata drain directly into the basilar plexus. It was found that during expiration more cranial venous blood exits the cranium via the basilar vertebral plexus compared with the internal jugular veins.[3] This becomes even more vital when considering arteriovenous fistulas and secondary increases in venous blood pressure with pooling of blood.[15]

Eckenhoff[16] has pointed out that the basilar plexus is important because of its connection to the internal vertebral venous plexus of Batson, so that during expiration, more cranial venous blood exits the cranium via the basilar/vertebral plexus compared with the internal jugular veins. McDougall et al.[17] and Ernst et al.[18] postulated that the basilar plexus is linked to the occipital sinus via the intervening marginal sinuses encircling the foramen magnum. In an earlier study, we found that the marginal sinus communicated with the basilar venous plexus in 80% of specimens.[7] Rhoton[19] stated that the venous plexus of the hypoglossal canal communicates the basilar venous plexus with the marginal sinus. Liebeskind[20] depicted a basilar plexus that ran in parallel with the inferior petrosal sinus and connected the cavernous sinus and jugular bulb together.

The internal vertebral (rachidian) venous plexus in humans is already well developed at 4 months of gestation.[21] This is the primary channel for cerebral venous drainage in an upright posture[22] and can provide for the entire drainage of venous blood from the cranial cavity.[23] Groen et al.[24] described the basilar venous plexus as a continuation of the cranial part of the anterior internal vertebral venous plexus. However, San MillánRuíz et al.[8] found connections between these two plexuses in only 37.5% of studied sides. We found visible connections between the internal vertebral plexus and the basilar plexus in the minority of our specimens. Padget[25] commented that the basilar plexus is a secondary anastomosis between bilateral embryonic channels near the midline. This plexus is most likely derived from the primary head vein.[26] Okudura et al.[27] postulated that the development of posterior fossa dural sinuses partly occurs in the postnatal period after postural changes.

The basilar plexus is found in other species such as the baboon.[28] In fact, the basilar plexus is more extensive in many primates and coalesces into two paired sphenoidal sinuses that drain caudally into the basisphenoid sinus of these species.[28] Studies involving the inferior petrosal sinuses have depicted these sinuses as not communicating with the basilar plexus. Doppman et al.[29] demonstrated that the basilar plexus receives few branches from the ipsilateral inferior petrosal sinus and connects inferiorly with the anterior spinal epidural plexus. We found that this basilar plexus communicated with the left and right inferior petrosal sinuses freely in all of our specimens and formed the main route for venous egress of the basilar plexus out of the cranium.

The basilar plexus may be visualized with dynamic computerized tomography and is seen best on postcontrast axial and sagittal MRI.[30] The basilar plexus can be sizable. Coskun et al.[31] found ipsilateral basilar plexus enlargement in a patient with carotid-cavernous fistula. The transvenous embolization of a dural arteriovenous fistula at the right jugular bulb has been described as being approached through the basilar plexus via the left inferior petrosal sinus. Halbachet al,[32] in one patient, approached a carotid-cavernous fistula using the basilar plexus. The basilar plexus may occasionally be a source of erroneous blood sampling of ACTH if used instead of the inferior petrosal sinus for lateralization of pituitary microadenomas.[29] We found that the basilar plexus was more or less confluent with the inferior petrosal and cavernous sinuses in all specimens. Interestingly, Pernkopf[33] has depicted and distinguished the more superior basilar "plexus" communicating between the inferior petrosal sinuses from the more inferior basilar "sinus" shown as a single, midline, small, vertical channel extending into the vertebral canal. We did appreciate a depreciating gradient as the basilar plexus descended inferiorly over the clivus but never identified a single inferior channel as shown by Pernkopf.[33]

The role of the basilar plexus in providing venous collateral drainage remains to be fully understood. Anderson[34] found that after injection of contrast, the superior sagittal sinus, confluence of sinuses, and straight and petrosal sinuses are well filled but only a portion of the basilar plexus was outlined. The anastomoses between the intracranial and vertebral venous plexus, the so-called cerebrospinal venous system (CSVS) (Tobinick, 2006)[35] may contribute to pressure homeostasis of the intracranial venous system with changes in posture and intracranial pressure values.[9,35] Classically, postulated that these anastomoses may serve to spread tumors, infection, or emboli from the pelvis or spine to the brain. Enhanced venous outflow via the basilar plexus may also result in the formation of spinal epidural varices in such cases as internal jugular vein thrombosis/stenosis or superior vena cava obstruction. As the basilar plexus is located cephalad to the internal vertebral venous plexus and is connected to the other intracranial venous sinuses, one may hypothesize that it is, developmentally, an intermediate portion of the CSVS. The development of a vascular network is mainly the work of local hemodynamic forces that result in the selection and persistence of a particular group of channels and the formation of complex vascular variations. We found only very small connections between the basilar plexus and internal vertebral plexus. This could be because of the very small diameter of the vessels contributing to this latter venous system.

EMBRYOLOGY

Development of the venous pattern of the skull base is very complex compared with the arterial. Within the literature, it is understood that the inferior petrosal sinuses develop from the ventral myeloencephalic vein and communicates with the cavernous sinus which itself is developed from prooticsinus. The basilar venous plexus, however, is a known continuation of the prevertebral venous plexus.[36] Hashimoto et al.[37] mentioned the presence of the basilar venous plexus at around the 70-mm stage (12weeks of gestation). This is the time when the cavernous sinus finally communicates posteriorly to meet the basilar venous plexus. As seen on venography, the sinus spears as a faint cluster of small vessels connecting with the ophthalmic vein anteriorly, inferior petrosal sinus posteriorly, and pterygoid venous plexus inferiorly. However, the plexus grows abruptly in size after the 225-mm stage.[37] Development of the posterior cranial fossa dural venous sinuses continues into the postnatal period after responses to postural changes. Because it is located cephalad to the internal vertebral venous plexus and is connected to other intracranial venous sinuses, the basilar venous plexus is developmentally considered an intermediate portion of the CSVS. This in turn may contribute to pressure homeostasis of the intracranial venous system in response to changes in posture and intracranial pressures.[3]

The basilar plexus is also said to be derived from the primary head vein and is considered to be a secondary anastomosis. During development, the basilar plexus develops a secondary anastomosis between bilateral embryonic channels near the midline.[3,25] It is structurally similar to the intercavernous sinuses, which is also considered a secondary anastomosis.[25]

According to Swedenborg,[38] the plexus basilaris is perfectly developed in children where it consists of two layers of intertwined vessels; one of which is superficial and composed of more delicate vessels, whereas the deeper layer has much thicker veins. These vessels continue downward near the foramen magnum in an anterior direction and eventually terminating underneath the margin of the sella. In adults, however, this plexus is sunken in and more perforated. Through enlargement and time, the netlike structure became sinuous and gives rise to extensive common lacunae, which is traversed by fibrous trabeculae.[38]

VARIATIONS

Multiple names have been given to the basilar venous plexus throughout the literature: sinus transversus, sinus basilaris, sinus fossa basilaris (Breschet), and plexus basilaris (Virchow). According to Swedenborg,[38] the plexus does not form a separate and distinct canal as it has been described before. Instead, it is a network of anastomosing veins placed between the layers of the dura mater covering the clivus. The involving veins include the inferior petrosal sinuses, the receptaculum, the cavernous sinus, and anterior rachidian veins.[38] Because of the vast number of veins which participate in the plexus, there have been many studies to quantify this. In a study by Ruíz,[39] 37.5% of cases involved a connection with the anterior vertebral venous plexus present at the C1 and C2 vertebral levels. Six cases (25%) were also reported that involved a small plexiform anastomosis with the anterior condylar vein.

Overall, the basilar venous plexus was present in all the cases, which were reviewed in a similar study. The only difference to note was that 24 of the 32 displayed a heterogeneous image without a defined vascular pattern, whereas the other 8 were a summation of the transversal, irregular vascular channels at the level of the dorsum sellae. There has also been another venous structure described, which was independent from the basilar plexus and posterior intercavernous sinus known as the dorsum sellaesinus.[40] The basilar venous plexus, inferior petrosal sinuses, and the anterior condylar veins come together in the craniocervical region as the extradural neural axis compartment. This venous confluence has a clinically significant role in dural arteriovenous fistulas of the anterior condylar vein.[39]

Imaging

Visualization of the basilar venous plexus can be performed through a wide array of techniques. However, the best method is on postcontrast axial and sagittal MRI. Within the literature, dynamic CT has also been a method of choice for proper visualization of the basilar venous plexus.[3]

Pathology

Within the literature, there are very few pathologies described that involve the basilar venous plexus. The pathologies that are discussed involve formation of arteriovenous fistulas with secondary connections to the plexus. In a case report by Horiuchi et al.,[15] a 27-year-old was found to have a congenital external carotid jugular arteriovenous fistula. From the MRI, severe venous congestion was noted in the inferior petrosal sinus as well as the basilar plexus, which was a result of the increased jugular venous pressure. This presented in the patient clinically as ataxia before admission in the emergency room.[15] A similar case was also reported by Takahashi et al.,[12] which involved a patient who presented with a dural arteriovenous fistula of the cavernous sinus. Secondary to the fistula, there was substantial venous reflux into the lateral mesencephalic vein as well as the cerebellar hemispheres because of the connection between the basilar plexus and bridging veins. The overall outcome of the patient improved with proper embolization technique.[12]

Finally, there was a very unique case of a 57-year-old man who suffered from sudden onset severe nuchal pain after reporting a postural headache. On CT, a subarachnoid hemorrhage in the basal cistern with findings of bilateral subdural fluid retention was noted. RIcisternogram and CT-myelogram were performed to locate the cause of cerebrospinal fluid leakage, and it was discovered that the region of interest was most likely to be at the retrospinal area of C1–C2. Postoperatively, the site of CSF leakage was sealed with appropriate resolution of the orthostatic headache. The authors later speculated that the cause of the SAH was likely secondary to a rupture of congested basilar plexus or bridging veins caused by a decrease in intracranial CSF pressure.[41]

Surgery

Because the incidence of overall pathology related to the basilar venous plexus is quite low, the amount of research on surgical intervention tends to follow suit. The usage of the basilar venous plexus was mentioned in a study of 13 patients who were undergoing embolization of cavernous dural fistulas. Eight patients had embolization through the inferior petrosal sinus, but because of inadequate access, the other five needed a route through the basilar plexus. Embolization through both routes was successful with significant improvement clinically of all patients except one.[32]

REFERENCES

1. Schmidek H, Auer L, Kapp J. The cerebral venous system. *Neurosurgery*. 1985;17:663–678.
2. Curé J, Tassel P, Smith M. Normal and variant anatomy of the dural venous sinuses. *Semin Ultrasound CT MRI*. 1994;15:499–519.
3. Tubbs RS, Hansasuta A, Loukas M, et al. The basilar venous plexus. *ClinAnat*. 2007;20:755–759.
4. Schaeffer JP. *Morris' Human Anatomy a Complete Systematic Treatise*. New York: The Blakiston Co; 1953.
5. Krayenbühl H, Yasargil M, Huber P. Cerebral angiography. In: *Georg ThiemeVerlag*. Stuttgart: Thieme; 1982:228–229.
6. Benndorf G. Dural cavernous sinus fistulas: diagnosis and endovascular therapy. In: Baert AL, Knauth M, Sartor K, eds. *Medical Radiology - Diagnostic Imaging*. Berlin: Springer-Verlag; 2010:42–43.
7. Tubbs RS, Ammar K, Liechty P, et al. The marginal sinus. *J Neurosurg*. 2006;104:429–431.
8. San MillánRuíz D, Gailloud P, Rüfenacht DA, Delavelle J, Henry F, Fasel JHD. The craniocervical venous system in relation to cerebral venous drainage. *AJNR*. 2002;23:1500–1508.
9. Arnautovic KI, al-Mefty O, Pait TG, Krisht AF, Husain MM. The suboccipital cavernous sinus. *J Neurosurg*. 1997;86:252–262.
10. Hollinshead WH, Rosse C. *Textbook of Anatomy*. Philadelphia: Harper & Row; 1985.
11. Wackenheim A, Braun JP. *The Veins of the Posterior Fossa, Normal and Pathologic Findings*. Berlin Heidelberg New York: Springer-Verlag; 1978.
12. Takahashi S, Kato K, Tomura N, Mizoi K. Dural arteriovenous fistula of the cavernous sinus with cortical venous reflux of the posterior fossa via a bridging vein. *Radiat Med*. 2001;19:219–222.
13. Oehmke HJ. Die bedeutung des canalisbasilaris und seine darstellungimröntgenbild. *GegenbaursMorpholJahrb*. 1963;104:459–475.
14. Lang J. *Floor of the Posterior Cranial Fossa in Clinical Anatomy of the Posterior Cranial Fossa and its Foramina*. New York: Thieme; 1991:2–8.
15. Horiuchi M, Kamo T, Sagihara H, et al. An adult case of congenital external carotid-jugular arteriovenous fistula with reversible circulatory insufficiency in the cerebellum and lower brain stem. *AJNR*. 2001;22:273–276.
16. Eckenhoff JE. The vertebral venous plexus. *Can Anaesth Soc J*. 1971;18:487–495.
17. McDougall CG, Halbach VV, Dowd CF, Higashida RT, Larsen DW, Hieshima GB. Dural arteriovenous fistulas of the marginal sinus. *AJNR Am J Neuroradiol*. 1997;18(8):1565–1572.
18. Ernst R, Bulas R, Tomsick T, van Loveren H, Aziz KA. Three cases of dural arteriovenous fistula of the anterior condylar vein within the hypoglossal canal. *AJNR*. 1999;20:2016–2020.
19. Rhoton AL Jr. The foramen magnum. *Neurosurgery*. 2000;47(suppl 3):S155–S193.
20. Liebeskind DS. Collateral circulation. *Stroke*. 2003; 34(9):2279–2284.
21. Okudera T, Huang YP, Ohta T, et al. Development of posterior fossa dural sinuses, emissary veins, and jugular bulb: morphological and radiologic study. *AJNR Am J Neuroradiol*. 1994;15(10):1871–1883.
22. Falk D, Conroy GC. The cranial venous sinus system in *Australopithecusafarensis*. *Nature*. 1983;306:779–781.
23. GIUS JA, GRIER DH. Venous adaptation following bilateral radical neck dissection with excision of the jugular veins. *Surgery*. 1950;28(2):305–321.
24. Groen RJ, Groenewegen HJ, van Alphen HA, Hoogland PV. Morphology of the human internal vertebral venous plexus: a cadaver study after intravenous Araldite CY 221 injection. *Anat Rec*. 1997;249(2):285–294.
25. Padget D. The cranial venous system in man in reference to development, adult configuration and relation to the arteries. *Am J Anat*. 1956;98:307–355.
26. de Caro R, Parenti A, Capitanio G, Ori C, Bracco F, Ricchieri GL. Basilar arterio-venous pseudoparallelism due to persistence of embryonal venous pattern. *Acta Neurochir (Wien)*. 1990;104(1-2):73–76.

27. Okudera T, Huang YP, Ohta T, et al. Development of posterior fossa dural sinuses, emissary veins, and jugular bulb: morphological and radiologic study. *AJNR Am J Neuroradiol*. 1994;15(10):1871–1883.
28. Lake AR, Van Niekerk IJ, Le Roux CG, Trevor-Jones TR, De Wet PD. Angiology of the brain of the baboon Papio ursinus, the vervet monkey Cercopithecus pygerithrus, and the bushbaby Galago senegalensis. *Am J Anat*. 1990;187(3):277–286.
29. Doppman JL, Krudy AG, Girton ME, Oldfield EH. Basilar venous plexus of the posterior fossa: a potential source of error in petrosal sinus sampling. *Radiology*. 1985;155(2):375–378.
30. Gebarski SS, Gebarski KS. Inferior petrosal sinus: imaging-anatomic correlation. *Radiology*. 1995;194(1):239–247.
31. Coskun O, Hamon M, Catroux G, Gosme L, Courthéoux P, Théron J. Carotid-cavernous fistulas: diagnosis with spiral CT angiography. *AJNR Am J Neuroradiol*. 2000;21(4):712–716.
32. Halbach V, Higashida R, Hieshima G, Hardin CW, Pribram H. Transvenous embolization of dural fistulas involving cavernous sinus. *AJNR*. 1989;10:377–383.
33. Pernkopf E. *Atlas of Topographical and Applied Human Anatomy*. Vol. 1. Philadelphia: W. B. Saunders; 1963:73.
34. Anderson R. Diodrast studies of the vertebral and cranial venous systems to show their probable role in cerebral metastases. *J Neurosurg*. 1951;8(4):411–422.
35. Tobinick E, Vega CP. The cerebrospinal venous system: anatomy, physiology, and clinical implications. *MedGenMed*. 2006;8(1):53.
36. Samii M, Knosp E. *Approaches to the Clivus: Approaches to No Man'sLand*. Berlin: Springer-Verlag; 1992.
37. Hashimoto M, Yokota A, Yamada H, Okudera T. Development of the cavernous sinus in the fetal period: a morphological study. *Neurol Med Chir*. 2000;40:140–150.
38. Swedenborg E. In: Tafel RL, ed. *The Brain Considered Anatomically, Physiologically and Philosophically*. London: James Speirs; 1887.
39. Ruíz D. *Systèmesveineux De La Base Du Crâneet De La Junction Cranio-Cervicale: Anatomiemacroscopique Et Radiologique Et Implications Cliniques*. Thèse de doctorat: Univ. Genève; 2006:59–76.
40. Aquini M, Marrone A, Schneider F. Intercavernous venous communications in the human skull base. *Skull BaseSurg*. 1994;4:145–150.
41. Tomokiyo M, Nishihara K, Nakazawa K. A case of subarachnoid hemorrhage associated with spontaneous intracranial hypotension. *Noshinkeigeka*. 2002;30:847–851.

FURTHER READING

1. Iaconetta G, Fusco M, Samii M. The sphenopetroclival venous gulf: amicroanatomical study. *J Neurosurg*. 2003;99:366–375.

CHAPTER 14

The Marginal Sinus

R. SHANE TUBBS

Most standard texts of anatomy either do not mention the marginal sinus (Figs. 14.1 and 14.2) or merely say that this sinus is found in the vicinity of the foramen magnum. This dural venous sinus also known as the sinus of Kölliker or sinus of Meckel is located between the layers of the dura mater and more or less rims the internal aspect of the foramen magnum.

EMBRYOLOGY

The cephalic venous drainage system in the early human embryo arises from three dural venous plexuses (anterior, middle, and posterior). In the adult, the marginal sinus constitutes an inconstant remnant of the embryonic posterior venous plexus that anastomoses with the distal part of the sigmoid sinus, thus communicating with the internal jugular system.[1] The occipital and marginal sinuses are established as a concomitant of the caudal expansion of the cerebrum over the midbrain and the cerebellum during fetal growth. The marginal sinus is already developed by the sixth fetal month, and before this (during the third and fourth month), it and the occipital sinus are plexiform in nature and extend from the tentorium cerebelli inferiorly toward the foramen magnum.[2] The marginal sinus tends to be enlarged in cases in which the occipital sinuses are large.[3] Some have considered these instances of enlarged marginal/occipital sinuses as persistence of the fetal prototype of posterior venous sinus formation.[3] Interestingly, some have reported that the occipital/marginal sinus system in the human neonate has a capacity equivalent to that of the transverse sinuses.[4]

Using injected fetal brains, Okudera et al.[2] showed that the marked increase in venous flow from the rapidly growing cerebral hemispheres leads to ballooning of the transverse sinuses in the absence of an increase in the inner diameters of the sigmoid and jugular sinuses. This ballooning also results in the formation of the occipital and marginal sinuses.[2]

ANATOMY

The marginal sinus communicates anteriorly with the basilar venous plexus on the superior surface of the inferior clivus and posteriorly with the occipital sinus.[5] The marginal sinuses may also connect the distal portions of the sigmoid sinuses (via small connections that pass across the intracranial surface) and communicate with the veins of the hypoglossal canal (anterior condylar confluence of Trolard or Luschka) via the condylar sinus of Labbé.[5] Distally, the marginal sinus drains freely into the vertebral venous plexus.[1] The occipital sinus begins at the junction of the left and right posterior parts of the marginal sinus.[6] However, the occipital sinus may not connect to the marginal sinus.[7]

In 15 adult cadavers, Tubbs et al.[8] identified the marginal sinus in all specimens. Sinuses were found to lie between the leaves of the dura mater at the superior margin of the foramen magnum in all specimens. The maximal vertical height of the sinuses ranged from 7 to 15 mm (mean 10 mm), and in all specimens, it was located at or near the foramen magnum where the accessory nerve crossed in route to the jugular foramen. In all specimens, the sinus was noted to taper to 3–5 mm as it traveled both anteriorly and posteriorly toward the basion and opisthion. The marginal sinus communicated with the basilar venous plexus in 12 of 15 specimens (80%) and with the occipital sinus in all specimens. Of 15 specimens, 14 (93%) were found to have drainage into the veins of the hypoglossal canal. The hypoglossal nerve rootlets were noted to pierce the sinus and its tributaries in 11 of 15 specimens (73%). Venous communication to the sigmoid sinus was seen in all specimens. The vertebral artery was found to course through the marginal sinus as it pierced the posterior atlantooccipital membrane on all left sides and 13 of 15 (87%) of right sides. Caruso et al.[9] have reported that the marginal sinus had a mean diameter of 2 mm in 14 patients undergoing magnetic resonance imaging.

Anatomy, Imaging and Surgery of the Intracranial Dural Venous Sinuses. https://doi.org/10.1016/B978-0-323-65377-0.00014-3

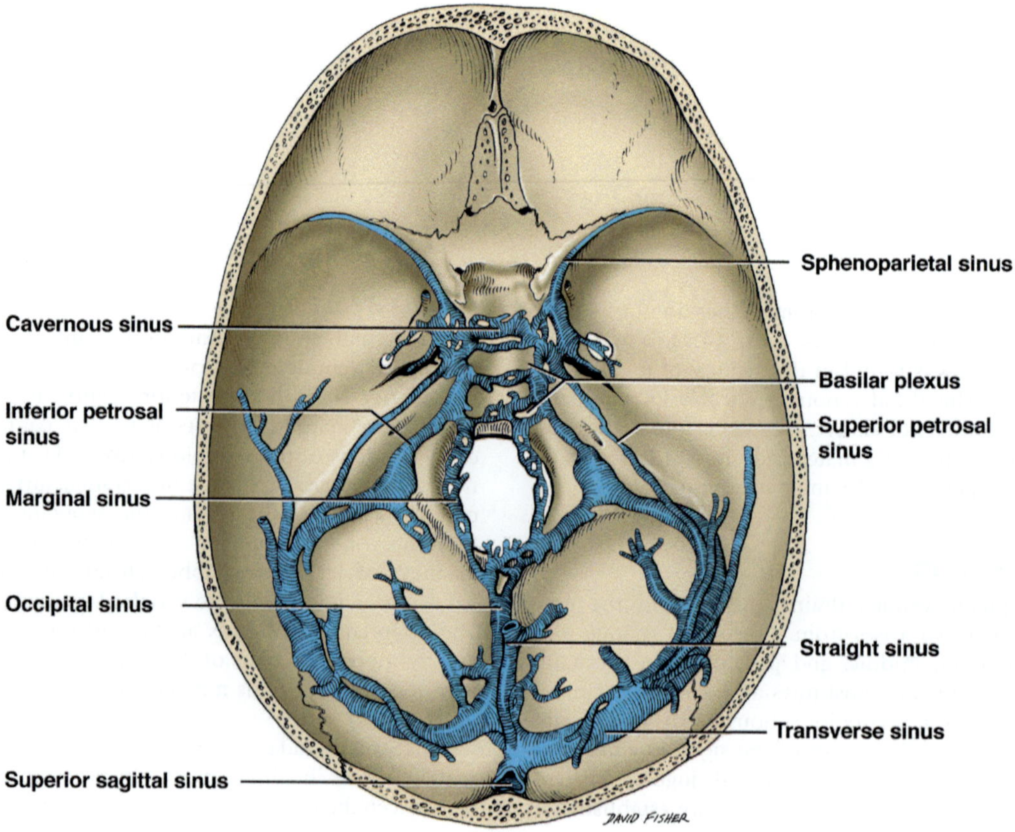

FIG. 14.1 Schematic drawing of the dural venous sinuses of the skull base including the marginal sinus seen here at the level of the foramen magnum.

BLOOD FLOW

Falk[10] has studied ancient hominid skulls and found that the early bipeds (*Australopithecus afarensis*) and the robust australopithecine were characterized by enlarged occipital and marginal sinus systems. This author suggested that selection for bipedalism initially resulted in epigenetic adaptations for routes to deliver blood to the vertebral plexus, including an enlarged marginal sinus, but that the pressures underlying these adaptations relaxed as bipedalism became established. Other routes for delivering blood to the vertebral plexus of veins were either directly or indirectly selected for, perhaps in conjunction with a changing architecture of the skull. The specimens examined by Falk[10] were also found to have marginal sinus/occipital sinus bony grooves that were much larger than the grooves for the transverse/sigmoid sinuses, thus presumably usurping their role as the main venous outflow of the cranium.

In modern adult humans, the marginal sinus does not provide for the main venous outflow of the cranium but rather serves as an alternative route for venous drainage to occur, particularly in cases of internal jugular vein obstruction, whether positional or pathologic.[5,11,12] However, some have stated that this sinus coupled with the vertebral venous plexus provides the majority of cranial venous drainage in the upright position of monkeys and humans.[9]

PATHOLOGY

Clinically, dural arteriovenous fistulas involving the marginal sinus have been reported.[11] These are often found after basilar skull fractures and may involve the occipital, posterior meningeal, or posterior auricular arteries. McDougall et al.[11] found that the ascending pharyngeal artery was most often involved with fistulas involving

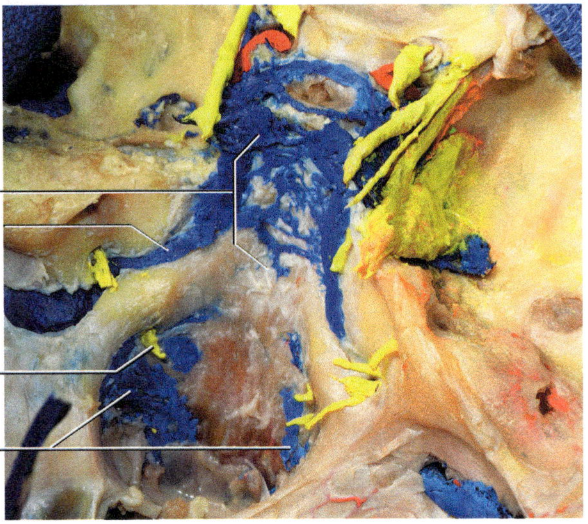

FIG. 14.2 Cadaveric dissection of the skull base venous sinuses. Note the marginal sinus and its relationship to the hypoglossal nerve rootlets.

the marginal sinus. Further, these authors stated that great care must be taken when treating these fistulas so as to not occlude the arterial supply to the lower cranial nerves: one of their patients incurred a transient hypoglossal nerve palsy following an embolization procedure. Surgically, entrance into the subdural space deep to the foramen magnum necessitates traversing the marginal sinus, such as in posterior cranial fossa decompression for Chiari I malformations or for posterior fossa tumors.

REFERENCES

1. Kimbel WH. Variation in the pattern of cranial venous sinuses and hominid phylogeny. *Am J Phys Anthropol.* 1984;63:243–263.
2. Okudera T, Huang YP, Ohta T, et al. Development of posterior fossa dural sinuses, emissary veins, and jugular bulb: morphological and radiologic study. *Am J Neuroradiol.* 1994;15:1871–1883.
3. Browder J, Kaplan HA. *Cerebral Dural Sinuses and Their Tributaries.* Springfield: Ch C Thomas; 1976.
4. Woodhall B. Variations of the cranial venous sinuses in the region of the torcular herophili. *Arch Surg.* 1936;33:297–314.
5. de Oliveira E, Rhoton AL, Peace D. Microsurgical anatomy of the region of the foramen magnum. *Surg Neurol.* 1985;24:293–352.
6. Go RT, Suzuki Y, Schapiro RL, Christie JH. The scintigraphic features of the occipital sinus. *Radiology.* 1974;112:635–638.
7. Dora F, Zileli. Common variations of the lateral and occipital sinuses. *Neuroradiology.* 1980;20:23–27.
8. Tubbs RS, Ammar K, Liechty P, et al. The marginal sinus. *J Neurosurg.* 2006;104:429–431.
9. Caruso RD, Rosenbaum AE, Chang JK, Joy SE. Craniocervical junction venous anatomy on enhanced MR images: the suboccipital cavernous sinus. *Am J Neuroradiol.* 1999;20:1127–1131.
10. Falk D. Evolution of cranial blood drainage in hominids: enlarged occipital/marginal sinuses and emissary foramina. *Am J Phys Anthropol.* 1986;70:311–324.
11. McDougall CG, Halbach VV, Dowd CF, Higashida RT, Larsen DW, Hieshima GB. Dural arteriovenous fistulas of the marginal sinus. *Am J Neuroradiol.* 1997;18:1565–1572.
12. Rhoton AL. *The Foramen Magnum in Rhoton Cranial Anatomy and Surgical Approaches.* Schaumburg: Congress of Neurological Surgeons; 2003:587–625.

CHAPTER 15

The Cavernous Sinus

AMIN DEMERDASH • R. SHANE TUBBS

HISTORY

Jacques Bénigne Winslow (1669–1760) coined the term cavernous sinus (sinus cavernosi, sinus ellipticus, sinus coronaries, clinoid sinus) in the 18th century; however, 250 years later, it is considered a misnomer.[1] Winslow considered that the cavernous sinus was similar to the corpus cavernosa of the penis, as he thought that both were made of a large single trabeculated venous cavern and thus misled many anatomists. Morgagni called this sinus the receptacula of Vieussens and Ortlob, in 1697, termed it the transverse or conciliatory sinus. Bell referred to the cavernous sinus as "a great irregular center of communication with the lesser sinuses in the base of the skull." Some authors have suggested a more precise name, such as "parasellar plexus of veins in the lateral sellar compartment."[2]

ANATOMY

The cavernous sinuses (Figs. 15.1–15.8) are a pair of intradural venous compartments that lay between the periosteal and meningeal layers of the dura.[3] They are located centrally within the skull in the anteromedial portion of the middle cranial fossa and are bordered medially by the pituitary gland and the body of the sphenoid bone. The cavernous sinus is a four-walled structure with a roof, and medial, lateral, and posterior walls in the shape of a "boat" as Rhoton described. The superior wall or the roof of the sinus consists of an anterior portion that is formed by the dural lining of the clinoid process and a posterior portion formed by the "oculomotor triangle," which is a dural patch through which the oculomotor penetrates the sinus. The lateral wall is formed of two dural layers: a thick external layer and an internal, semitransparent layer. It extends from the superior orbital fissure anteriorly to the medial border of Meckel's cave posteriorly and from the lower border of the carotid sulcus inferiorly to the anterior petroclinoid ligament superiorly. The medial wall consists of two parts, sellar and spheroidal, both of which consist of one dural layer. The borders of the medial wall extend from the superior orbital fissure anteriorly to the lateral border of the dorsum sellae posteriorly, and from the lower border of the carotid sulcus inferiorly to the interclinoid ligament superiorly. The posterior wall consists of two dural layers, the periostic and meningeal. The cavernous sinus shares part of its wide posterior wall with the lateral border of the basilar sinus, and the remaining portion of that wall can be divided into upper, lower, medial, and lateral margins. The upper margin lays at the level of the petroclinoid ligament, whereas the lower is located at the upper border of the petroclival fissure above the petrous apex. The medial margin of the posterior wall of the cavernous sinus lays at the lateral aspect of the dorsum sellae, whereas the lateral margin is located medial to the porus of Meckel's cave.[4,5]

The cavernous sinus is more than just a compartment filled with venous blood; in fact, it is a complex neurovascular structure in which fibrous and adipose tissues fill the space. Four cranial nerves are related directly to the cavernous sinus: the oculomotor (CN III), trochlear (CN IV), trigeminal (CN V), and the abducens nerve (CN VI). The lateral wall of the cavernous sinus contains CNs III and IV in its upper part, and both the ophthalmic and maxillary branches of the trigeminal (V_1 and V_2) in the lower part of the wall. The posterior wall is related directly to CN VI, whereas the roof of the cavernous sinus has the trigeminal triangle through which CN III pierces the dura, joins CNs IV, V_1, and VI, and exits the cranium through the superior orbital fissure, which leaves V_2 as the only cranial nerve that exits the skull through the foramen rotundum.[4–6] The internal carotid artery (ICA) is another significant component of the cavernous sinus neurovascular complex. The cavernous ICA is an S-shaped vessel that lies within the dural layers that form the sinus; its short course begins with its ascent toward the posterior clinoid process to form an upward convexity before it perforates the dural layers of the superior wall medial to the anterior clinoid process. In its short journey through the cavernous sinus, the ICA gives rise to three branches: the meningohypophyseal artery that provides branches to regional cranial nerves and walls of

Anatomy, Imaging and Surgery of the Intracranial Dural Venous Sinuses. https://doi.org/10.1016/B978-0-323-65377-0.00015-5

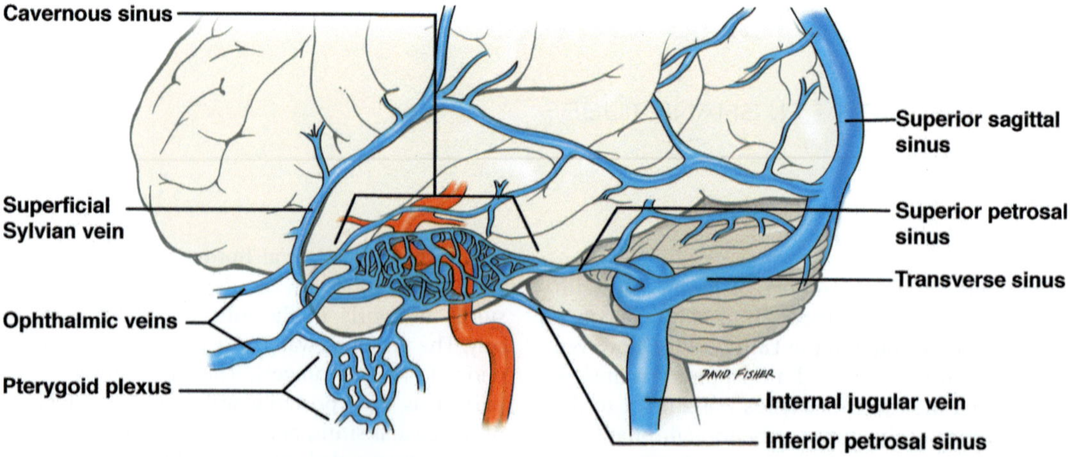

A

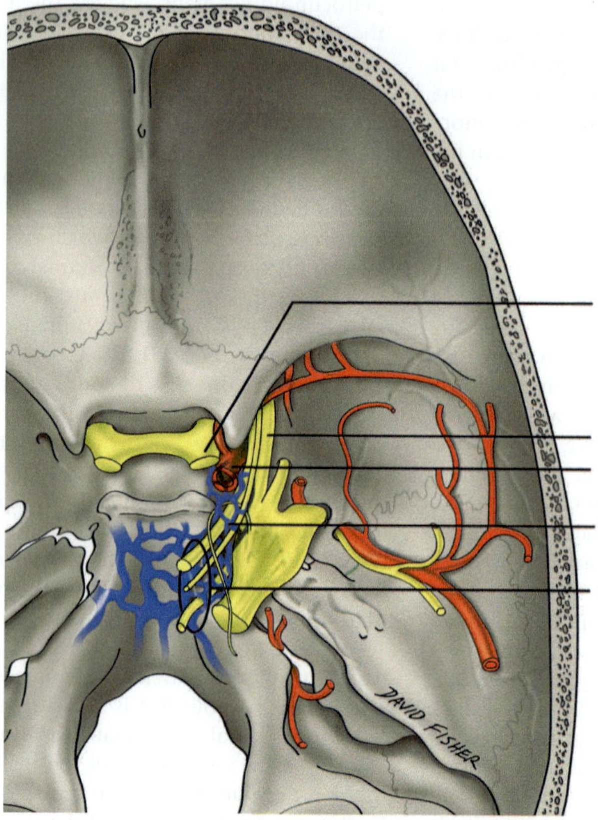

B

FIG. 15.1 **(A)** Schematic drawing of the position and relationships of the cavernous sinus at the skull base, lateral view. **(B)** Schematic drawing of the position and relationships of the cavernous sinus at the skull base, superior view.

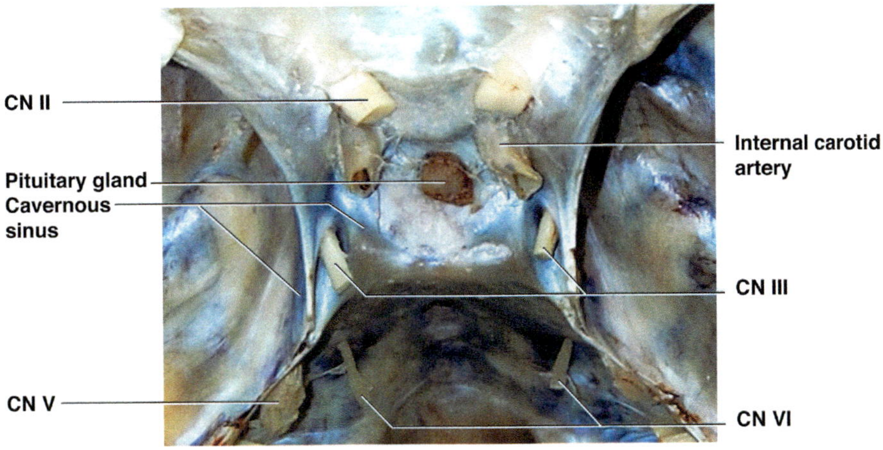

FIG. 15.2 Cadaveric dissection of the cavernous sinus after removal of the brain but before opening of the dura mater.

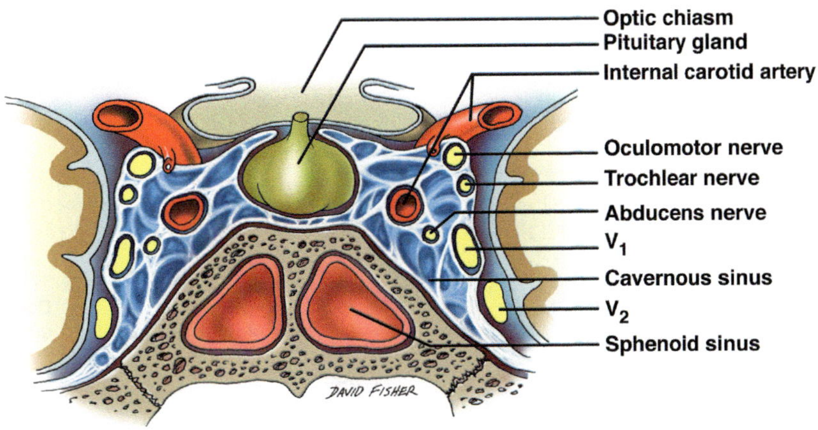

FIG. 15.3 Schematic drawing of the cavernous sinus and its contents in coronal section.

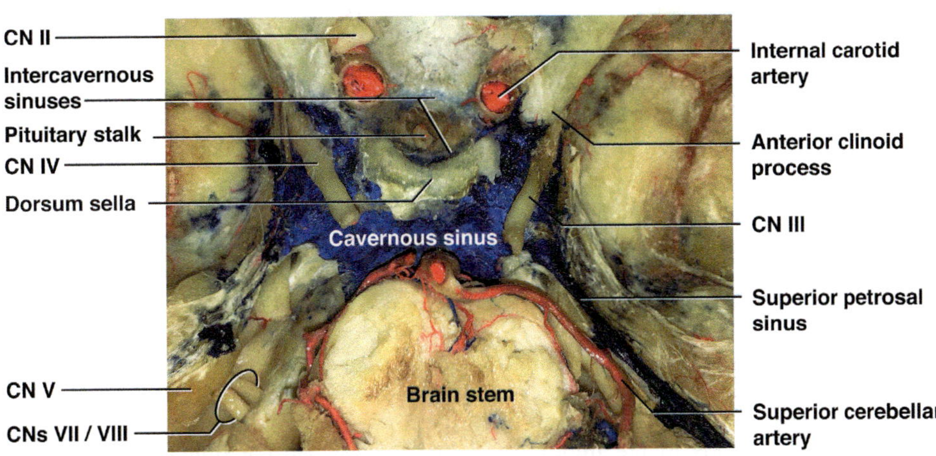

FIG. 15.4 Cadaveric dissection of the cavernous sinus and surrounding brain/cranial nerves after blue latex injection into the internal jugular veins. The brain has been sectioned at the pons.

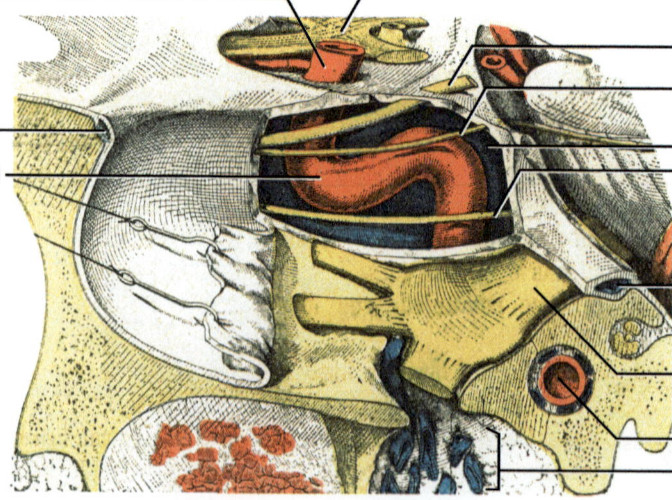

FIG. 15.5 Drawing of a lateral view of the cavernous sinus and its contents after Testut.

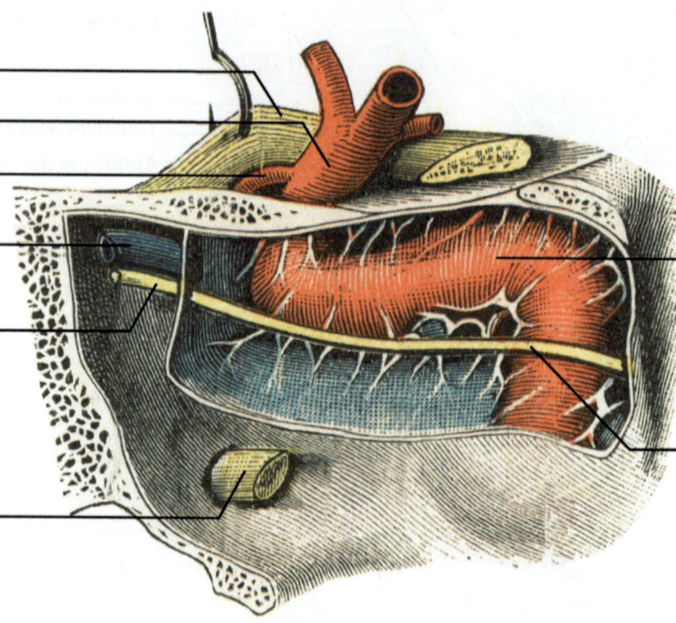

FIG. 15.6 Drawing of a lateral view of the cavernous sinus and its contents after Testut. Note the intracavernous trabeculae and relationship of the abducens nerve to the internal carotid artery.

the sinus, the inferior cavernous sinus artery, and the capsular arteries.[7]

The cavernous sinus has several venous connections that add further clinical significance to the plexus of veins in the lateral sellar compartment and can be considered the venous crossroads in the middle of the skull. The middle meningeal veins connect the cavernous sinus to the dura, whereas the ophthalmic veins connect it to the facial veins. The cavernous sinus is associated directly with other sinuses as well; it communicates with the transverse sinus via the superior petrosal sinus and to the internal jugular vein through the inferior petrosal sinus. The superior and inferior ophthalmic veins connect the cavernous sinus to the

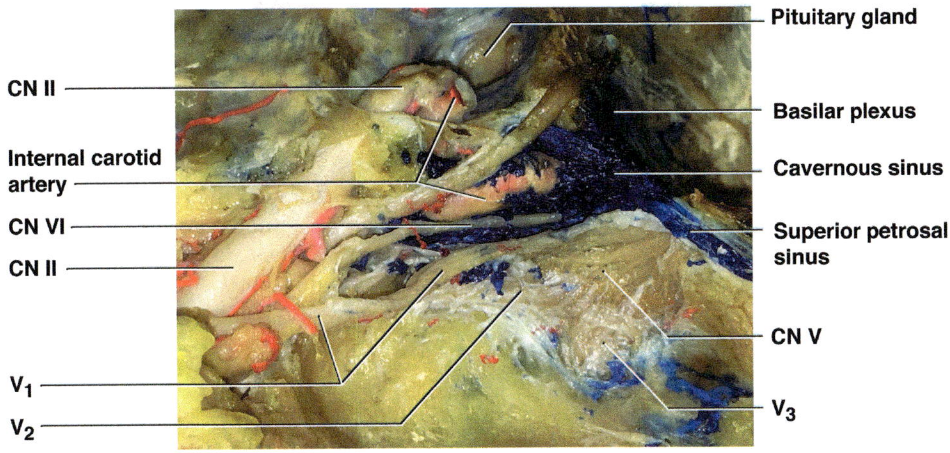

FIG. 15.7 Cadaveric dissection of the lateral view of the left cavernous sinus and its contents.

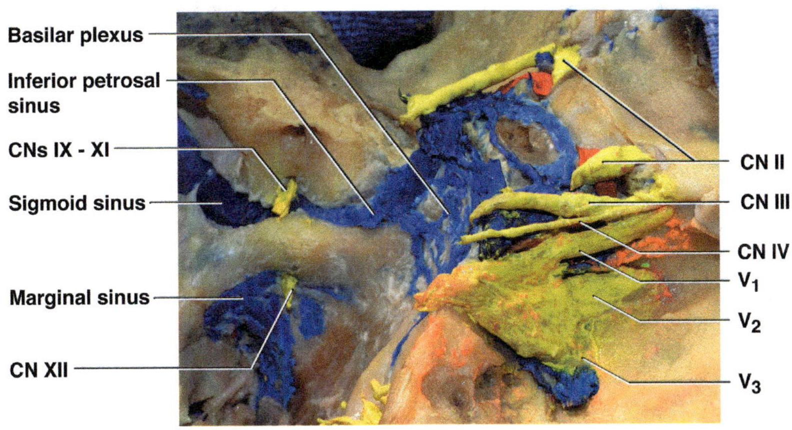

FIG. 15.8 Cadaveric dissection of the superolateral view of the right cavernous sinus and its contents.

orbit, the middle and inferior cerebral veins connect it to the cerebral hemispheres, and the retinal veins link the sinus to the retina. The emissary veins perforate the skull to give the cavernous sinus an opportunity to communicate with the outside world by connecting it to the pterygoid venous plexus, which drains eventually into the facial vein. The small anterior and posterior intercavernous sinuses and the basal plexus veins connect both cavernous sinuses at the midline.[6,8]

Tubbs et al.'s[9] study showed that the maxillary division of the trigeminal (V2) is not part of the cavernous sinus. Their study, which used 10 fresh cadaveric heads, found no evidence that V2 travels within the sinus itself; however, they demonstrated that the emissary veins travelling with V2 could cause that confusion.

Emanuel Swendenborg gave one of the most detailed accounts of the cavernous sinus in the 19th century. Swendenborg referred to the cavernous sinuses as the "receptacles of the sphenoid bone" because they filled the grooves of the sphenoid bone. The clinoid processes—the anterior and the posterior sinuses—block the sinuses on each side. The sinuses resemble the cavernous substance of the spleen and the urethra, which probably led to the name that other authors disputed later. He also mentioned the presence of CNs III, IV, and VI, as well as part of the carotid artery within the cavernous sinus. Swendenborg also outlined the accounts of several "modern" authors. Vieussens made a very important observation of the presence of a connection between the cavernous sinuses on both sides, which he discovered by injecting liquor on one side and then finding it on the other. On the other hand, Ridley did not agree with many of Vieussens' observations and suggested that the circular sinus was responsible for returning the blood to the circulation rather than the veins accompanying the carotid artery. Furthermore, Swendenborg highlighted Winslow's comments that we mentioned earlier, in which he described the cavernous sinus as a spongy substance filled with blood.[10]

EMBRYOLOGY

Anatomic studies using autopsied fetuses have been conducted to investigate the development of the cavernous sinus. Beginning at 6 weeks of gestation, an S-shaped structure referred to as the anterior dural plexus is found to receive tributaries from the pituitary region, the eye, and the trigeminal branches, after which it forms the primary head vein by joining the posterior and medial dural plexuses that are surrounded by primitive mesenchyme. A rapid significant development of the meninges begins at 7–8 weeks of gestation and becomes more prominent and differentiated at 10 weeks. By the 11th week, most of the small venous channels begin to degenerate and only one large venous compartment can be observed that is not bounded by any definitive lateral or medial walls; however, the hypophysis borders it superiorly and medially. During weeks 13–18, the cavernous sinus appears to consist of fine venous spaces that some authors have referred to as the venous canals of Krivosic, which are made of a single layer of endothelial cells with no smooth muscles. At the beginning of the 23rd week, the venous canals begin to dilate and join the degenerated primitive mesenchyme to form the gaps between the canals, and at 28 weeks, collagen fibers begin to provide a supporting framework for the developing venous space. With respect to the venous connections, it has been observed that the cavernous sinus is connected anteriorly to the common ophthalmic vein after 13 weeks of gestation, as well as the basilar venous plexus posteriorly, which appears as a faint group of small vessels. The cranial nerves related to the cavernous sinus begin to assume an adult configuration beginning in the 13th week, and by the age of 23 weeks, CNs III, IV, V_1, and V_2 approach the meningeal layer of the dura. The development of the ICA within the cavernous sinus occurs from 13 to 15 weeks of gestation, as it enters the venous space inferolateral to the developing cartilaginous sphenoid and then runs straight medial to the anterior clinoid process.[11,12]

HISTOLOGY

The morphology of the cavernous sinus under the microscope shows that its building blocks are adipose tissue and networks of collagen fibers. The adipose tissue, which consists of typical adipocytes, fills in the spaces between the different structures of the cavernous sinus and is continuous with the adipose tissue outside the sinus. Arachnoidal epithelium is found to cover the root of CN V, as well as the internal wall of Meckel's cave, thus separating the cerebrospinal fluid from the blood of the cavernous sinus. The venous canals within the cavernous sinus are composed of endothelial cells that cover a thin fibrous layer surrounded by the adipose tissue without any smooth muscles.[13]

VARIATIONS

Studies have shown that the cavernous sinus has many variants and different appearances among the population (Fig. 15.9); it might be relatively small, or in fact, may be absent completely.[14,15]

The superficial middle cerebral vein (SMCV) has been an area of interest among anatomists who have studied the variations of the cavernous sinus. It has been demonstrated that the relation between the SMCV and the cavernous sinus can be classified into four different variants: Type 1—SMCV enters the cavernous sinus from its anterolateral aspect; hence the name (cavernous type); Type 2—(paracavernous sinus type)—courses outside the cavernous sinus and enters the foramen or the superior petrosal sinus; Type 3—(laterocavernous type)—runs through the layers of the lateral wall and enters the pterygoid plexus of veins, which causes a decrease in its diameter along its course, and Type 4, in which the SMCV is absent.[16] Another study also classified the SMCV into four different types: Type A—SMCV connects with the proximal sphenoparietal sinus and flows into the frontal aspect of the cavernous sinus; Type B—the SMCV connects independently with the lateral aspect of the cavernous sinus; Type C—SMCV connects with the pterygoid venous plexus through the middle cranial fossa, and Type D—the SMCV runs across the pyramidal ridge and connects with the superior petrosal sinus or transverse sinus via the tentorial sinus.[17]

The structure of the cavernous sinus' medial wall has been the subject of controversy. Some studies have stated that the medial wall, which also serves as the lateral wall of the pituitary capsule, is composed of loose fibrous tissue. Other authors have indicated that the medial wall consists of a single thin layer of dura that may allow direct extension.[18] Another study showed that, in fact, both the loose fibrous network and the meningeal dura contribute to the formation of the medial wall of the cavernous sinus.[19]

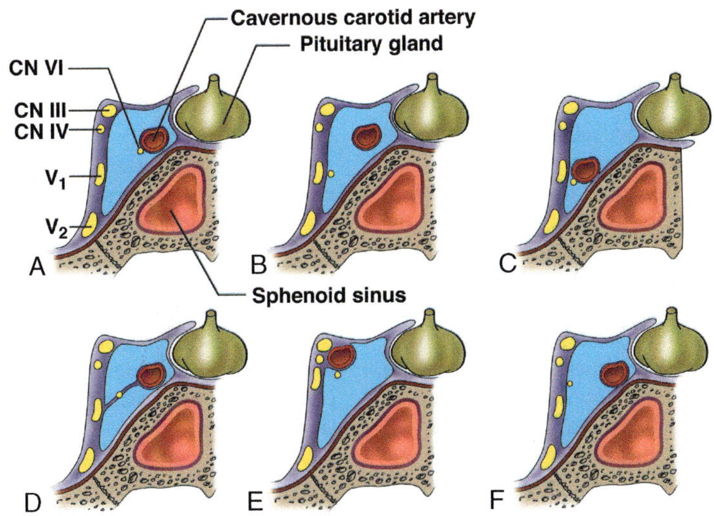

FIG. 15.9 Variations of the cavernous sinus after Testut.

Another area that exhibits variation in the lateral sellar compartment is the intercavernous sinus, which anatomists have investigated in several studies. Whereas some authors have discussed the different sizes of the anterior and posterior intercavernous sinuses, others actually have found that the transverse veins that connect the two sides of the cavernous sinus can be missing.[3,14,20,21]

Using a sample of 35 cadavers, Tubbs et al.[22] demonstrated that the anterior and posterior intercavernous sinuses can be classified into four different types: Type I (80%) had both an anterior and posterior intercavernous sinus; Type II (25% of Type I) had a circular connection between the anterior and posterior intercavernous sinuses; Type III (17%) had only an anterior intercavernous sinus, and Type IV (2.9%) had only a posterior intercavernous sinus. The study also showed variations in the size of the anterior, posterior, and inferior intercavernous sinuses.

Some authors have mentioned that a single intercavernous vein may be found below the pituitary body, and hence, have referred to it as the inferior intercavernous sinus.[14] Aquini et al.[21] observed the inferior intercavernous sinus in 96.9% of their specimens by serial section and 75% by X-ray studies. The inferior intercavernous sinus presented in three different ways on the sella turcica floor: plexus type, venous lake type, and mixed type. A basilar plexus was found in 100% of cases.

The cavernous sinus' lateral wall has been found to enclose a dural sinus within its layers to which authors have referred as the laterocavernous sinus. When present, the sinus appears as a slitlike venous sinus that runs parallel to the cavernous sinus and is separated from it by the medial layer of the lateral wall of the cavernous sinus. The sinus that receives blood from the SMCV and to a lesser extent, the deep middle cerebral vein, has three draining pathways, either isolated or combined: the superior petrosal and the cavernous sinuses, and the pterygoid venous plexus. The laterocavernous sinus is connected to the cavernous sinus through an opening in the posterior aspect of the lateral, through small fenestrations in the medial layer of the lateral wall, or via small anastomotic channels at the base of the skull.[23–25]

Dynamic CT scanning, which is better than is MRI in terms of its dynamic properties and spatial resolution, is another way to demonstrate the cavernous sinus' true nature. Bonneville et al.[26] used dynamic CT to provide a better understanding of the venous structures within the lateral sellar compartment. In a sample of 680 patients, they observed that a "true cavernous sinus," that is, a vascular space containing ICA and CNs, was found only in four patients (0.6%). The venous structure of the cavernous sinus in the remaining patients showed considerable variations: the veins of the cavernous sinus lateral wall were observed in 98% of the patients; the inferolateral venous group was present in 92%; the vein of the carotid artery sulcus was found in 65%, and the medial vein was present in 20%–30% of the sample.

IMAGING

Studies have used MRI and CT scans to visualize the appearance of the cavernous sinus and its contents.

The most significant structures found on a coronal or axial MRI are ICA, CNs III, IV, V_1, V_2, and VI, lateral wall of the cavernous sinus, and Gasserian ganglion in Meckel's cave. A coronal section through the posterior section of the cavernous sinus will show the ICA medial to CNs III and IV, as well as Meckel's cave, which has an oval shape and a slightly more intense signal than does the cerebrospinal fluid. The images also show that the artery has a fixed relation to the nerves: CN III is superolateral, CN IV is lateral, and the ophthalmic nerve and CN VI are inferolateral to the artery. On a partial saturation 3–5 mm coronal section slice, the cranial nerves appear as small hyperdense areas in the cavernous sinus that match the intensity of the corpus callosum signal. On the other hand, an axial cut will not help differentiate the cranial nerves and a hyperdense CSF signal can be observed lateral to the lateral wall of the cavernous sinus.[27]

On coronal CT scan images with contrast enhancement, the cranial nerves appear as low-attenuated structures within the cavernous sinus, which is represented as an area of high attenuation lateral to the sella turcica. The sinus can be divided into three different compartments: anteriorly at the level of the clinoid process where CN III runs below the process and CN VI can be viewed beneath the sinus, a middle compartment where V_1 can be seen in the inferior part of the lateral wall and CN III runs superiorly along the wall, and a posterior section where the Gasserian ganglion can be seen. The ICA cannot be seen on CT scans unless the vessel is calcified or surrounded by a tumor. Axial CT scans show that the cavernous sinus occupies the parasellar region but do not distinguish its components, even with contrast enhancement.[28]

PATHOLOGY

The cavernous sinus has acquired clinical significance because of the various pathologic conditions that develop in the lateral sellar compartment. Cavernous sinus syndrome is the term used to indicate the suite of signs and symptoms that are associated with a lesion that affects the sinus, including infections, tumors, inflammation, and thrombosis.[29]

Cavernous sinus thrombosis (CST) is still reported even today despite the advancements in imaging and antibiotics and is a condition that poses a serious risk of morbidity and mortality. Early detection of its signs and symptoms is crucial to prevent the life-threatening circumstances associated with this condition. The causes of CST can be classified as infectious and noninfectious. The infectious causes of CST include sinusitis, otitis, and facial skin infections, whereas the noninfectious causes are traumatic and postsurgical. Direct spread of the infection is the most frequent cause of CST; however, it also can occur after propagation of a thrombus or a septic embolus.

The clinical appearance of these patients has been discussed in many case reports; symptoms of sepsis, including hypotension, rigor, tachycardia, and confusion, have been described in patients with CST. Headache and nuchal rigidity have also been found in several cases, but ophthalmic symptoms are the hallmarks of CST. Most patients demonstrate the typical triad of chemosis, periorbital edema, and proptosis, which occurs primarily in the ipsilateral eye before the contralateral side shows symptoms 2 days later. Other eye symptoms include impairment of extraocular muscles that CNs III and IV supply, in which their anatomic position puts them at greater risk than in the case of CN VI, and deteriorating vision to the extent of total blindness has been reported in some cases. Extensive brain infection can follow untreated CVT, and the condition may develop into meningitis, brain abscess, or encephalitis that may lead to coma and eventually death. Based on the anatomy of the cavernous sinus, the pituitary gland could be affected easily, and it has been reported in a handful of cases that showed hypopituitarism. A recent report compared the current mortality rate of 13% and morbidity of 23% with the 80% mortality and 75% morbidity of the 19th and 20th centuries and gave credit to the new treatment modalities that lead to CST patients' better outcomes today.[30]

The ICA is one of the most important structures within the cavernous sinus and adds further clinical significance to the sinus. Carotid-cavernous fistula (CCF) is a pathologic connection between the artery and the sinus that requires endovascular intervention. There are two distinct types of CCFs: the direct type (dCCF), which is a defect in the cavernous ICA wall primarily, or a consequence of a ruptured aneurysm, and the indirect type (iCCF) that can be viewed as a dural arteriovenous fistula. iCCF can be classified further into three subtypes based on the blood supply: arterial supply by meningeal ICA branches, by meningeal external carotid artery (ECA) branches, and by meningeal branches of both the ICA and ECA. As is the case for any shunt system in the body, the flow of arterial blood into the cavernous sinus causes an increase in sinus pressure that leads to a classic clinical appearance.[31]

Fistulas can also be classified as traumatic or spontaneous depending on their etiology: The traumatic type occurs after a tear in the cavernous ICA that leads to the formation of high-flow, high-pressure that never resolves on its own. The spontaneous type can occur for idiopathic reasons, tends to occur in middle-aged women, and generally is a low-flow type of fistula, most of which resolve spontaneously.[32]

The rise in intercavernous pressure is transmitted to the inferior petrosal sinus and the ipsilateral orbit, the latter of which is responsible for the triad of exophthalmos, conjunctival chemosis, and to a lesser extent, cephalic bruit. Other ophthalmic complications include double vision and even blindness after retinal ischemia.[31–33]

INTERVENTIONAL RADIOLOGY

Diagnosing CCF can be established using cerebral angiography via femoral access on the side contralateral to the lesion. The fistulas can be differentiated into high- and low-flow using angiographic criteria. A high-flow fistula will show rapid filling of the cavernous sinus and the efferent veins, whereas the intracranial ICA will fill in part or not be visualized at all. A low-flow fistula shows slow filling of the venous system. Barrow et al.[32] mentioned that the duration between the first onset of symptoms and the appearance of radiographic evidence could be as long as 18 months. It is important to study the arterial and venous circulation of the brain to detect any other lesions, such as pseudoaneurysms and venous thrombosis and reflux, and most importantly, to study the flow rate of the CCF that determines the treatment modalities. Indirect CCFs that have low blood flow present with mild symptoms, and thus, can be managed conservatively by manual compression of the jugular vein and carotid artery, as well as monitoring visual acuity and the intraocular pressure closely. The endovascular approach has been tested widely and proven to be safe in managing CCF using either arterial or venous routes to perform embolization procedures using coils, inflatable balloons, and liquid embolic solutions.[31]

SURGERY

Given its clinical significance, surgeons have approached the cavernous sinus using a variety of modalities and techniques. Inoue et al.[34] described the various methods that have been used to perform surgical procedures within the cavernous sinus. The variations in its anatomy require surgeons to adopt different approaches, including the following: (1) The superior intradural approach through the roof of the sinus after a frontotemporal craniotomy, which can include further an extradural approach to excise the clinoid process and expose the orbit and optic canal; (2) intradural and extradural lateral approaches, and (3) superomedial and inferomedial approaches.

The skull base is a technically difficult space for neurosurgeons, and many of the surgical approaches to this area have yet to be perfected. The normal anatomy of the four cavernous triangles, four middle fossa triangles, and two paraclival triangles is very important in approaching surgical lesions around the cavernous sinus, petrous and cavernous carotid, internal auditory canal, and labyrinth.[35,36] Parkinson was the first to describe a triangle in the lateral wall of the cavernous sinus in the mid-1960s. Dolenc[37,38] elaborated further on direct microsurgical approaches with respect to anatomy and surgery within the corridors of the cavernous sinus. Since then, oculomotor, Glassock's, and Kawase's triangles have been documented,[39,40] but details of the other triangles remain to be reported. There also is incongruity in naming and describing the triangular spaces.[41–43] This chapter will review the anatomic borders, average dimensions, and surgical implications of these triangles, as well as provide illustrations to aid in our understanding of the locations of all of them.

Other triangles in the skull base are equally important as the cavernous sinus triangles and are associated with a new level of safety in skull base surgery, as well as some level of procedural standardization.

Cavernous Sinus Triangles

Clinoidal triangle

Drilling the anterior clinoid process either extradurally or intradurally exposes the clinoidal or anteromedial triangle area. This is bordered by the optic nerve medially, CN III laterally, and tentorial edge, which extends between CN II and III at the base. The average measurements of the medial and lateral borders, base, and area are 9.5, 13.3, and 7.2 mm, and 32.3 mm^2, respectively.[43] These dimensions have been explored further via microsurgical techniques on cadaveric dissections, and the average sizes of the medial and lateral borders, base, and area were 7.34, 13.89, and 8.53, and 26.25 mm^2, respectively.[44] Day et al.[41] and Fukushima[42] indicated that the lateral border of the optic nerve, the medial wall of the superior orbital fissure dura, and the dural ring surrounding the ICA define the anterior triangle as it enters the subarachnoid space. They measured the dimensions of these borders as 6.30 posteriorly, 6.88 medially, and 8.72 mm laterally. Although different authors' measurements vary, they agree about the triangle's contents—the clinoidal segment of the ICA in the middle, the optic strut anteriorly, and the roof of the cavernous sinus posteriorly. To access the clinoidal

ICA, the anterior clinoid process can be pneumatized to expose an interdural space beyond which the clinoidal ICA can be visualized.[45] The anterior clinoid process can also be drilled to obtain access to the sphenoidal sinus corridor. An osseous bridge between the anterior and middle clinoid process surrounds the subclinoidal ICA occasionally, and it has been reported that removing this process in one piece damages the ICA.[46] Furthermore, when a meningioma invades the anterior clinoid process, it is necessary to perform intradural resection by approaching the clinoidal triangle.[47]

The clinoidal triangle can be exposed with the endoscopic supraorbital extradural approach. Following a supraorbital craniotomy and drilling the sphenoidal ridge, orbital roof, and the greater and lesser sphenoid wings, the floor of the middle cranial fossa can be exposed by lifting the temporal dura slightly. At this point, the anterior clinoid process can be removed to allow visualization of the clinoidal triangle.[48] Komatsu et al.[49] proposed that the clinoidal triangle, together with the anteromedial and anterolateral triangles, is a possible route to the middle cranial fossa in the endoscopic endonasal approach.

Oculomotor triangle

The oculomotor, medial, or Hakuba triangle is approached to explore CN III and the horizontal segment of the ICA.[50] The oculomotor is one of the few triangles formed via the superior wall of the cavernous sinus and dural folds—medially by the interclinoid, laterally by the petroclinoid, and at the base by the posterior petroclinoid fold. The average measurements of the medial, lateral, and base sides are 10.4, 16.1, and 12.2 mm, respectively. The oculomotor triangle plays a significant role in accessing tumors located in the medial cavernous sinus, and interpeduncular lesions. Day et al.[41] observed that this triangle has different corners—the subclinoidal carotid segment, posterior clinoid process, and porus oculomotorius. The dimensions of the medial triangle vary by several millimeters, 9.6 × 16.6 × 13.8 mm.[45,51] The horizontal portion of the cavernous ICA can be explored through this triangle's window to locate various vascular pathologies. It also has a very important relation with aneurysms that form at the junction of the ICA and the posterior communicating artery.[52] The posterosuperior venous space of the cavernous sinus, the posterior bend of the intracavernous ICA with the origin of the meningohypophyseal trunk, the initial intracavernous course of CN VI, and the interclinoid ligament also can be visualized.[45]

CNs III and IV enter the cavernous sinus in this area of the superior wall. The average distance from the dural foramen of the occipital nerve to the anterior clinoid process was 7.2 mm, and to the posterior clinoid process 8.5 mm. The dural opening for the Meckel nerve was, on average, 16.04 mm and was 12.74 mm from the anterior and posterior clinoid processes, respectively.[45]

Supra-Meckel triangle

After the posterior bend of the ICA, allows entrance to the supra-Meckel or paramedian triangle. CN III is this triangle's medial border, and the lateral border is Meckel's cave with the base formed by the tentorial edge extending between CNs III and IV. In addition to its origin in the meningohypophyseal trunk, the inferolateral trunk, and less commonly, the medial loop of the ICA, can be found in this space.[41,53] The dimensions of the medial, lateral, and base are 13.18, 14.27, and 5.51 mm, respectively. These measurements correlate with Watanabe et al.'s[43] documentation of 10.9, 14.0, and 7.0 mm, respectively. This triangle is used to explore the medial loop of the intracavernous ICA and the meningohypophyseal trunk and is accessed to clip cavernous aneurysms.

Parkinson's triangle Parkinson[35,54] described the infra-Meckel or Parkinson's triangle originally as a way to enter the cavernous sinus directly. It is limited medially by the Meckel nerve, laterally by the ophthalmic division of CN V, and at the base by the tentorial edge of these two nerves. Although few other studies mention variations in the measurements, Watanabe et al. documented the dimensions as 13.1, 16.4, and 6.2 mm for the medial, lateral, and base of the Parkinson's space, respectively.[35,54] Watanabe et al.[43] and Day et al.[41] referred to it as the superolateral space.[55,56] This triangular area is relatively narrow, but its space can be enlarged during surgical approaches via retraction or dissection of the Meckel nerve medially and trigeminal laterally.[57] Opening this space further allows exploration of the entire intracavernous segment of the ICA from the lateral ring to proximal ring and also permits complete exposure of CN VI from its entry through Dorello's canal to its exit through the superior orbital fissure.[57] Thus, this triangle plays a role in surgical management of vascular abnormalities along the ICA, as well as cranial nerve mass lesions. Furthermore, Knosp et al.[58] discussed the way Parkinson's triangle can be used to access and resect meningiomas in the cavernous sinus.[58]

After exposing the lateral wall of the cavernous sinus via the endoscopic supraorbital extradural approach, Parkinson's triangle can be seen by slight temporal retraction. The number of structures that can be visualized via this approach reflects its great utility in microsurgery. The posteroinferior part of the cavernous sinus can be exposed through this triangle, as well as lateral views of the posterior vertical segment, posterior bend, horizontal segment of the ICA and its branches, and the posterior wall of the cavernous sinus.[48]

The literature discusses the parasellar region in infants rarely. Virtually all of the information available on this region has come from studies of adult specimens. Weninger et al.[66] (1999) used 49 specimens from human infants aged 0–9 months in their study of the parasellar region. Along the upper rim of CN V, the side of Parkinson's triangle was 7.33 mm and along the clivus, its side was 3.77 mm long. The average height at the level of the posterior clinoid process was 3.48 mm. In 50% of the cases examined, the meningohypophyseal trunk, its branches, the site of its origin from the ICA, and the medial wall of the upper posterior portion of the parasellar region can be approached through this triangle in infants.

Anteromedial triangle

Also referred to as the Mullan's triangle, the ophthalmic division of the trigeminal medially and the maxillary division of the trigeminal laterally form the boundaries of the anteromedial triangle.[59] The base of the triangle consists of the anterolateral wall of the bony middle cranial fossa formed by a line connecting the superior orbital fissure and foramen rotundum. The length of these limits is 11.7 × 7.8 × 12.0 mm.[43] This corridor is suited well to expose several important structures, including the superior orbital vein, ophthalmic vein, sphenoid sinus, and CN VI. Further dissection within Mullan's space allows ready access to the CCFs. Slight temporal retraction is necessary to expose this triangle during endoscopic surgery via the supraorbital extradural approach.[48]

Cranial nerve deficits postintracavernous surgical interventions are not uncommon and can be attributable to direct manipulation of the nerves or disturbance of their blood supply. The superior orbital fissure artery, which branches from the inferolateral trunk typically, runs immediately under the reticularis layer of the anteromedial triangle in the lateral wall of the cavernous sinus. This artery supplies CNs III, IV, VI, and VI, and the ophthalmic division of the CN V. Hence, any procedure that interrupts the anatomy of the cavernous sinus' lateral wall at the anteromedial triangle puts the vascular supply of these nerves at risk, although collaterals exist.[60]

Anterolateral triangle

The anterolateral, also referred to as the lateral triangle, is formed medially by the maxillary division and laterally by the mandibular division of the trigeminal.[44] The identification of the base is via a bony line connecting the foramen rotundum and foramen ovale. The border dimensions of the medial, lateral, and base of the triangle are 13.9, 15.5, and 7.6 mm, respectively.[43] This space is used to expose the lateral sphenoid wing, sphenoidal emissary vein, and the cavernous-pterygoid venous anastomosis, through which lesions located in the lateral part of the cavernous sinus are revealed.

Kodera et al.[61] demonstrated that access sufficient to resect tissue from intracavernous lesions can be gained via the anterolateral triangle with a frontotemporal interdural approach without zygomatic or orbitozygomatic osteotomy. This approach requires only minimal dissection of the dura propria and inner layer, thereby avoiding excessive retraction of the temporal lobe.

Posteromedial triangle

Possibly the largest of all of the triangles, Kawase et al.[40] were first to describe this rhomboid-shaped space referred to as the posteromedial or Kawase triangle. The lateral margin of the greater superficial petrosal nerve medially and the lateral edge of CN V at the crest of the petrous apex laterally bound this area. The base consists of a line connecting the posterior border of the mandibular division of the trigeminal and crest of the petrous apex to the center of the geniculate ganglion. Watanabe et al.[43] documented this triangle's dimensions as 16.1 × 13.9 × 12.5 mm and commented further on the consistency of its shape. Removing the bone in this triangle permits exposure of the petrous apex or petroclival area and internal auditory canal. In addition, the corridor through Kawase's space allows access to the vertebrobasilar junction and anterolateral brain stem.

Tripathi et al.[62] conducted a volumetric analysis of 12 dried temporal bones using laser technology. They defined the bounds of the Kawase triangle as follows: (1) the junction of the greater superficial petrosal nerve with the lateral border of the mandibular division of the trigeminal (V3); (2) the lateral margin of the porus trigeminus, and (3) the anteromedial margin of the arcuate eminence. They compared the dimensions of this triangle with that of a modified Dolenc-Kawase rhomboid with the following boundaries: (1) the lateral margin of V3 after medial mobilization of CN V; (2) the bony surface just lateral to the petroclival ligament, and (3) the arcuate eminence and the intersection of a line drawn along the axes of the GSPN and the arcuate eminence. Tripathi et al. went on to show that the area of Kawase's triangle averaged 269.13 mm^2 with a mean volume of 666.61 mm^3. In the MDK approach, the average area was 408.09 mm^2 with a corresponding mean volume of 1349.272 mm^3. Compared with Kawase's triangle, the MDK approach boasts larger areas and volumes through which middle cranial fossa pathologies, such as large sphenopetroclival lesions can be accessed.

Posterolateral triangle

The posterolateral triangle is relatively inconsistent in size. Also referred to as Glasscock's triangle, it is bound laterally by a line from the foramen spinosum to the arcuate eminence of the petrous bone, and medially by a line between where the greater superficial petrosal nerve crosses under the mandibular division of CN V and the foramen spinosum.[39] Its base is the greater superficial petrosal nerve itself.[44] Glasscock defined the corners originally as the posterior rim of the foramen ovale, the apex of the cochlea, and the posterior border of the mandibular division of CN V.[39] Rhoton[63] defined this triangle by the lateral surface of the trigeminal and the anterior margin of the petrosal nerve. Contrary to Watanabe et al.'s[43] and Dolenc's[53] measurements, Isolan et al.[44] documented the dimensions as 14.7 × 7.04 × 15.3 mm, with an area of 49.2 mm^2 area. Day et al.'s[41] measurements indicated that the medial border was larger than were Isolan et al.'s[44] and Watanabe et al.'s,[43] and the lateral border was less attributable to differences in the anatomic points among the authors. Glasscock's triangle is known not only for its variations in size but also for its contents, which include the greater and lesser petrosal nerves, tensor tympani muscle, Eustachian tube, middle meningeal artery, foramen spinosum, infratemporal fossa, and most importantly, the horizontal petrous ICA.[57] Drilling away Glasscock's triangle exposes the horizontal intrapetrosal segment of the ICA for proximal control in a bypass graft or anastomosis and also allows access to the cavernous sinus for tumor resections.[64]

Inferomedial triangle

The inferomedial paraclival triangle is defined medially by a line connecting the dural entrance of CN VI at Dorello's canal to the posterior clinoid process, laterally by a line connecting the dural entrance of CNs IV and VI, and at the base by the petrous apex. According to Isolan et al.,[44] it measures 16.2 × 11.4 × 7.3, with an area of 34.9 mm^2, which correspond to measurements in other cadaveric studies.[43] The inferomedial space extends into the posterior cavernous sinus wall, and drilling the medial aspect of this space exposes the lateral edge of the dorsum sellae, petroclival fissure, and Dorello's canal. Furthermore, this triangle contains CN VI, the posterior genu of the ICA, dorsal meningeal branch of the meningohypophysial trunk, basilar venous plexus and overlying dura, posterior petroclinoid fold, and Gruber's or the petrosphenoid ligament.

Inferolateral triangle

Similarly, the inferolateral paraclival triangle is defined medially by a line between the dural entrance of the Meckel nerve into the tentorium cerebelli to the dural entry of CN VI and laterally by a line between the dural entry point of CN VI and petrosal vein. This triangle shares the same base as the inferomedial triangle—the petrous apex. Isolan et al.[44] measured it as 11.4 mm medially × 15.0 mm laterally × 7.9 mm at the base, with an area of 34.9 mm^2.[43] Dolenc divided this space by a line between the entry point of the petrosal vein and the entry point of CN V into the tentorial triangle above and the osseous triangle below.[37,53,65] Access to the tentorial artery, superior petrosal sinus, and Meckel's cave is obtained through the tentorial triangle, and CN V is accessed from the osseous triangle.

REFERENCES

1. Thakur JD, Sonig A, Khan IS, et al. Jacques Benigne Winslow (1669–1760) and the misnomer cavernous sinus. *World Neurosurg*. 2014;81:191–197.
2. Parkinson D. Lateral sellar compartment O.T. (cavernous sinus): history, anatomy, terminology. *Anat Rec*. 1998;251:486–490.
3. Browder J, Kaplan HA. *Cerebral Dural Sinuses and Their Tributaries*. Springfield: Charles Thomas; 1976.
4. Rhoton Jr AL. In: Dolenc V, Rogers L, eds. *The Middle Cranial Base and Cavernous Sinus*. Vienna: Springer; 2009:3–25.
5. Campero A, Campero AA, Martins C, et al. Surgical anatomy of the dural walls of the cavernous sinus. *J Clin Neurosci*. 2010;17:746–750.
6. Bakan AA, Alkan A, Kurtcan S, et al. Cavernous sinus: a comprehensive review of its anatomy, pathologic conditions, and imaging features. *Clin Neuroradiol*. 2015;25:109–125.
7. Wallace S, Goldberg HI, Leeds NE, et al. The cavernous branches of the internal carotid artery. *Am J Roentgenol*. 1967;101:34–46.
8. Keller JT, Leach JL, van Loveren HR, et al. Venous anatomy of the lateral sellar compartment. In: Dolenc V, Rogers L, eds. Vienna: Springer; 2009:35–51.
9. Tubbs RS, Hill M, May WR, et al. Does the maxillary division of the trigeminal nerve traverse the cavernous sinus? An anatomical study and review of the literature. *Surg Radiol Anat*. 2008;30(1):37–40.
10. Swedenborg E. *The Brain Considered Anatomically, Physiologically and Philosophically*. Vol. 2. James Speirs; 1887.

11. Kehrli P, Maillot C, Wolff MJ. The venous system of the lateral sellar compartment (cavernous sinus): an histological and embryological study. *Neurol Res*. 1996;18: 387–393.
12. Hashimoto M, Yokota A, Yamada H, et al. Development of the cavernous sinus in the fetal period. A morphological study. *Neurol Med*. 2000;40:140–150.
13. Krivosic I. In: Dolenc V, ed. *Histoarchitecture of the Cavernous Sinus*. Vienna: Springer; 1987:117–129.
14. Knott JF. On the cerebral sinuses and their variations. *J Anat*. 1881;16:27–42.
15. Bergman RA, Thompson SA, Afifi AK, et al. *Compendium of Human Anatomic Variation: Catalog, Atlas and World Literature*. Baltimore, MD, Munich: Urban & Schwarzenberg; 1988.
16. Takahashi S, Sakuma I, Otani T, et al. Venous anatomy of the sphenoparietal sinus: evaluation by MR imaging. *Intervent Neuroradiol*. 2007;13:84–89.
17. Tanoue S, Kiyosue H, Okahara M, et al. Para-cavernous sinus venous structures: anatomic variations and pathologic conditions evaluated on fat-suppressed 3D fast gradient-echo MR images. *Am J Neuroradiol*. 2006;27:1083–1089.
18. Goncalves MB, de Oliveira JG, Williams HA, et al. Cavernous sinus medial wall: dural or fibrous layer? Systematic review of the literature. *Neurosurg Rev*. 2012;35:147–153; discussion 153–4.
19. Diao Y, Liang L, Yu C, et al. Is there an identifiable intact medial wall of the cavernous sinus? macro- and microscopic anatomical study using sheet plastination. *Neurosurgery*. 2013;73:120–125.
20. Renn WH, Rhoton AL. Microsurgical anatomy of the sellar region. *J Neurosurg*. 1975;43:288–298.
21. Aquini MG, Marrone AC, Schneider FL. Intercavernous venous communications in the human skull base. *Skull Base Surg*. 1994;4:145–150.
22. Tubbs RS, Griessenauer C, Loukas M, et al. The circular sinus: an anatomic study with neurosurgical and neurointerventional applications. *World Neurosurg*. 2013;82:e475–e478.
23. San Millan Ruiz D, Gailloud P, de Miquel MA, et al. Laterocavernous sinus. *Anat Rec*. 1999;254:7–12.
24. Gailloud P, San Millan Ruiz D, Muster M, et al. Angiographic anatomy of the laterocavernous sinus. *AJNR Am J Neuroradiol*. 2000;21:1923–1929.
25. Lv X, Feng W, Li Y, et al. Cavernous region dural fistulas with venous drainage of laterocavernous sinus. *Neurol India*. 2011;59:190–194.
26. Bonneville JF, Cattin F, Racle A, et al. Dynamic CT of the laterosellar extradural venous spaces. *AJNR Am J Neuroradiol*. 1989;10:535–542.
27. Daniels DL, Pech P, Mark L, et al. Magnetic resonance imaging of the cavernous sinus. *Am J Roentgenol*. 1985;144:1009–1014.
28. Kline L, Acker J, Post M, et al. The cavernous sinus: a computed tomographic study. *Am J Neuroradiol*. 1981;2:299–305.
29. Lee JH, Lee HK, Park JK, et al. Cavernous sinus syndrome: clinical features and differential diagnosis with MR imaging. *AJR Am J Roentgenol*. 2003;181:583–590.
30. Desa V, Green R. Cavernous sinus thrombosis: current therapy. *J Oral Maxillofac Surg*. 2012;70:2085–2091.
31. Ducruet AF, Albuquerque FC, Crowley RW, et al. The evolution of endovascular treatment of carotid cavernous fistulas: a single-center experience. *World Neurosurg*. 2013;80:538–548.
32. Barrow DL, Spector RH, Braun IF, et al. Classification and treatment of spontaneous carotid-cavernous sinus fistulas. *J Neurosurg*. 1985;62:248–256.
33. Tjoumakaris SI, Jabbour PM, Rosenwasser RH. Neuroendovascular management of carotid cavernous fistulae. *Neurosurg Clin*. 2009;20:447–452.
34. Inoue T, Rhoton Jr AL, Theele D, et al. Surgical approaches to the cavernous sinus: a microsurgical study. *Neurosurgery*. 1990;26:903–932.
35. Parkinson D. A surgical approach to the cavernous portion of the carotid artery. Anatomical studies and case report. *J Neurosurg*. 1965;23:474–483.
36. Parkinson D. Transcavernous repair of carotid cavernous fistula. Case report. *J Neurosurg*. 1967;26:420–424.
37. Dolenc VV. A combined epi- and subdural direct approach to carotid-ophthalmic artery aneurysms. *J Neurosurg*. 1985;62:667–672.
38. Dolenc VV. Surgery of vascular lesions of the cavernous sinus. *Clin Neurosurg*. 1990;36:240–255.
39. Glassock III ME, Jackson CG, Dickins JR, Wiet RJ. Panel discussion: glomus jugulare tumors of the temporal bone. The surgical management of glomus tumors. *Laryngoscope*. 1979;89:1640–1654.
40. Kawase T, Toya S, Shiobara R, Mine T. Transpetrosal approach for aneurysms of the lower basilar artery. *J Neurosurg*. 1985;63:857–861.
41. Day JD, Fukushima T, Giannotta SL. Innovations in surgical approach: lateral cranial base approaches. *Clin Neurosurg*. 1996;43:72–90.
42. Fukushima T. Direct operative approach to the vascular lesions in the cavernous sinus: summary of 27 cases. *Cerebrovasc Dis*. 1988;6:169–189.
43. Watanabe A, Nagaseki Y, Ohkubo S, et al. Anatomical variations of the ten triangles around the cavernous sinus. *Clin Anat N Y N*. 2003;16:9–14.
44. Isolan GR, Krayenbühl N, de Oliveira E, Al-Mefty O. Microsurgical anatomy of the cavernous sinus: measurements of the triangles in and around it. *Skull Base Off J North Am Skull Base Soc Al*. 2007;17:357–367.
45. Umansky F, Valarezo A, Elidan J. The superior wall of the cavernous sinus: a microanatomical study. *J Neurosurg*. 1994;81:914–920.
46. Yasuda A, Campero A, Martins C, et al. Microsurgical anatomy and approaches to the cavernous sinus. *Neurosurgery*. 2005;56:4–27; discussion 4–27.
47. Al-Mefty O. *Operative Atlas for Meningiomas*. Philadelphia: Lippincott-Raven; 1998.
48. Komatsu F, Komatsu M, Inoue T, Tschabitscher M. Endoscopic supraorbital extradural approach to the cavernous sinus: a cadaver study: laboratory investigation. *J Neurosurg*. 2011;114:1331–1337.

49. Komatsu F, Shinri O, Masami S, et al. Endoscopic endonasal approach to the middle cranial fossa through the cavernous sinus triangles: anatomical considerations. *Neurol Med -Chir*. 2014;54:1004–1008.
50. Hakuba A, Tanaka K, Suzuki T, Nishimura S. A combined orbitozygomatic infratemporal epidural and subdural approach for lesions involving the entire cavernous sinus. *J Neurosurg*. 1989;71:699–704.
51. Umansky F, Nathan H. The lateral wall of the cavernous sinus. With special reference to the nerves related to it. *J Neurosurg*. 1982;56:228–234.
52. González-Darder JM, Quilis-Quesada V, Talamantes-Escribá F, et al. Microsurgical relations between internal carotid artery–posterior communicating artery (ICA-PComA) segment aneurysms and skull base: an anatomoclinical Study. *J Neurosurg Part B Skull Base*. 2012;73:337.
53. Dolenc V. Direct microsurgical repair of intracavernous vascular lesions. *J Neurosurg*. 1983;58:824–831.
54. Parkinson D. Collateral circulation of cavernous carotid artery: Anatomy. *Can J Surg/J Can Chir*. 1964;7:251–268.
55. Miyazaki Y, Yamamoto I, Shinozuka S, Sato O. Microsurgical anatomy of the cavernous sinus. *Neurol Med -Chir*. 1994;34:150–163.
56. Sekhar LN, Burgess J, Akin O. Anatomical study of the cavernous sinus emphasizing operative approaches and related vascular and neural reconstruction. *Neurosurgery*. 1987;21:806–816.
57. Dolenc VV. Introduction: surgery of the central skull base. *Neurosurg Focus*. 2008;25:E1.
58. Knosp E, Perneczky A, Koos WT, Fries G, Matula C. Meningiomas of the space of the cavernous sinus. *Neurosurgery*. 1996;38:434–444.
59. Mullan S. Treatment of carotid-cavernous fistulas by cavernous sinus occlusion. *J Neurosurg*. 1979;50:131–144.
60. Dalgiç A, Boyaci S, Aksoy K. Anatomical study of the cavernous sinus emphasizing operative approaches. *Turk Neurosurg*. 2010;20:186–204.
61. Kodera T, Hiroaki T, Hidetaka A, et al. Microsurgical findings of Tolosa-Hunt syndrome. *World Neurosurg*. 2013;79:594-e1.
62. Tripathi M, Rama Chandra D, Ashish S, et al. Quantitative analysis of the Kawase versus the modified Dolenc-Kawase approach for middle cranial fossa lesions with variable anteroposterior extension. *J Neurosurg*. 2015;143:14–22.
63. Rhoton Jr AL. The cavernous sinus, the cavernous venous plexus, and the carotid collar. *Neurosurgery*. 2002;51:S375–S410.
64. Suri A, Ahmad FU, Mahapatra AK. Extradural transcavernous approach to cavernous sinus hemangiomas. *Neurosurgery*. 2007;60(3):483–489.
65. Dolenc VV. *Anatomy and Surgery of the Cavernous Sinus*. Wien, New York, NY: Springer-Verlag; 1989.
66. Weninger WJ, Müller GB. The parasellar region of human infants: cavernous sinus topography and surgical approaches. *J Neurosurg*. 1999;90:484–490. https://doi.org/10.3171/jns.1999.90.3.0484.

CHAPTER 16

The Intercavernous Sinuses

R. SHANE TUBBS

The cavernous sinuses are located on and around the sides of the sella turcica. The internal carotid artery and various cranial nerves traverse this venous structure.[1,2] The intercavernous sinus was first described in 1645 and referred to as the "circular" sinuses (of Ridley).[2] Unfortunately, many have confused the circular sinus with the marginal sinus at the foramen magnum.

ANATOMY

The intercavernous sinuses (Figs. 16.1–16.3) connect the left and right cavernous sinuses and occupy the meningeal dural layer covering the pituitary gland and the endosteal layer covering the floor of the sella turcica.[3–5] These can be further classified as anterior, posterior, and inferior.

Ridley described then as the following:

> *By having first injected the veins with wax, I discovered another sinus running round the pituitary gland on its upper side forwards, within a duplicature of the dura mater backwards between the dura mater and pia mater. Here it is somewhat loosely stretched over the subjacent gland itself, and laterally it is a sort of canal, made up of the dura mater above, and the carotid artery on each outer side of the land, which by being fastened to the dura mater above, and below at the basis of the skull too, leaves only a little interstice between itself and the gland, thereby constituting a cavity communicating with the aforesaid arteries (from whence the above-mentioned four small sinuses descend) by a visible continuity, on each side, from a little beneath the hinder process of the sella turcica.*

The anterior intercavernous sinus is said to be present in most cases and may cover the entire anterior aspect of the sella turcica.[3,6] Various reports have described it as being larger[4,7] and longer[8] than the posterior intercavernous sinus, which is located along the superior border of the dorsum sellae. One study found this structure in sagittal sections of all studied anatomic specimens.[3] Some authors have suggested that the posterior intercavernous sinus is more variable and less frequently present and, under nonpathologic conditions, difficult to distinguish from the basilar plexus.[9–11] An inferior intercavernous sinus may be present;[7] however, one venographic study did not identify this structure.[12] The intercavernous sinuses are important clinically and surgically. Kaplan et al.[7] emphasized the possible complications of encountering a sizable intercavernous sinus with transsellar approaches to the sella turcica. Additionally, these interconnecting sinuses may be involved with fistulas between the internal carotid artery and cavernous sinus,[13] may convey infection to the contralateral cavernous sinus,[14] and can be canulated so that its blood is evaluated for increased hormone levels indicative of various neurologic pathologies such as tumors of the pituitary gland.[15] We[15a] previously studied 35 cadaveric specimens and classified the different forms as types 1–4 (Fig. 16.4) and found a coexistent anterior and posterior intercavernous sinus 80% and classified this as a type I configuration. Of the 80% of specimens with both sinuses, a circular connection between these was found in 25% and termed a type II configuration. In six cadavers, only the anterior intercavernous sinus was found (17%), and this morphology was termed a type III configuration. In 2.9%, a posterior intercavernous sinus was found in isolation, and this was termed a type IV configuration. Knott[2] did not identify the posterior intercavernous sinus in 45.4% of cadaveric specimens. At least one of the intercavernous sinuses was present, that is, no specimen had absence of both. In most, the anterior intercavernous sinus was larger in size than the posterior intercavernous sinus. In 17% of specimens, an inferior intercavernous sinus was found (Fig. 16.5). When present, these sinuses were typically much smaller than the anterior or posterior intercavernous sinuses. None of the intercavernous sinuses ran in the free edge of the diaphragma sellae. The mean diameter of the anterior intercavernous sinus was 4.9 mm (range 2–6 mm), and the mean diameter of the posterior intercavernous sinus was 3 mm (range 1.5–4.8 mm). Lastly, if a large basilar plexus was present, then the intercavernous sinuses were smaller in size.

Anatomy, Imaging and Surgery of the Intracranial Dural Venous Sinuses. https://doi.org/10.1016/B978-0-323-65377-0.00016-7

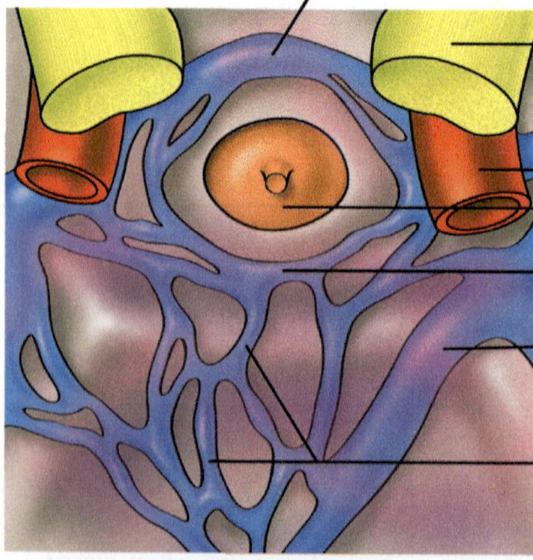

FIG. 16.1 Schematic drawing of the intercavernous sinuses.

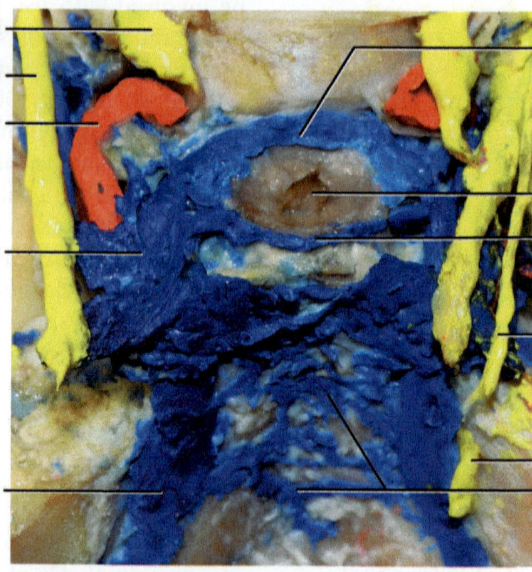

FIG. 16.2 Cadaveric dissection after blue latex injection into the cavernous sinuses and their relationship to the pituitary gland and region nerves.

CLINICAL

When an intercavernous sinus is present, these can explain certain pathologic events, such as septic cavernous sinus thrombosis,[14] and the manifestations of anomalous arteriovenous malformations, such as a carotid cavernous fistula. For example, contralateral eye findings in patients with carotid cavernous fistulas imply an intercavernous connection.[16,17] Kurata et al.[13] reported two thirds of carotid cavernous fistulas that they studied drained into an intercavernous sinus,[13] and a study by Kiyosue et al.[18] reported that 38% of carotid cavernous fistulas drained into the intercavernous sinuses.

Identification of one or all of the intercavernous sinuses on imaging can be one finding of cavernous sinus fistulas, although these sinuses can also sometimes be seen on imaging of normal individuals.[13,19–21]

The anatomic configuration of the intercavernous sinuses can change in the presence of certain pituitary pathologies. For example, pituitary tumors may compress and obliterate the intercavernous sinuses.[15] With

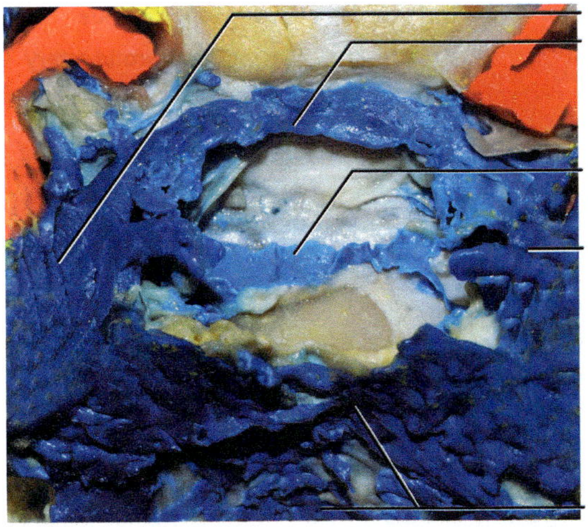

FIG. 16.3 Cadaveric dissection after blue latex injection into the cavernous sinuses and removal of the pituitary gland noting well-formed anterior and posterior intercavernous sinuses.

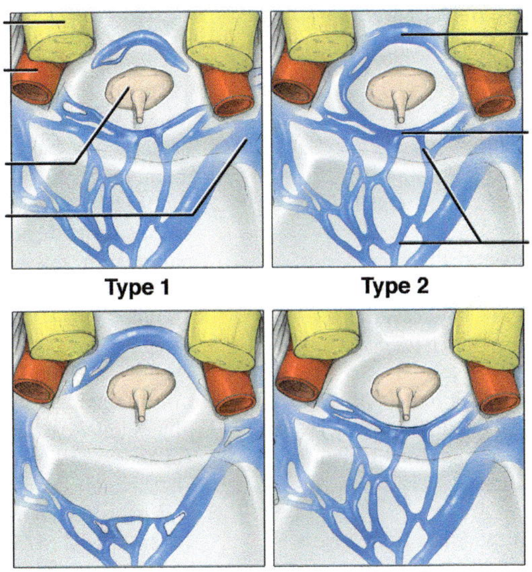

FIG. 16.4 Schematic drawing of the types of intercavernous sinus identified during a previous study of ours.

adenomas of the pituitary gland, the intercavernous sinuses, particularly in Cushing's disease, are frequently enlarged.[5] One study determined that the sensitivity of intercavernous sinus venography for diagnosing pituitary microadenomas was roughly 83%.

Alcaide-Leon et al.[22] reported a visible inferior intercavernous sinus in 50% of patients with intracranial hypotension and that such a finding should not be mistaken for a pituitary lesion.

During transsphenoidal approaches to pituitary lesions, understanding the intercavernous sinuses is important as hemorrhage from these venous structures can be difficult to control. Compression, suturing, cautery, and hemostatic agents have been all been used to control intercavernous sinus bleeding during such approaches.[23] Hong et al.[5] used titanium clips to occlude a prominent anterior intracavernous sinus during operation.[5] Lastly, Newfield et al.[24] found evidence

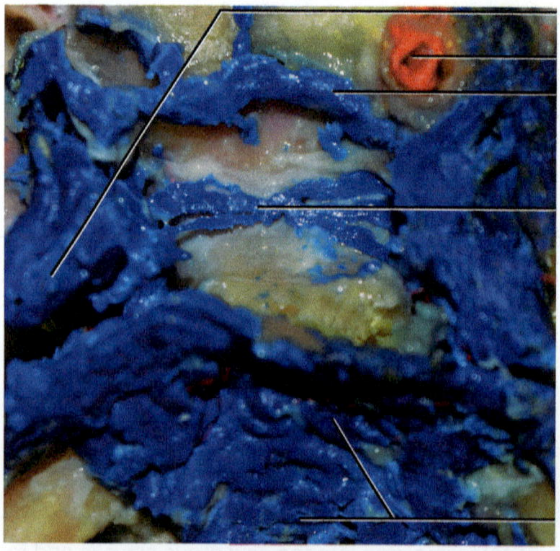

FIG. 16.5 Cadaveric dissection after blue latex injection into the cavernous sinuses and removal of the pituitary gland and dura covering the floor of the sella turcica and noting an inferior intercavernous sinus.

of venous air embolism in approximately 10% of transsphenoidal surgeries and believed this was due to the intercavernous sinuses.

REFERENCES

1. Bedford MA. The "cavernous" sinus. *Br J Ophthalmol.* 1966;50:41–46.
2. Knott JF. On the cerebral sinuses and their variations. *J Anat Physiol.* 1881;16:27–42.
3. Aquini MG, Marrone AC, Schneider FL. Intercavernous venous communications in the human skull base. *Skull Base Surg.* 1994;4:145–150.
4. Dolenc VV. *Cavernous Sinus.* New York: Springer; 2009.
5. Hong Y, Chen S, Guo S, Yu J, Wu Q, Zhang J. A new technique for management of intercavernous sinus bleeding with titanium clips in transsphenoidal surgery. *Neurol India.* 2010;58:847–851.
6. de Divitiis E, Spaziante R, Iaccarino V, Stella L, Genovese L. Phlebography of the cavernous and intercavernous sinuses. *Surg Neurol.* 1981;15:306–312.
7. Kaplan HA, Browder J, Krieger AJ. Intercavernous connections of the cavernous sinuses: the superior and inferior circular sinuses. *J Neurosurg.* 1976;45:166–168.
8. Krayenbuehl H, Yasargil MG, Huber P. *Cerebral Angiography.* 2nd ed. New York: Thieme; 1982.
9. Renn WH, Rhoton Jr AL. Microsurgical anatomy of the sellar region. *J Neurosurg.* 1975;43:288–298.
10. Schnitzlein HN, Murtagh FR, Arrington JA, Parkinson D. The sinus of the dorsum sellae. *Anat Rec.* 1985;213:587–589.
11. Theron J, Chevalier D, Delvert M, Laffont J. Diagnosis of small and micro pituitary adenomas by intercavernous sinus venography: a preliminary report. *Neuroradiology.* 1979;18:23–30.
12. Waga S, Kikuchi H, Handa J, Handa H. Cavernous sinus venography. *Am J Roentgenol Radium Ther Nucl Med.* 1970;109:130–137.
13. Kurata A, Suzuki S, Iwamoto K, et al. Dural arteriovenous fistulas in the cavernous sinus: clinical research and treatment. *ISRN Neurol.* 2011;453834:2011.
14. Kiddee W, Preechawai P, Hirunpat S. Bilateral septic cavernous sinus thrombosis following the masticator and parapharyngeal space infection from the odontogenic origin: a case report. *J Med Assoc Thail.* 2010;93:1107–1111.
15. Tanabe S, Sato O, Hasunuma M, Sohma H, Nakagawa T. Diagnosis of pituitary microadenoma by magnification carotid angiography and intercavernous sinus venography. *Noshinkeigeka.* 1984;12:815–822.

15a. Tubbs RS, Griessenauer C, Loukas M, Cohen-Gadol AA. The circular sinus: an anatomic study with neurosurgical and neurointerventional applications. *World Neurosurg.* 2014;82(3–4):e475–e478.

16. Miller NR, Hoyt WF. *Walsh and Hoyt's Clinical Neuro Ophthalmology.* 6th ed. Philadelphia: Lippincott Williams & Wilkins; 2005.
17. West CG. Bilateral carotid-cavernous fistulae: a review. *Surg Neurol.* 1980;13:85–90.
18. Kiyosue H, Mori H, Sagara Y, et al. Basal cerebral venous drainage from cavernous sinus dural arteriovenous fistulas. *Neuroradiology.* 2009;51:175–181.
19. Elster AD, Chen MY, Richardson DN, Yeatts PR. Dilated intercavernous sinuses: an MR sign of carotid-cavernous and carotid-dural fistulas. *Am J Neuroradiol.* 1991;12:641–645.
20. Kurata A, Miyasaka Y, Kunii M, et al. The value of long-term clinical follow-up for cases of spontaneous carotid cavernous fistula. *Acta Neurochir.* 1998;140:65–72.

21. Loumiotis I, Cloft HJ, Lanzino G. Intercavernous sinus dural arteriovenous fistula successfully treated with transvenous embolization. a case report. *Interv Neuroradiol*. 2011;17:208–211.
22. Alcaide-Leon P, Coblentz A, Kucharczyk W, Bharatha A, de Tilly LN. Prominent inferior intercavernous sinus on sagittal T1-weighted Images: a sign of intracranial hypotension. *Am J Roentgenol*. 2016;206:817–822.
23. Kim EH, Ahn JY, Chang JH, Kim SH. Management strategies of intercavernous sinus bleeding during transsphenoidal surgery. *Acta Neurochir*. 2009;151:803–808.
24. Newfield P, Albin MS, Chestnut JS, Maroon J. Air embolism during trans-sphenoidal pituitary operations. *Neurosurgery*. 1978;2:39–42.

CHAPTER 17

The Sphenoparietal Sinus

CHIRAG PATEL • R. SHANE TUBBS

EMBRYOLOGY

The middle meningeal vein arises from the primitive middle meningeal sinus, which is the lateral tributary of the prootic sinus. This is the precursor of the cavernous and inferior petrosal sinus. Primitive middle meningeal sinus developed as an extrachondrocranial vessel around 400 mm stage and is involved in the vascularization of membranous bones within the cranial vault. Sylvian veins drain along the deep middle cerebral veins and the primitive tributaries of the basal vein into the primitive tentorial sinus. Cerebral hemispheres develop in the 60–80 mm stage, which subsequently leads to the caudal deviation of the transverse sinuses. The caudal end of the tentorial sinus migrates cranially and ventrally toward the junction between the sigmoid and transverse sinus. In adults, the remnant becomes either incorporated into the cavernous sinus, within the lateral wall of the cavernous sinus, or remains on the floor of the middle cranial fossa as a paracavernous sinus. The portion that persists anterior to the cavernous sinus is what becomes the sphenoparietal sinus. Uniquely, the sinus is a novelty restricted to hominoids.[1] According to Chung and Weon,[2] the sphenoparietal sinus is the most frequent type of anatomic variation of the SMCV in adults, regardless of the presence of an anastomosis with the cavernous sinus. The embryonic tentorial sinus should be entirely regressed by the growing hemispheres except only in the preservation of the cranial remnant. As noted in their study, more were seen without an anastomosis with the cavernous sinus than with.[2]

According to Padget,[3] the sphenoparietal sinus is partially meningeal and partially diploic. Usually, it is not apparent in the younger subject and, as the name implies, has a longer course than what is usually portrayed. As stated above, the sinus is derived from the embryonic prootic sinus, specifically the anteroparietal meningeal sinus. The upper end may be continuous in large part with the anteroparietal (temporal) diploic vein, which creates a channel that either deeply grooves the bone or partially passes through it (diploic).[3] Padget also mentioned that the ophthalmomeningeal sinus may be continuous with the ventral end of the adult sphenoparietal sinus.

ANATOMY

Breschet introduced the term sphenoparietal sinus (*sinus alae parvae*) (Figs. 17.1–17.4) in the early 19th century as the sinus found within the limits of the anterior and medial portions of the base of the skull, which occupies a transversally oriented gutter that runs inward into the cavernous sinus. This sinus receives several braches from the skull bones, the dura mater, and the diploic vein of the temporal bone.[4] The sinus has been identified under the lesser sphenoid wing, which connects to the cavernous sinus medially. Near the pterion, the sphenoparietal sinus connects with the anterior branch of the middle meningeal vein, which courses from the foramen spinosum along the vascular groove in the floor of the middle cranial fossa.[5,6] Overall, the sinus receives contributions from the orbital, medial anterior temporal (uncal) and inferior frontal veins as well. Occasionally, the superior ophthalmic vein communicates posteriorly with sphenoparietal sinus instead of with the cavernous sinus.[7] The sinus can be best visualized with the removal of the dura mater from the anterior part of the middle cranial fossa with an anterior viewing perspective (Figs. 17.3 and 17.4). In a study by Tubbs et al.,[1] 15 adult cadavers were visualized, all of which had both a left and right sphenoparietal sinus. The sinuses measured on average 2.5 and 3 mm for the left and right sides, respectively.[1]

Frigeri et al.[8] described that the central lobe is drained directly into 1 of 3 sinuses: superior sagittal, transverse, and sphenoparietal. The lower one-third of the lateral surface most commonly drains to the superficial sylvian veins and from there to the transverse sinus via the vein of Labbé or anteriorly to the sphenoparietal sinus via the superficial sylvian veins. Inferior one-third of the precentral gyrus drained to the sphenoparietal sinus in 50% of their specimens, the transverse sinus 40%, and the superior sagittal sinus 10% of the time. Finally, the lower portion of the postcentral drained to the sphenoparietal sinus in 35% of the specimens, the transverse sinus in 45%, and the superior sagittal sinus via the vein of Trolard in the final 20% of specimens.[8]

A point of controversy, which came up in the literature, is the drainage of the superficial middle

Anatomy, Imaging and Surgery of the Intracranial Dural Venous Sinuses. https://doi.org/10.1016/B978-0-323-65377-0.00017-9

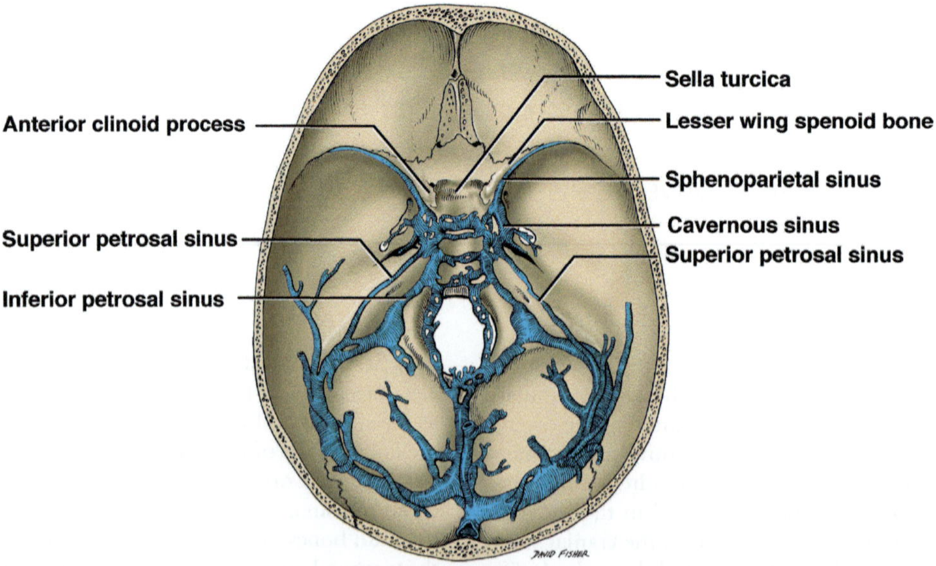

FIG. 17.1 Schematic drawing of the venous sinuses of the skull base. Note the sphenoparietal sinus and its relationship with the cavernous sinus.

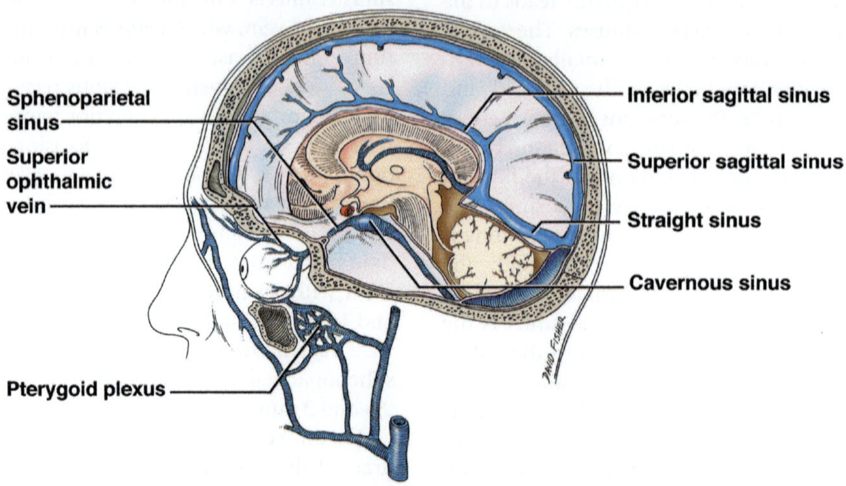

FIG. 17.2 Schematic view of the sphenoparietal sinus, lateral view.

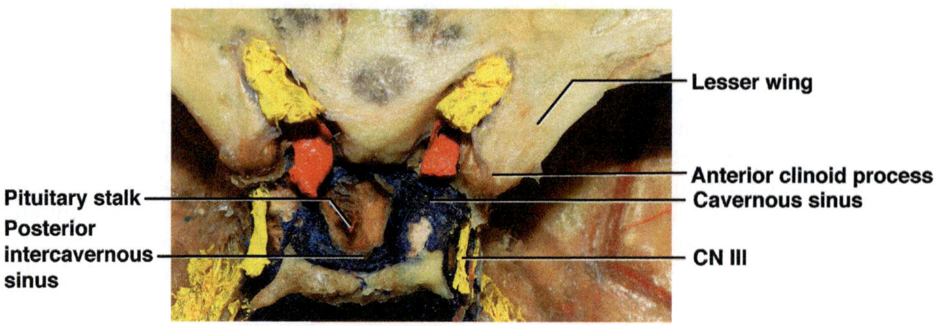

FIG. 17.3 Cadaveric dissection of the venous sinus of the skull base following latex injection into the internal jugular veins. Here, the intercavernous sinuses are well seen.

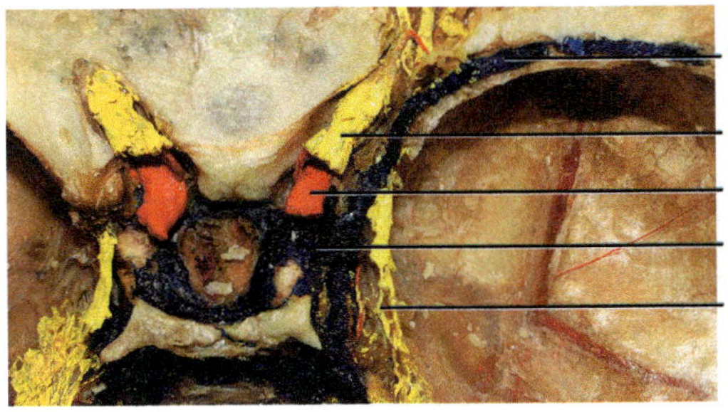

FIG. 17.4 Following removal of the lesser wing of the sphenoid of Fig. 17.3, the underlying sphenoparietal sinus is seen.

cerebral vein. In a study by Suzuki and Matsumoto,[9] 250 patients were evaluated via CT angiography to evaluate the drainage of the SMCV. They concluded that the SMCV entered the sphenoparietal sinus in 54% of their patients.[9] In a similar study by Takahashi et al.,[6] drainage of the SMCV into the sphenoparietal sinus occurred in 67.1% of their patients. Opposition to these findings has come from Ruíz et al.,[4] who in a study of 15 nonfixed human specimens found no connections between the SMCV and the anterior branch of the middle meningeal vein or the sinus of the lesser sphenoid wing.[4]

VARIATIONS

In the literature, there have been three different drainage patters defined in regard to the sphenoparietal sinus. A true sphenoparietal sinus is only when the sphenoidal component anastomoses with the parietal component, the latter consisting of the dural veins that accompany the middle meningeal artery.[10] As mentioned previously, the medial extension of the superficial middle cerebral (Sylvian) vein can travel beneath the lesser wing and drain directly into the cavernous sinus, which is known as the cavernous type. Otherwise, it can drain into the pterygoid plexus via the basal emissary veins in what is called the paracavernous or sphenobasal pattern. Finally, it can travel posteriorly along the floor of the middle cranial fossa after rounding the tip of the temporal lobe to drain into the superior petrosal sinus or transverse sinus[1,4,10,11] (Fig. 17.5). Such a variant as this is probably the same as what has been described as the sinus of Kelch, ophthalmopetrous sinus of Hyrtl and accessory sinus of Verga. In a study by Takahashi et al.,[6] it was observed that the cavernous type of SMCV drainage was equal to the SMCV being completely absent in 35.4% of the specimens. The paracavernous type was present in 10.4% and the laterocavernous was present in 16.7% of the specimens.[6]

Tubbs et al.[12] presented a case report in which a 69-year-old male cadaver was found to have a sinus, which was 5 mm in width and traveled from the sphenoparietal sinus to the veins draining into the foramen spinosum. Known as the accessory venous sinus of Hyrtl (see above), it begins near the superior orbital fissure, the sphenoparietal sinus, and travels posteriorly into the transverse sinus.[12]

IMAGING

Currently, the most definitive diagnostic tool is the digital subtraction angiography. It is both highly specific and sensitive, allowing to better visualize the sphenoparietal sinus without an excess of contraindications. The major disadvantages of DSA are the extended postprocedure hospital stay and radiation exposure, with possible allergic or nephrotoxic effects of iodinated contrast medium.[13] Throughout the literature, CT has been used to identify any associated hemorrhage, yet angiography is the mainstay for visualizing the dural sinuses.[2,7,9,13–15] CT cerebral venography and MR venography have been considered comparable in terms of visualization. However, when performing a CT, the patient needs to be exposed to ionizing radiation as well as the iodinated contrast material. Comparatively, MR can visualize the dural sinus without the use of invasive techniques or ionizing radiation. The only real major contraindication for MR is in individuals with implanted electronic devices, including cochlear implants, cerebral clips, and mechanical valves.[13] According to Scott and Farb,[13] gadolinium-enhanced 3-dimensional MRA is increasing in clinical acceptance as of late. Gadolinium increases the signal intensity of blood with no saturation effects, which allows the contrast between blood and stationary tissue to be relatively flow independent.[13]

PATHOLOGY

Within the literature, there have been very few reports of arteriovenous fistulas and malformations involving

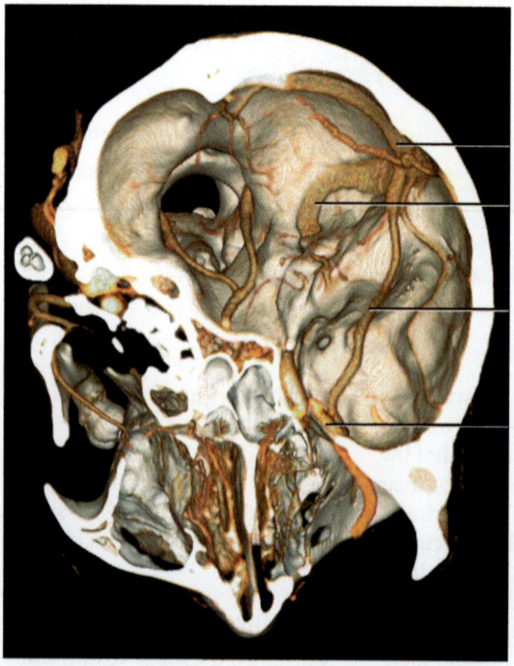

FIG. 17.5 3D CTA noting an anomalous connection between the sphenoparietal sinus anteriorly and the junction of the left transverse and sigmoid sinuses posteriorly. Such a vessel is probably equivalent to what has historically been termed the accessory sinus of Kelch, ophthalmopetrous sinus of Hyrtl, and accessory sinus of Verga. (Courtesy Dr. Joel Curé.)

the sphenoparietal sinus.[1,14–18] A dural arteriovenous fistula is defined as an abnormal connection between an arterial feeder and a dural venous sinus or leptomeningeal vein with the nidus located within the dural leaflets.[19] A majority of these fistulas seem to present secondary to a traumatic event, usually associated with an underlying skull fracture.[14,15,19,20] Nomura et al.[17] goes on to state that sphenoparietal sinus dural AVFs are known to be associated with pulsatile exophthalmos, whereas sphenopetrosal sinus involvement may present with tinnitus or even no obvious symptoms. In a report by Smith et al.,[15] there were two cases of middle meningeal vein and sphenoparietal sinus AVF, both of which were associated with a demonstrable skull fracture. Similarly, Bitoh et al.[16] presented a 14-year-old boy who also developed a dural arteriovenous malformation in the region of the sphenoparietal sinus, which was associated with a dilated dural sinus. In this case, the arterial supply was solely via the meningeal braches of the left external carotid artery with venous drainage through dilated venous channels into the superior ophthalmic vein and pterygoid venous plexus.[16] Arteriovenous fistulas do not occur solely after traumatic injury, but they can also present postoperatively. In a case report by Tsutsumi et al.,[18] there was a postoperative middle meningeal AVF found after craniotomy on a patient who previously had a surgical repair of an aneurysm.

In a large-scale study by Kakarla et al.,[19] 53 patients were identified with high-risk dural arteriovenous fistulas (DAVFs). Of the 53 fistulas identified, only 3 involved the sphenoparietal sinus; however, each was associated with an intracranial hemorrhage. After proper endovascular therapy including arterial embolization, all patients had a Glasgow outcome scale score of 5 on their final follow-up appoint.

SURGERY

Dural arteriovenous fistulas account for 10%–15% of all intracranial AV shunts. The fistula is dependent on the venous drainage pattern. If the intracranial DAVF drains anterograde into a major dural sinus, then the course is usually benign, whereas if the flow is retrograde into arterialized leptomeningeal veins, then there tends to be a more aggressive course.[21] According to Nelson et al.,[22] ligation of the proximal feeding artery alone by using endovascular or surgical methods is insufficient as the arterial supply of the fistula is invariably reestablished. For this reason, transvenous embolization has proven useful in treating many DAVFs by obliterating the fistula and sacrificing the recipient venous structure.[22] In the study of three sphenoparietal sinus AVFs, two underwent preoperative embolization and one required a temporal or frontotemporal craniotomy to ligate the fistulous site.[19]

The middle meningeal artery and the orbitomeningeal arteries may be interrupted extradurally; however, arterial embolization of the fistula endovascularly may reduce the risk of a surgical approach. Usually, a lack of transvenous or transarterial access can prevent effective endovascular management of the fistula. With simple exposure of the sinus, a craniotomy or craniectomy can provide access and enable complete endovascular obliteration of the fistula.[19] In a case report by Kattner et al.,[21] after an attempted arterial embolization of a sphenoparietal DAVF, a cranial base technique was used. Initially, the embolization was unsuccessful because the feeding artery could not be safely cannulated. To combat this issue, the fistula was approached via a standard pterional craniotomy, an extradural approach. The sphenoid bone was removed, which allowed exposure of the left ophthalmic artery as it entered the sphenoparietal sinus. The artery was coagulated and cut at this location, which kept the sinus from being resected. Transarterial or transvenous endovascular approach is usually the first-line treatment with a good long-term obliteration rate. However, the redirection of flow may result in postoperative hemorrhage.[21]

Another approach to treating complex DAVFs could also include a wedge microcatheter and a liquid embolic agent.[23] In a study of 21 patients, one patient had a DAVF, which involved the sphenoparietal sinus. All patients were treated using transarterial *N*-butyl cyanoacrylate (NBCA) with the aid of a wedge catheter. This approach established an effective embolization point closer to the fistula, thereby facilitating both delivery of the liquid across the fistula site and permeation of the perifistulous collateral network. After 16 months of follow-up, the patient with a sphenoparietal AVF was found to have normal functioning and a Glasgow outcome scale of 5. No residual fistula or arteriovenous malformation was noted postoperatively.[22]

REFERENCES

1. Tubbs RS, Salter E, Wellons III J, Blount JB, Oakes WJ. The sphenoparietal sinus. *Neurosurgery*. 2007;60:1–5.
2. Chung J, Weon Y. Anatomic variations of the superficial middle cerebral vein: embryologic aspects of the regressed embryonic tentorial sinus. *Interv Radiol*. 2005;11:115–122.
3. Padget D. The cranial venous system in man in reference to development, adult configuration and relation to the arteries. *Am J Anat*. 1956;98:307–355.
4. Ruíz D, Fasel J, Rufenacht D, Gailloud P. The sphenoparietal sinus of Breschet: does it exist? An anatomic study. *AJNR Am J Neuroradiol*. 2004;25:112–120.
5. Nagata T, Ishibashi K, Metwally H, et al. Analysis of venous drainage from sylvian veins in clinoidal meningiomas. *World Neurosurg*. 2011;79:116–123.
6. Takahashi S, Sakuma I, Otani T, et al. Venous anatomy of the sphenoparietal sinus: evaluation by MR imaging. *Intervent Neuroradiol*. 2007;13:84–89.
7. Morris P. *Practical Neuroangiography*. 2nd ed. Philadelphia: Lippincott and Wilkins; 2007:276–278.
8. Frigeri T, Paglioli E, Olivera E, Rhoton A. Microsurgical anatomy of the central lobe. *J Neurosurg*. 2015;122:483–498.
9. Suzuki Y, Matsumoto K. Variations of the superficial middle cerebral vein: classification using three-dimensional CT angiography. *AJNR Am J Neuroradiol*. 2000;21:932–938.
10. Curé Van Tassel P, Smith T. Normal and variant anatomy of the dural venous sinuses. *Semin Ultrasound CT MRI*. 1994;15:499–519.
11. Browder J, Kaplan H. *Cerebral Dural Sinuses and Their Tributaries*. Springfield: Charles C Thomas; 1998:85–87.
12. Tubbs RS, Loukas M, Shoja MM, Oakes WJ. Accessory venous sinus of Hyrtl. *Folia Morphol*. 2007;66:198–199.
13. Scott J, Farb R. Imaging and anatomy of the normal intracranial venous system. *Neuroimaging Clin*. 2003;13:1–12.
14. Sakata H, Nishimura S, Mino M, et al. Serial angiography of dynamic changes of traumatic middle meningeal arteriovenous fistula. *Neurol Med -Chir*. 2009;49:462–464.
15. Smith J, Epps J, Press H, Adair L. Traumatic arteriovenous fistula between the middle meningeal artery and the sphenoparietal sinus: a case report and review of the world literature. *J Natl Med Assoc*. 1981;73:274–278.
16. Bitoh S, Arita N, Fujiwara M, Ozaki K, Nakao Y. Dural arteriovenous malformation near the left sphenoparietal sinus. *Surg Neurol*. 1980;13:345–349.
17. Nomura S, Anegawa S, Nakagawa S, Tomokiyo M, Koga H, Hayashi T. Subarachnoid hemorrhage caused by dural arteriovenous fistula of the sphenobasal sinus. *Neurol Med -Chir*. 2002;42:255–258.
18. Tsutsumi K, Shiokawa Y, Kubota M, Aoki N, Mizutani H. Postoperative arteriovenous fistula between the middle meningeal artery and the sphenoparietal sinus. *Neurosurgery*. 1990;26:869–871.
19. Kakarla U, Deshmukh V, Zabramski J, Albuquerque FC, McDougall CG, Spetzler RF. Surgical treatment of high-risk intracranial dural arteriovenous fistulae: clinical outcomes and avoidance of complications. *Neurosurgery*. 2007;61:447–459.
20. Unterhofer C, Chemelli A, Waldenberger P, Bauer R, Ortler M. Traumatic fistula between the middle meningeal artery and the sphenoparietal sinus. *Acta Neurochir*. 2009;151:1301–1304.

21. Kattner K, Roth T, Nardone E, Giannotta S. The treatment of complex dural arteriorvenous fistulae through cranial base techniques. *Neurol India*. 2004;52:325–331.
22. Nelson PK, Russell SM, Woo HH, Alastra AJ, Vidovich DV. Use of a wedge microcatheter for curative transarterial embolization of complex intracranial dural arteriovenous fistulas: indications, endovascular technique and outcomes in 21 patients. *J Neurosurg*. 2003;98:498–506.
23. Osbun J, Kim L, Spetzler R, McDougall C. Aberrant venous drainage pattern in a medial sphenoid wing dural arteriovenous fistula: a case report and review of the literature. *World Neurosurg*. 2013;80:381–386.

CHAPTER 18

The Lateral Lacunae

R. SHANE TUBBS

There is scant and conflicting information in the literature, including the neurosurgical literature, regarding the lateral lacunae (lateral lakes of Trolard) (Figs. 18.1–18.6). The lacunae may be synonymous with the glandulae conglobatae as described by Pacchioni. Interestingly, this author believed these structures secreted lymph that lubricated the sliding movements between the brain and meninges.[1]

Crosby[2] stated that the parameningeal veins empty into the lacunae and that in the young adult, there are three of these structures on either side, but they tend to coalesce later on to form one or two. These authors also stated that the lacunae as well as the Pacchionian granulations (large arachnoid granulations) are absent at birth. Le Gros Clark[3] identified the lacunae as increasing in size with age and as developing pari passu with the growth of the arachnoid granulations. However, this author identified the lacunae as forming before the granulations and as being responsible for the depressions of the inner table of the skull found overlying them. O'Connell[4] stressed that few granulations are found projecting into the venous sinuses and that the vast majority (up to four times the amount found in the cranial venous sinuses)[5] project into the lacunae, which in the adult are carpeted with arachnoid granulations. Rhoton[6] stated that the arachnoid granulations project into the floor and walls of the lacunae. Of note, parasagittal meningiomas usually arise from the arachnoid granulations of the lacunae.[6]

Woodburne[7] stated that these venous lakes are found only at parietal levels and that many of the cerebral veins empty into them. Clemente[8] also thought that most of the cerebral veins open into the lacunae, but O'Connell[4] found that these dilatations do not receive drainage from cortical veins. Hollinshead[9] reported that the lacunae are irregular expansions, and Clemente[8] published that the lacunae are usually three in number on each side of the sagittal sinus. This author described these as a small frontal, a large parietal, and an occipital, which was intermediate in size.

O'Connell[4] found that the lacunae develop after birth from a plexus formed by the union of the meningeal and diploic veins and that after middle age, they become reduced to a single pair, one on each side of the superior sagittal sinus.

Tubbs et al.[10] studied 35 adult cadavers and found a mean of 1.9 lacunae (range 0–3) were found on right sides and a mean of 1.4 (0–3) lacunae were seen on left sides. Although there tended to be slightly more lacunae on right sides, this did not reach statistical significance ($P > .05$). The average length of the lacunae was 3.2 cm (range 1.5–6 cm) for right sides and 2.0 cm (range 1.1–3.2 cm) for left sides. The mean width of these venous lakes was 1.5 cm for right sides (range 0.8–3.4 cm) and 0.8 cm for left sides (range 0.4–1.2 cm). Lacunae were variably positioned but tended to cluster near the vertex of the skull. No lacunae were identified posterior to the lambdoid sutures, and only five lacunae were found to lie anterior to the coronal suture with four of these located on the right ($P < .05$). When lacunae were identified anterior to the coronal suture, they were generally 5–6 cm from this structure. The vast majority of lacunae could be identified between the coronal and lambdoid sutures and within 3 cm of the midline.

Some have described a venous plexus that exists alongside the superior sagittal sinus in newborn infants and adults.[3,4] These could represent remnants of the embryologic superior sagittal sinus, which begins as two parallel structures that then coalesce.[11] Fox et al.[12] questioned whether or not large channels identified in infants greater than 37 weeks' gestation were lacunae. They hypothesized that these channels may "evolve" into the lacunae. Gómez et al.[13] found that the lacunae develop in a frontal direction.

Functionally, Portnoy et al.[14] found that the lacunae act as a Starling resistor and control venous outflow resistance and thus aide in autoregulation of blood flow. Shakhnovich et al.[15] posited that obstruction to venous outflow at the level of the lacunae and bridging veins may contribute to benign intracranial hypertension.

In regard to variation, Crosby[2] stated that sometimes the sphenoparietal sinus continues lateralward and upward, accompanying an anterior branch of the

Anatomy, Imaging and Surgery of the Intracranial Dural Venous Sinuses. https://doi.org/10.1016/B978-0-323-65377-0.00018-0

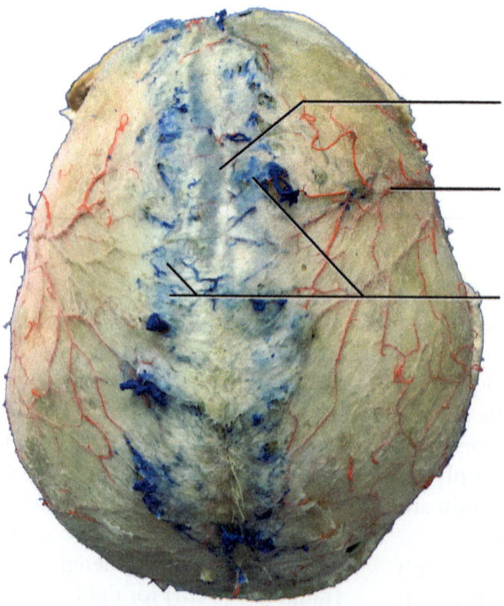

FIG. 18.1 Removed cadaveric dura mater following latex injection of the dural venous sinuses.

middle meningeal artery, to communicate with the superior sagittal sinus via the lacunae.[16] Rhoton[6] found that the lacunae receive predominantly the drainage from the meningeal veins and that contrary to some authors,[3] he did find sites of communication between cortical veins and the lacunae although these usually passed inferior to rather than emptying directly into the lacunae to reach the superior sagittal sinus. Additionally, some lacunae were found to share a common opening into the sinus with cortical veins. Interestingly, O'Connell[4] observed that thrombus was never found in the lacunae at postmortem examination.

Topographically, Rhoton[6] found that the lacunae are largest and most constant in the parietal and posterior frontal regions and that smaller lakes are seen in the occipital and frontal regions and on occasion, separate lacunae are replaced by a single lacuna on each side of the superior sagittal sinus. This is opposed to the description of others that found the lacunae as mostly related to the posterior part of the superior sagittal sinus.[13] This author further described the lacunae as extending as far as 3 cm lateral to the midline and spread out over the upper extent of the precentral, central, and postcentral gyri. O'Connell[4] described these structures as having an average length and width of 15 and 3 cm, respectively. Callander[17] has said that the most important of these lacunae overlie the anterior and posterior central convolutions and that the arachnoid granulations almost completely fill the lacunae and by pressure atrophy even cause depressions on the undersurface of the cranium. This author stated further that operative intervention may be attended by serious hemorrhage because it is difficult to remove the bone from the dura mater without tearing the thinned-out dura overlying these lacunae.

Operatively, Rhoton[6] found that entering or occluding a lacuna at operation does not necessarily result in occlusion of adjacent cortical veins or the superior sagittal sinus. Hollinshead[18] stated that "the position of the superior sagittal sinus, its enlargement as it runs posteriorly, and the occurrence of the lacunae in connection with it must be taken into account in trephine operations upon the calvaria." This author concluded that "the lacunae so increase its (superior sagittal sinus) width that in trephining over the posterior half of the parietal region, where the lacunae are largest and most constant, the medial edge of the trephine should be not much closer than 2 cm to the midline." In a previous report, we[19] found that the superior sagittal sinus deviated up to 1.1 cm lateral to the overlying sagittal suture usually on right sides. With our study on the lateral lacunae, we found that the lateral lacunae were on average approximately 3 cm lateral to the sagittal suture for both left and right sides. Surgically and if an option, the operator could tailor incisions and bone removal between the coronal and lambdoid sutures and greater than 3 cm lateral to the midline and, based on our findings, avoid the majority of these lateral lacunae.

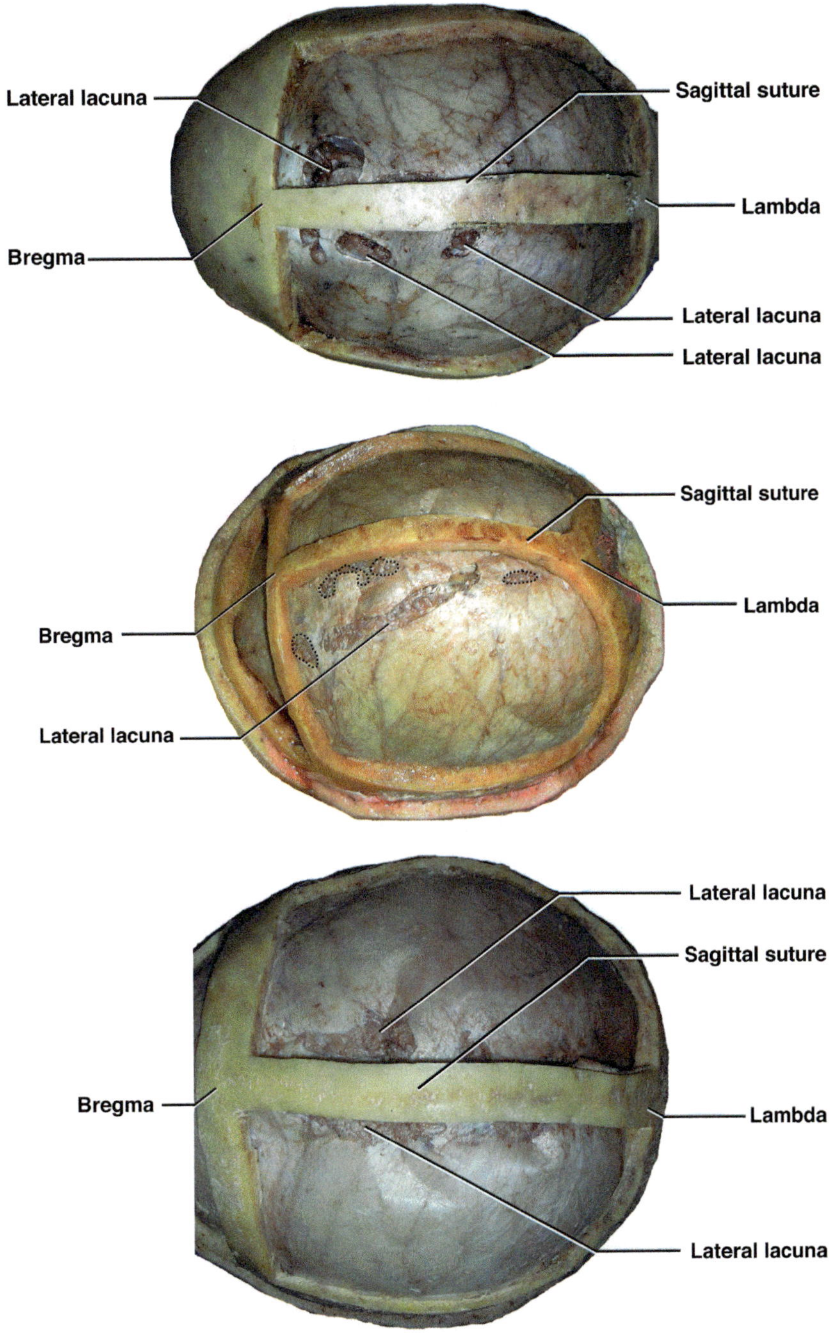

FIGS. 18.2–18.6 Cadaveric dissections following removal of most of the calvaria but leaving the sutures so that the underlying lateral lacunae and their relationships to these bony structures can be seen.

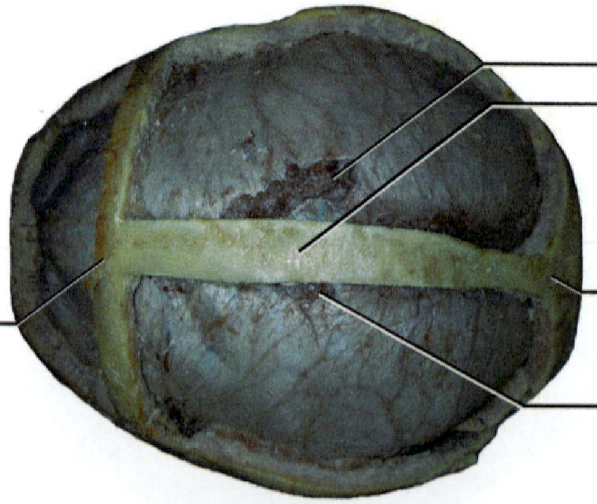

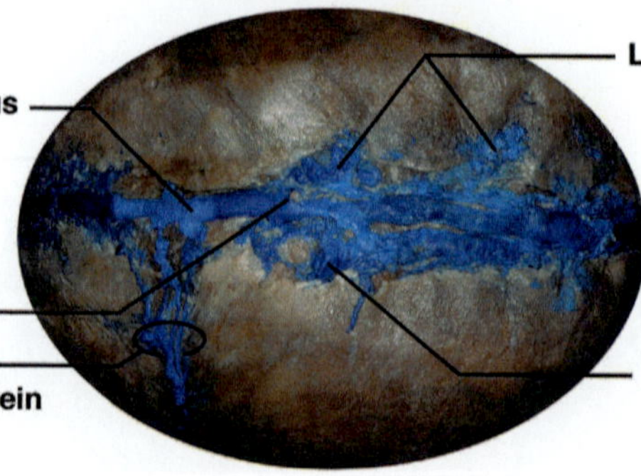

FIGS. 18.2-18.6, cont'd

These structures could also be further localized with preoperative imaging (e.g., skull radiographs in which the bony depression caused by the lacuna can be identified).[20]

Regarding connections to the cerebral veins and superior sagittal sinus, our findings echoed those of Rhoton[6] with only occasional connections found between these structures and the lateral lacunae. Therefore, one would not expect the majority of patients to experience sequelae from hemostasis used to treat a bleeding lateral lacuna.

REFERENCES

1. Brunoir A, Vagnozzi R, Giuffrè R. Antonio Pacchioni (1665–1726): early studies of the dura mater. *J Neurosurg*. 1993;78:515–518.
2. Crosby EC. *Correlative Anatomy of the Nervous System*. New York: The Macmillan Company; 1962:568.
3. Le Gros Clark WE. On the pacchionian bodies. *J Anat*. 1920;55:40–48.
4. O'Connell JEA. Some observation of the cerebral veins. *Brain*. 1934;57:484–503.
5. Browder J, Browder A, Kaplan HA. Anatomical relationships of the cerebral and dural venous systems in the parasagittal area. *Anat Rec*. 1973;176:329–332.
6. Rhoton AL. The cerebral veins. *Neurosurgery*. 2002;51:159–205.
7. Woodburne RT. *Essentials of Human Anatomy*. New York: Oxford University Press; 1978:275.
8. Clemente C. *Gray's Anatomy*. 30th ed. Philadelphia: Lea& Febiger; 1985:809.
9. Hollinshead WH. *Anatomy for Surgeons*. New York: Harper & Row; 1954:12.
10. Tubbs RS, Loukas M, Shoja MM, Apaydin N, Ardalan MR, Oakes WJ. Lateral lakes of Trolard: anatomy, quantitation, and surgical landmarks. Laboratory investigation. *J Neurosurg*. 2008;108:1005–1009.
11. Tubbs RS, Loukas M. Duplication of the superior sagittal sinus. *Clin Anat*. 2006;19:728.
12. Fox RJ, Walji AH, Mielke B, Petruk K, Aronyk KE. Anatomic details of intradural channels in the parasagittal dura: a possible pathway for flow of cerebrospinal fluid. *Neurosurgery*. 1996;39:84–91.
13. Gómez DG, Di Bendetto AT, Pavese AM, Firpo A, Hershan DB, Potts DG. Development of arachnoid villi and granulations in man. *Acta Anat*. 1981;111:247–258.

14. Portnoy HD, Branch C, Castro ME. The relationship of intracranial venous pressure to hydrocephalus. *Childs Nerv Syst*. 1994;10:29–35.
15. Shakhnovich AR, Razumovsky AY, Gasparjan SS, Ozerova VI. Venous and cerebrospinal fluid outflow in patients with brain swelling and oedema. *Acta Neurochir*. 1990;51:357–361.
16. Tubbs RS, Salter EG, Wellons 3rd JC, Blount JP, Oakes WJ. The sphenoparietal sinus. *Neurosurgery*. 2007;60:9–12.
17. Callander CL. *Surgical Anatomy*. 2nd ed. Philadelphia: W. B. Saunders Company; 1939:30–31.
18. Hollinshead WH. *Anatomy for Surgeons*. 2nd ed. New York: Harper & Row; 1968:13–14.
19. Tubbs RS, Salter G, Elton S, Grabb PA, Oakes WJ. Sagittal suture as an external landmark for the superior sagittal sinus. *J Neurosurg*. 2001;94:985–987.
20. Meschan I. *An Atlas of Anatomy Basic to Radiology*. Philadelphia: WB Saunders; 1975.

CHAPTER 19

The Petrosquamosal Sinus

DIEGO SAN MILLÁN

ABBREVIATIONS

EJV	External jugular vein
IJV	Internal jugular vein
PSS	Petrosquamosal sinus
PTCS	Pseudotumor cerebri
VVS	Vertebral venous system

BACKGROUND

In humans, most of the cerebral venous drainage reaches the posterior fossa before being directed primarily toward the internal jugular veins (IJVs) or the vertebral venous system (VVS), the latter comprising the internal vertebral venous plexus (epidural venous plexus), the vertebral artery venous plexus, and the deep cervical veins.[1] There is a postural dependency of the encephalic drainage toward the IJV and the VVS, with dominance toward the IJV in the supine position and transfer of the IJV outflow to the VVS when standing upright.[2–5]

The external jugular veins (EJVs) in humans are primarily involved in the venous drainage of the viscero- and neurocranium, with a variable, but generally limited, participation in the cerebral venous drainage itself, mainly as an effluent of the pterygoid plexus. Schematically, encephalic drainage therefore occurs through three descending venous drainage pathways on each side of the neck: the IJV, the VVS, and the EJV.

Two possible pathways connecting the cerebral drainage to the EJV system exist. The most common pathway involves the drainage of the superficial and deep middle cerebral veins (SMCV and DMCV) into the pterygoid plexus by way of the cavernous, laterocavernous, or paracavernous sinuses and their outflow through the emissary veins of the middle cranial fossa.[6,7] The second pathway involves a connection between the rostral portion of the transverse sinus and the veins of the temporal fossa through a petrosquamosal sinus (PSS).[8–12] This pathway normally regresses during fetal and early postnatal life and may be absent in the human adult. Whereas the drainage PSS-EJV pathway is prominent in strepsirrhines[a] and in most nonprimate mammals such as dogs, sheep, rabbits, and horses, it is rarely of any significance in humans, most catarrhine primates,[b] and some nonprimate mammals including cats and pigs, in whom the IJV and VVS represent the major venous outflow pathways.[13–15]

Since the early descriptions attributed to Rathke and Luschka, the embryology and morphology of the PSS have been extensively documented in humans, mostly in postmortem anatomic studies.[9–14,16–20] A phylogenetic role of the PSS has been suggested by several authors.[11,14] A radiologic description of the PSS was first provided by Marsot-Dupuch et al.[21] in 2001. Since then, various clinical reports have focused on the potential role of the PSS in humans and its clinical significance.

DEVELOPMENTAL CONSIDERATIONS

The development of the PSS and its connections to the EJV seem to be a constant feature in the early development of all mammalian embryos.[11] The degree of subsequent involution of the PSS is correlated to the growing dominance of the IJV over the EJV, which itself seems to be determined by the relative development of the brain over the face.[9] Conroy[14] corroborated this view, suggesting that the development of the telencephalon and its caudal expansion over the cerebellum, observed in catarrhine primates (including humans), is at the origin of the modifications taking place in the dural venous sinuses of the posterior and middle cranial fossae. The transverse sinus is, in the early human embryo as in most

[a]The suborder strepsirrhini includes the lemurs and lorises (Classification phylogénétique du vivant. Eds. Le Guyader H and Lecointre G. Paris: Belin 2001).

[b]The superfamily of catarrhini includes the cercopithecidae (Old World monkeys), hominidae (humans, gorilla, chimpanzee, bonobo, orangutan), and hylobatidae (gibbons) (Classification phylogénétique du vivant. Eds. Le Guyader H and Lecointre G. Paris: Belin 2001).

Anatomy, Imaging and Surgery of the Intracranial Dural Venous Sinuses. https://doi.org/10.1016/B978-0-323-65377-0.00019-2

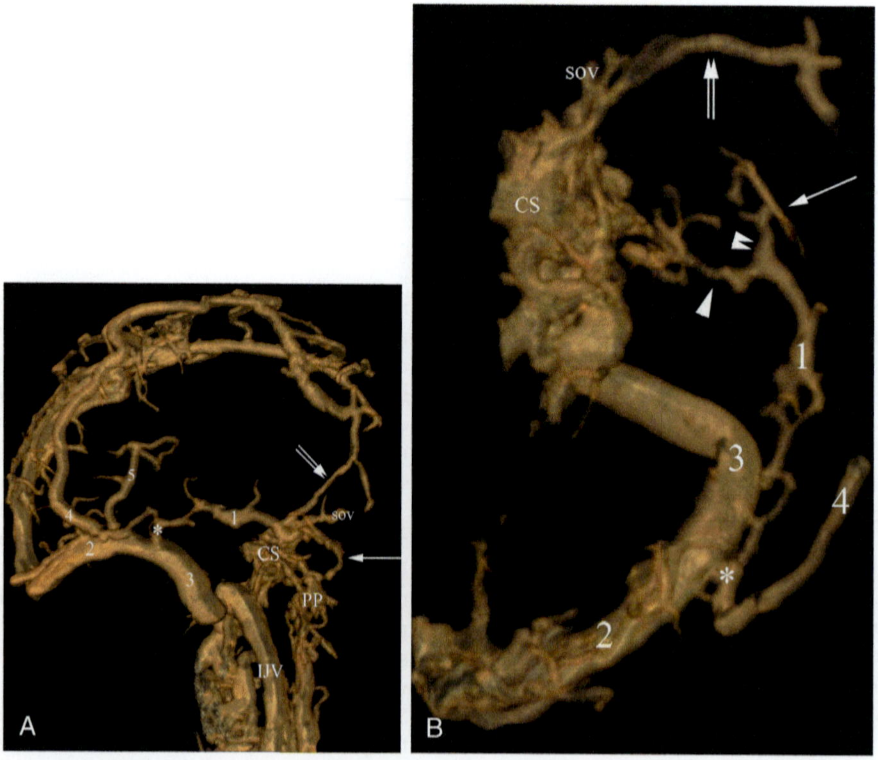

FIG. 19.1 3D images after reconstruction of a CT of a corrosion cast of the cranial venous system. The cortical veins have been virtually dissected. **(A)** Right lateral view showing a PSS. 1, the transverse sinus; 2, the sigmoid sinus; 3, the cavernous sinus (CS), a temporoparietal diploic vein; 4, the internal jugular vein (IJV), the pterygoid plexus (PP), and the superior ophthalmic vein (SOV). The PSS is connected to the transverse sinus/sigmoid sinus junction (asterisk). Close to this point, the PSS receives a posterior temporoparietal diploic vein. The *single arrow* points at a deep temporal vein. The *double arrow* represents the sphenoparietal sinus, which drained a large anterior parietal diploic vein into the cavernous sinus. **(B)** Superior view of the right middle cranial fossa. Same legend as 1**(A)**. The connection of the PSS with the emissary veins of the middle cranial fossa (foramen ovale) is marked by an *arrowhead*. The *double arrowhead* indicates the connection with the deep temporal vein through an SJF. The sphenoparietal sinus (*double arrow*) courses over the superior ophthalmic vein (SOV) and joins the anterior superior aspect of the cavernous sinus (CS). (From San Millan Ruiz D, Gailloud P, Yilmaz H, et al. The petrosquamosal sinus in humans. *J Anat.* 2006;209:711–720 reprint with permission.)

mammals, vertically oriented and follows a craniocaudal course. At this stage, the sigmoid sinus and the PSS have similar diameters. The caudal expansion of the telencephalon over the cerebellum will later displace the transverse sinus from a vertical to a horizontal position. Conroy[14] has suggested that this reorientation leads to the regression of the PSS, with the sigmoid sinus then becoming the major outflow pathway of the transverse sinus. Inversely, in animals with a lesser telencephalic development and a persistent verticality of the transverse sinus, the PSS is likely to be retained as the major outflow pathway of the transverse sinus. The crossroad in embryologic development during which the growth of the hemispheres will modify the orientation of the transverse sinus begins around stage 6 (embryos in horizons XX, XXI, 18–26 mm stage).[9] This is concomitant to the development of the definite EJV, which not only begins to drain the PSS but also takes over, to a variable degree, the primitive facial tributaries of the IJV.

ANATOMY

The PSS arises in the temporal bone at or in the vicinity of the transverse sinus (TS) and its junction with the superior petrosal sinus (SPS)/sigmoid sinus (SS) (Figs. 19.1–19.3). It runs anteriorly along or in the vicinity of the petrosquamosal fissure, either within an osseous groove or a complete canal referred to as the temporal canal of Vergi[13] (Fig. 19.2).

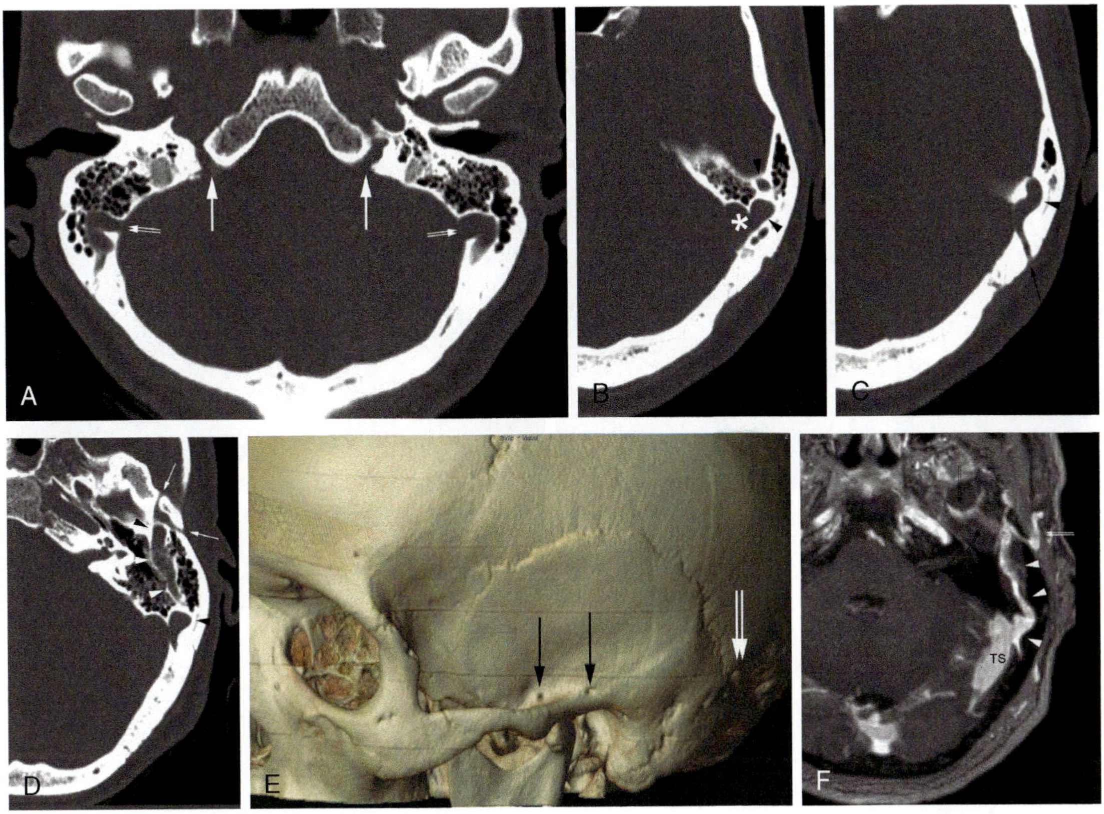

FIG. 19.2 43-year-old woman presenting with vertigo. Bilateral aplasia of the distal sigmoid sinus, which terminates into a prominent mastoid emissary vein on each side (**A**, *double arrow*). The pars vascularis of the jugular foramen is absent (**B**, *arrow*). On the left, a relatively large complete PSS (**B** and **D**, *arrowheads*). A few millimeters from its origin **(C)**, the PSS gives a posteriorly coursing branch corresponding to an anomalous mastoid emissary vein (*black arrow*) that exits the skull at the upper portion of the mastoid; all connect ultimately to the EJV (see **G** and **H**). Anteriorly, the PSS connects with the temporal veins by way of two SJFs at the base of the zygomatic process of the temporal bone (**D** and **E**, *arrows*). The orifice of the anomalous mastoid emissary vein draining the PSS posteriorly is also visible on the volume-rendered reconstruction of the skull (**E**, *double arrow*). The anteromedial (*black double arrows*) and anterolateral (*white double arrows*) portions of the PSS (*arrowheads*) are demonstrated on (**F**).

The PSS thus generally shares characteristics of both meningeal and a diploic vein in some portion of its course. In its full persistent form, the PSS maintains two venous connections with the EJV:

1. anterolaterally with the deep temporal veins through an emissary canal located around the glenoid fossa, called the postglenoid foramen (PGF) or the spurious jugular foramen (SJF), the preferred term hereafter[8–11,13,14,19] (Figs. 19.1 and 19.2);
2. anteromedially, after coursing as a meningeal vein in the middle cranial fossa, generally with the emissary vein of the foramen ovale[12] or the foramen spinosum[22] to join the pterygoid plexus (Figs. 19.1 and 19.2).

The PSS in its full, persistent form presents less frequently than an incomplete PSS in which some portions have regressed completely. It would seem that the connection of the PSS with the middle meningeal veins and the transverse sinus persist more frequently than the lateral connection with the deep temporal veins through an SJF. In a venous corrosion cast study,[12] only one of the five identified PSS (Fig. 19.1) had retained a connection with the veins of the temporal fossa, although this could have been an underestimation because of imperfect venous filling in the remaining corrosion casts. The rare observation of temporal foramina in human skulls, reported in 8 of 1500 dry skulls (0.53%) by Boyd,[19] in 23 out of 2585 (0.88%) by Cheatle,[8] and in 5 of 200 dry skull sides (3.5%) by Wysocki,[13] is in accordance with the loss of the connection between the PSS and the deep temporal veins.

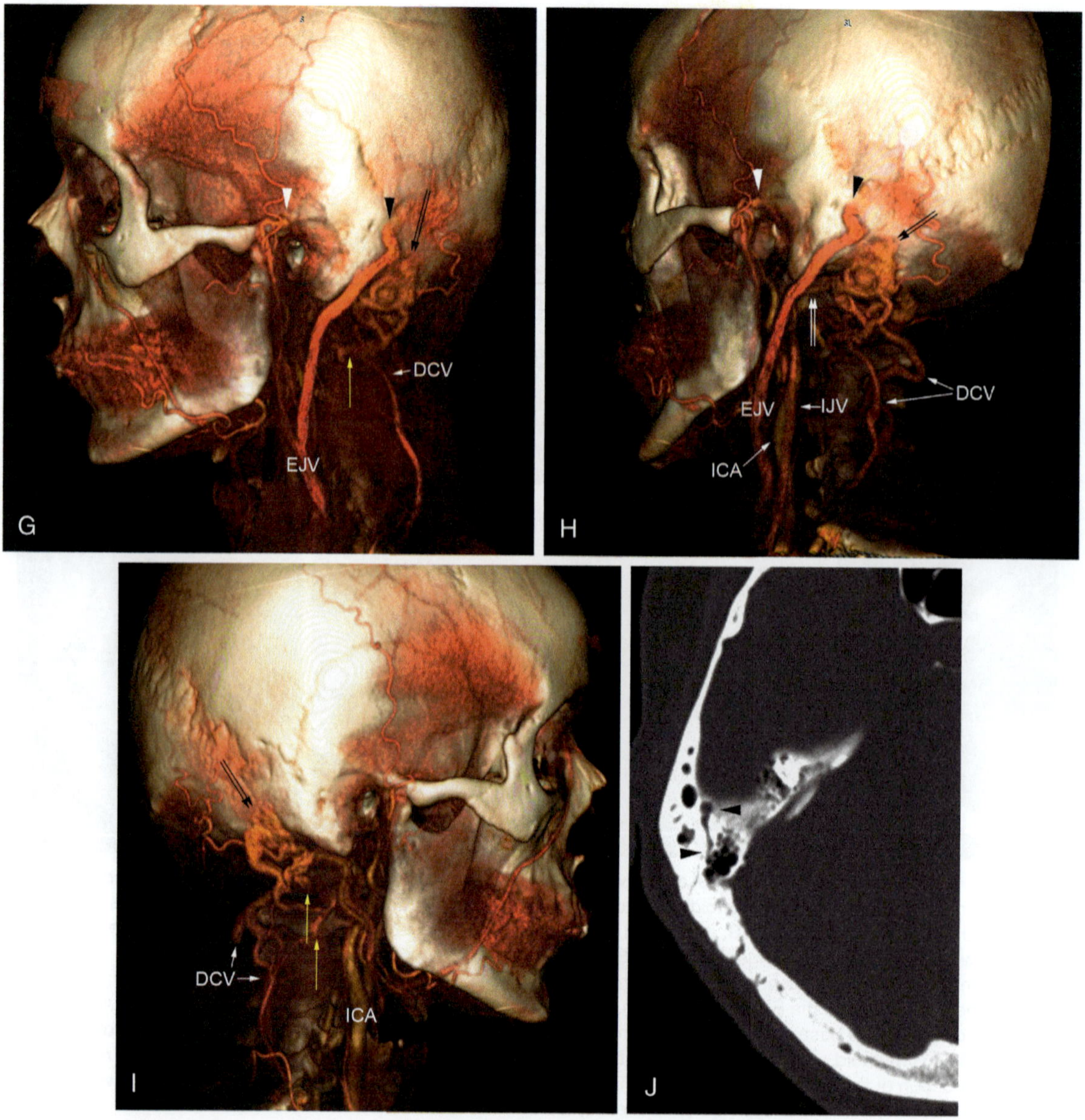

FIG. 19.2, cont'd The temporal (*white arrowhead*) and occipital (*black arrowhead*) veins that, respectively, drain the anterolateral and posterior branches of the left PSS are shown in (**G** and **H**); they both join the EJV system (EJV) in the neck. The internal carotid artery (ICA) is visible next to a rudimentary left IJV (IJV). The IJV was formed by the inferior petrosal sinus (not shown) and a connecting vein (*double white arrow*) with the mastoid emissary vein (*double black arrow*) in (**H**). The deep cervical veins (DCV), which are part of the VVS, participate in the drainage of the left mastoid emissary vein in (**G** and **H**). On the left side of the neck, no IJV is visible (**I**). The left mastoid emissary vein (*double black arrow*) is the only drainage pathway of the left sigmoid sinus, the terminal portion of which is aplastic (not shown). This prominent mastoid emissary drains into the deep cervical vein (DCV) and the vertebral artery venous plexus (*yellow arrows*). A small incomplete PSS was also noted on the right side (**J**, *black arrowheads*). In this patient, the only existing IJV was the left one, and it was not directly involved in encephalic drainage, as the terminal portion of the sigmoid sinus was absent. On the left, two descending venous drainage pathways existed, the EJV and the VVS. On the right, the VVS drained the bulk of the encephalic venous blood entering the transverse and sigmoid sinuses, although connections between the VVS and a small IJV were also present (**H**, *double white arrow*). The right EJV received no encephalic drainage as the SMCV/DMCV drained into a paracavernous sinus that joined the transverse sinus. The patient had no signs of PTCS or any symptoms attributable to this venous anomaly. **(A–D)** Axial noncontrast CT; **(E)** volume-rendered 3D reconstruction of noncontrast CT; **(F)** MRI, MIP axial reconstruction of gadolinium-enhanced 3DT1 MPRAGE; **(G–I)** CT angiography, volume-rendered 3D reconstruction; **(J)** axial noncontrast CT.

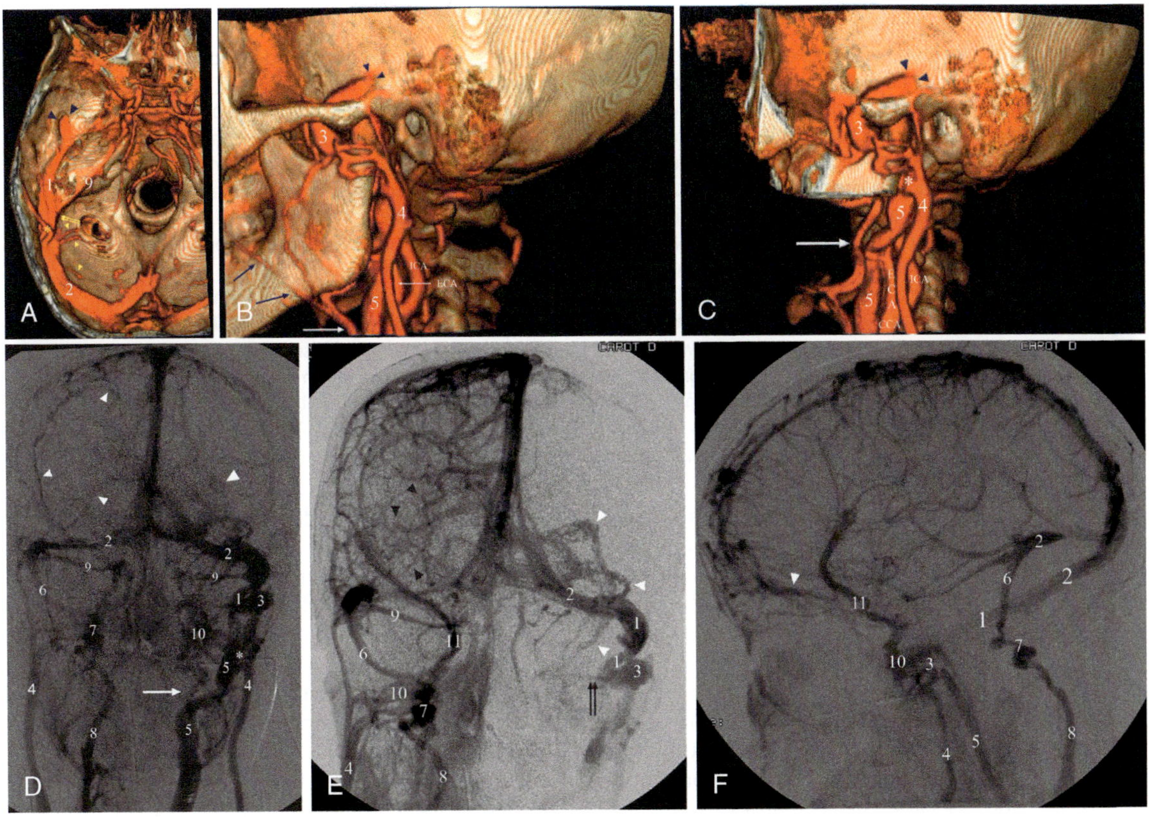

FIG. 19.3 A 7-year-old girl with history of cluster headache since the age of 3 years and new severe and constant of postural-dependant headache possibly related to cranial venous hypertension. **(A–C)** 3D reconstruction of angio-CT images. **(A)** Superior view of the left cranial fossa showing the left transverse sinus (2) draining anteriorly through a large PSS (1). The anterior-lateral branch of the PSS exits the middle cranial fossa through a PGF (*blue arrowheads*). The size of the PSS is identical to the transverse sinus. No left sigmoid sinus is observed. The transverse sinus receives several infratentorial veins (*yellow arrowheads*) and a lateral temporal vein (*yellow asterisk*). The superior petrosal sinus (9) joins the stem of the PSS (*double yellow arrows*). **(B and C)** Left lateral view centered on the external auditory canal before **(B)** and after virtual dissection of the left zygomatic process and ramus of the mandible **(C)**. The PSS opens into enlarged deep temporal veins (2) via an SJF (*blue arrowheads*). The deep temporal veins communicate with the external jugular vein (EJV) (4), and with a "hybrid jugular vein" that initially courses for a short distance in the carotid sheath and then terminates as an anomalous anterior jugular vein. A deep facial vein draining the pterygoid plexus is joined by a superficial facial vein (*blue arrows*) and forms a common facial vein (*white arrow*). The point at which the deep temporal veins join the EJV and the "hybrid jugular vein" is marked by a white asterisk. Note venous branches from the deep temporal veins going around the condyle of the mandible and forming a venous arch. The white arrow shows a left common facial vein, which was seen to drain caudally into the middle portion of the "hybrid jugular vein." *CCA*, common carotid artery. **(D–F)** Digital subtraction angiography (DSA). Aside from confirming the CTA findings, DSA disclosed signs of venous hypertension, partial obstruction of the superior sagittal sinus draining cortical veins from the left convexity (not shown), and compensatory collateral drainage through an enlarged system of diploic veins on both sides. **(D)** Late venous phase obtained after injection of contrast agent into the ascending aorta, anteroposterior view. Same legend as in previous figures. The absence of the left sigmoid sinus is confirmed. The right transverse sinus is hypoplastic and connects to a sigmoid sinus (6), the terminal portion of which is aplastic. The sigmoid sinus drains into a posterior condylar emissary vein (7) and into a deep cervical vein (8). Note the absence of a right IJV. The left pterygoid plexus (10) is prominent and drains into a large deep facial vein, which ultimately becomes a common facial vein (*white arrow*). Cortical veins have washed out at this stage,

continued

and only a few prominent diploic veins are recognizable (*white arrowheads*) on both sides, compatible with collateral venous flow. **(E)** Early venous phase after right ICA injection, anteroposterior view. There is simultaneous opacification of the transverse sinuses. Contralateral drainage into the PSS is conspicuous. The anterior-medial connection of the PSS with the middle meningeal veins (not seen here) is faintly opacified (*double black arrow*). A right laterocavernous sinus (11) transverses a prominent superficial middle cerebral vein and drains into a large pterygoid plexus (10). This drainage pattern was also seen on the left side (not shown). The cortical veins (*black arrowheads*) on the right display a "corkscrew" appearance, suggesting a certain degree of venous hypertension. Note that prominent diploic veins have already appeared on the left (*white arrowheads*). **(F)** Lateral view, right ICA injection, slightly earlier venous phase than **(E)**, confirming the absence of the left sigmoid sinus. The prominent left diploic veins seen in **(E)** are within the frontal bone and drain into the supraorbital veins by way of a large orbital diploic vein (*arrowhead*). The cavernous sinuses and the inferior petrosal sinuses were never observed. In this case, the descending venous drainage pathways of the neck are severely congenitally restricted, which, in association with possible old dural venous sinus thrombosis and right proximal transverse sinus hypoplasia, likely contributed to clinical signs of raised intracranial pressure. (From San Millan Ruiz D, Gailloud P, Yilmaz H, et al. The petrosquamosal sinus in humans. *J Anat.* 2006;209:711–720 reprint with permission.)

In adults, the remnants of the PSS can drain a posterior temporal diploic vein and superior tympanic veins[8,9,23] and are also involved in the meningeal venous drainage of the middle cranial fossa.[12]

INCIDENCE OF A PSS IN HUMANS

Remnants of the PSS in a partial form are not a rare finding in the human adult. Knott[24] found 19 unilateral and 7 bilateral PSS in 44 adult cadavers, representing 30% of the sides. Cheatle[8] stated that it was "the rule rather than the exception for remains of the sinus [the PSS] to be present in some form or another all through life." In a study based on venous corrosion casts of 13 adult human heads,[12] a PSS was found unilaterally in 19% of the sides (5 of 26 sides).

To the best of our knowledge, the incidence of PSS in the pediatric and adult population without temporal bone pathology, malformation, or otologic manifestations has not been reported in the surgical or radiologic literature. Imaging studies are generally based on a high-resolution CT, which can underestimate the incidence of a PSS because of an absent or inconspicuous bony canal, small size of the PSS, incomplete PSS, or a highly pneumatized temporal bone. A PSS was observed in 1.4% (6/440) skull base sides by Koesling et al.[25] based on a high-resolution CT of the temporal bone performed for hearing disorders (29%), inflammatory disorders (20%), trauma (13%), malformation (11%), tumor (10%), cochlear implant candidates (7%), tinnitus (5%), affections of the sixth and seventh cranial nerves, vestibular disorders, and/or vertigo (5%). Twenty-seven percent of the CT images were read on hard copies, which could have accounted for a lower incidence of PSS in the study of Koesling et al. Zhao et al.[23] found an incidence of 3.7% (39 PSS of 1064 sides) in 532 adult patients with no history of head trauma, skull-base surgery, or soft-tissue mass in the middle ear, investigated by CT angiography for pulsatile tinnitus. Finally, Hiraumi et al.[26] found a 10.3% and 45.7% incidence, respectively, of PSS in patients undergoing CT for Bell's palsy/Ramsay-Hunt syndrome and for chronic otomastoiditis. The authors suggested that the higher incidence of PSS in their chronic otomastoiditis patients was likely explained by the hypopneumatization and sclerosis of the petrous bone, rendering the PSS more conspicuous than in normal petrous bones.

An association between PSS and inner ear malformations has been suggested in the literature.[21,27,28] This association seems to be significant in patients with complete aplasia of the semicircular canals, where a PSS was found in 65% of the sides.[27] The incidence of a PSS and complete aplasia of the semicircular canal rose to 89% in patients who had CHARGE syndrome (58% of all the patients).[27] A PSS in association with complete aplasia of the semicircular canals and CHARGE syndrome was also found by Morimoto et al.[28] In the latter study, the PSS was present 11.5% of sides, which seems to correspond to the incidence of PSS remnants found in the normal adult population.

THE PSS AS A MAJOR VENOUS OUTFLOW PATHWAY

On rare occasions, when the sigmoid sinus is severely hypoplastic or absent (aplasia), the PSS may be very prominent and provide the major or only outflow pathway for the transverse sinus uni- or bilaterally (Figs. 19.2 and 19.3). In such cases, which are usually associated with a severely hypoplastic or absent IJV, the EJV becomes the main or only derivation pathway for encephalic venous drainage normally going through the posterior fossa.[12] In cases of complete sigmoid sinus aplasia, the connection toward the IJV (if present) and the VVS is not established, whereas with distal aplasia of the sigmoid sinus, the connection to the VVS is generally maintained by a mastoid emissary vein. Furstenberg[29] described a case of surgically proven "aseptic thrombus which could be traced for a considerable distance and removed from a persistent PSS of large proportions" in the absence of a sigmoid sinus. Marsot-Dupuch et al.[21] documented a case with HRCT and MR phlebography in which the transverse sinus drained anteriorly into the EJV system by way of a large PSS. Their case showed severe hypoplasia of the jugular foramen in keeping with the absence of a sigmoid sinus. San Millan Ruiz et al.[12] reported a case of a dominant left transverse sinus draining exclusively into a prominent, complete PSS with aplasia of the ipsilateral sigmoid sinus. The right transverse sinus was smaller and drained into a sigmoid sinus, the only outflow of which was a posterior condylar vein into a deep cervical vein.

SIZE OF THE PSS

The PSS is a small venous channel measuring 0.7–3 mm.[12,23] It can, however, be much larger if the PSS acts as the major outflow pathway of the transverse sinus, measuring up to 12.3 mm in diameter.[27]

SIGNIFICANCE OF THE PSS

As mentioned above, extreme anatomic variation involving the sigmoid sinus in association with a prominent, persistent PSS may reduce the number of existing descending venous drainage pathways in the neck. This may severely restrict venous outflow if present bilaterally. Bilateral venous outflow restriction may lead to elevation of the venous and CSF pressures and to pseudotumor cerebri syndrome (PTCS), which is well documented in cases of severe stenosis (by thrombosis or arachnoid granulations) in a normally developed transverse/sigmoid.[30] For PTCS to develop in cases of extreme anatomic variation likely requires, on the one hand, a severe congenital reduction of the number of available descending venous drainage pathways of the neck from three (IJV, VVS, and EJV) to one (EJV or VVS) on both sides and, on the other hand, such an additional factor as venous thrombosis or severe hypoplasia of a dural venous sinus (Fig. 19.3).

A PSS may represent a hemorrhagic hazard during middle ear or mastoid surgery or during translabyrinthine approaches to the posterior fossa or for cochlear implants.[22,26,27] Preserving a large PSS during such surgery may be challenging, but necessary, if the PSS represents the major or only outflow for the transverse sinus, particularly if the contralateral transverse/sinuses are hypoplastic (risk of pseudotumor cerebri syndrome). Preoperative knowledge of a PSS is therefore mandatory to prevent such complications.

Because of its proximity to the inner ear, a PSS may be a source of ipsilateral pulsatile tinnitus. Closure of the PSS in such cases can lead to the resolution of this condition.[31]

CONCLUSION

A PSS is not a rare or abnormal finding in humans, although only parts of its embryologic constituents usually persist into adult life. Rarely, the PSS may become the major or only outflow pathway of the transverse sinus when the sigmoid sinus is insufficiently developed or absent, in which case it persists as a conspicuous vessel. On such occasions, the EJV system becomes the major encephalic outflow pathway in the affected side, a drainage pattern observed in most mammals. Modern imaging techniques allow for in vivo recognition of the PSS, which, especially when large, may be of clinical importance, as it may represent a hazard during surgical procedures in the surrounding regions. Knowledge of the anatomy of the PSS and its various forms of persistence in adult humans is therefore relevant for anatomists and clinicians.

REFERENCES

1. San Millan Ruiz D, Gailloud P, Rufenacht DA, et al. The craniocervical venous system in relation to cerebral venous drainage. *AJNR Am J Neuroradiol*. 2002;23:1500–1508.
2. Epstein HM, Linde HW, Crampton AR, et al. The vertebral venous plexus as a major cerebral venous outflow tract. *Anesthesiology*. 1970;32:332–337.
3. Eckenhoff JE. The physiologic significance of the vertebral venous plexus. *Surg Gynecol Obstet*. 1970;131:72–78.
4. Theron J, Moret J. *Spinal Phlebography. Lumbar and Cervical Techniques*. Berlin Heidelberg: Springer-Verlag; 1978.
5. Valdueza JM, von Munster T, Hoffman O, et al. Postural dependency of the cerebral venous outflow. *Lancet*. 2000;355:200–201.
6. Hacker H. Superficial supratentorial veins and dural sinuses. In: newton THaPDG, ed. *Radiology of the Skull and Brain: Angiography*. Saint Louis: The C.V. Mosby Company; 1974:1851–1902.
7. San Millan Ruiz D, Gailloud P, de Miquel Miquel MA, et al. Laterocavernous sinus. *Anat Rec*. 1999;254:7–12.

8. Cheatle AH. On the anatomy and pathological importance of the petrosquamosal sinus. *Lancet*. 1899;II:611–612.
9. Padget DH. The development of the cranial venous system in man, from the viewpoint of comparative anatomy. *Contributions Embryol*. 1957;247:81–140.
10. Butler H. The development of certain human dural venous sinuses. *J Anat*. 1957;91:510–526.
11. Butler H. The development of mammalian dural venous sinuses with especial reference to the post-glenoid vein. *J Anat*. 1967;102:33–56.
12. San Millan Ruiz D, Gailloud P, Yilmaz H, et al. The petrosquamosal sinus in humans. *J Anat*. 2006;209:711–720.
13. Wysocki J. Morphology of the temporal canal and postglenoid foramen with reference to the size of the jugular foramen in man and selected species of animals. *Folia Morphol*. 2002;61:199–208.
14. Conroy G. A study of the cerebral vascular evolution in primates. In: Armstrong DaF D, ed. *Primate Brain Evolution*. New York: Plenum Press; 1982:247–261.
15. Hegedus SA, Shackelford RT. A comparative-anatomical study of the cranio-cervical venous systems in mammals, with special reference to the dog: relationship of anatomy to measurements of cerebral blood flow. *Am J Anat*. 1965;116:375–386.
16. Luschka H. Das foramen jugulare spurium and des Sulcus petrosquamosus des Menschen. *Zeitschr Rat Med*. 1859;3:72–81.
17. Streeter G. The development f the venous sinuses of the dura mater in the human embryo. *Am J Anat*. 1915;18:145–177.
18. Fisher MH. Le sinus pétro-squameux chez l'homme: un cas de communication de la veine jugulaire externe avec le sinus latéral. *Bulletin de l'Association des Anatomistes*. 1926;1:210–211.
19. Boyd GI. The emissary foramina of the cranium in man and the anthropoids. *J Anat*. 1930;65:108–121.
20. Waltner JG. Anatomic variations of the lateral and sigmoid sinus. *Arch Otolaryngol*. 1944;39:307–312.
21. Marsot-Dupuch K, Gayet-Delacroix M, Elmaleh-Berges M, et al. The petrosquamosal sinus: CT and MR findings of a rare emissary vein. *AJNR Am J Neuroradiol*. 2001;22:1186–1193.
22. An YH, Wee JH, Han KH, et al. Two cases of petrosquamosal sinus in the temporal bone presented as perioperative finding. *Laryngoscope*. 2011;121:381–384.
23. Zhao P, Wang Z, Xian J, et al. Persistent petrosquamosal sinus in adults: qualitative imaging evaluation on high-resolution CT venography. *Acta Radiol*. 2014;55:225–230.
24. Knott JF. On the cerebral sinuses and their variations. *J Anat*. 1882;16:27–42.
25. Koesling S, Kunkel P, Schul T. Vascular anomalies, sutures and small canals of the temporal bone on axial CT. *Eur J Radiol*. 2005;54:335–343.
26. Hiraumi H, Yamamoto A, Yamamoto N, et al. Detection of the petrosquamosal sinus in chronic otitis media using high-resolution CT. *Otolaryngol Head Neck Surg*. 2013;149:488–491.
27. Giesemann AM, Goetz GF, Neuburger J, et al. Persistent petrosquamosal sinus: high incidence in cases of complete aplasia of the semicircular canals. *Radiology*. 2011;259:825–833.
28. Morimoto AK, Wiggins 3rd RH, Hudgins PA, et al. Absent semicircular canals in CHARGE syndrome: radiologic spectrum of findings. *AJNR Am J Neuroradiol*. 2006;27:1663–1671.
29. Furstenberg AC. Septic thrombophlebitis of the sigmoid sinus. *Trans Am Acad Ophthalmol*. 1937;42:424–431.
30. Owler BK, Parker G, Halmagyi GM, et al. Pseudotumor cerebri syndrome: venous sinus obstruction and its treatment with stent placement. *J Neurosurg*. 2003;98:1045–1055.
31. Liu Z, Chen C, Wang Z, et al. Petrosquamosal sinus in the temporal bone as a cause of pulsatile tinnitus: a radiological detection. *Clin Imag*. 2013;37:561–563.

CHAPTER 20

The Emissary Veins

MAIA SCHUMACHER • R. SHANE TUBBS

The emissary veins (Fig. 20.1), named based on the position on the skull, connect the veins outside the cranium with the intracranial venous sinuses and can be seen at embryonic stage 7. The veins of the hypoglossal canal are the first emissary veins to form and the parietal emissary veins are the last. These structures are more commonly found in children, and not each individual may have a varied number of the various emissary veins.[1] Various authors have posited that these structures equalize intracranial pressure.[1–6] The foramina for these emissarial vessels tend to be larger during childhood[4] and may communicate with the diploic veins.[5] Louis et al.[6] found that emissary veins act as the primary outflow route for venous drainage in the upright position and may serve to cool venous blood circulating through the head.

Emissary veins can often be seen on magnetic resonance imaging, computerized tomography images, and angiograms.[2,6,7] Interestingly, an enlarged emissary foramen does not necessarily transmit a large emissary vein,[2] and fossil records indicate that there is an increasing frequency of some emissary veins in modern man such as the emissary veins of the parietal bone and mastoid part of the temporal bone.[8]

POSTERIOR CONDYLAR EMISSARY VEIN

The posterior condylar emissary vein connect either the sigmoid, marginal, or occipital sinuses with part of Batson's plexus, that is, internal vertebral venous plexus.[4,5,8,9] Irmak et al.[10] noted that a posterior condylar emissary vein may connect the sigmoid sinus with the suboccipital plexus of veins.[5] Observations have shown that the posterior condylar foramen (Fig. 20.2) is usually the largest emissary foramen in the retromastoid region.[2] Lang[11] found that this vein joined the hypoglossal plexus in 3.84%, and in another 3.84%, it joined the internal jugular vein.

Mastoid Emissary Vein

The mastoid emissary vein (Figs. 20.3–20.6) passes through the mastoid canal and connects the transverse or sigmoid sinus to the posterior auricular or occipital veins, which then join Batson's plexus.[2,5,8,10,12,13] Lang and Samii[14] observed that the mastoid emissary foramen (Fig. 20.4) exists less frequently in females than males and there is no clear laterality.[6] Cheatle[12] noted a potential association between the mastoid emissary veins and the petrosquamosal sinus. Several mastoid emissary veins may converge toward and enter a mastoid foramen of which multiple may exist.

Occipital Emissary Vein

The occipital emissary vein (Fig. 20.7) connects the torcular Herophili or transverse sinus to the occipital veins, which then drain blood to Batson's plexus.[4,8] The occipital emissary vein might join the transverse-sigmoid sinus complex.[15] Okudera et al.[16] have reported that when the occipital vein drains into the torcular Herophili, it is known as the vein of Sperino. Several occipital veins may drain into one occipital foramen.

Parietal Emissary Vein

The parietal emissary veins (Figs. 20.1, 20.8 and 20.9) connect the superior sagittal sinus with occipital veins, which then join Batson's plexus.[4,8] Diploic veins might also connect with the parietal emissary veins.

Petrosquamosal Sinus

Serving as the primary venous drainage of the brain in many animals such as primates, the petrosquamosal sinus (Fig. 20.10) is uncommonly found in humans and usually disappears before birth. It ranges in diameter from 2 to 4 mm and often originates at the transverse-sigmoid sinus junction, coursing anteriorly over the petrous part of the temporal bone.

Emissary Veins of the Foramen Ovale

As with the sphenoidal emissary veins, the veins of the foramen ovale (Fig. 20.11) connect the superiorly located cavernous sinus with the pterygoid venous plexus located in the infratemporal fossa.[17,18]

Anatomy, Imaging and Surgery of the Intracranial Dural Venous Sinuses. https://doi.org/10.1016/B978-0-323-65377-0.00020-9

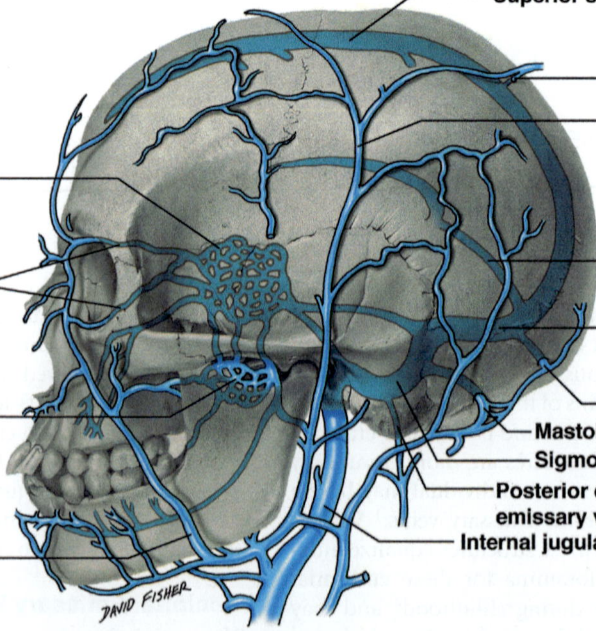

FIG. 20.1 Schematic drawing of many of the emissary veins and their connections to the underlying dural venous sinuses.

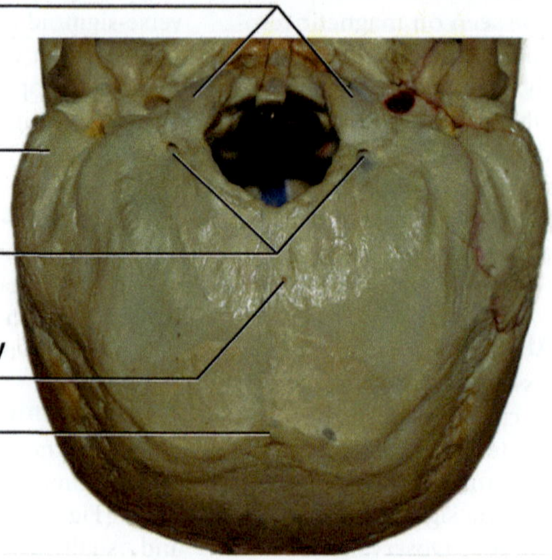

FIG. 20.2 Posteroinferior view of the skull illustrating the posterior condylar foramina. In addition, note a smaller and less constant midline foramen for the occipital emissary vein.

Ophthalmic Veins

The ophthalmic veins (Fig. 20.1) are considered by some to be emissary veins, as they join the exterior to the cavernous sinus and do not contain valves (Fig. 20.11).

The superior ophthalmic vein has two roots that form confluence with the supraorbital and angular veins within the superior orbit. The first segment extends from the roof of the orbit, via the trochlea of the superior oblique. It runs posteriorly in adipose tissue to the medial border of the superior rectus. The second segment enters the muscle cone and passes posterolaterally in connective tissue along the lateral

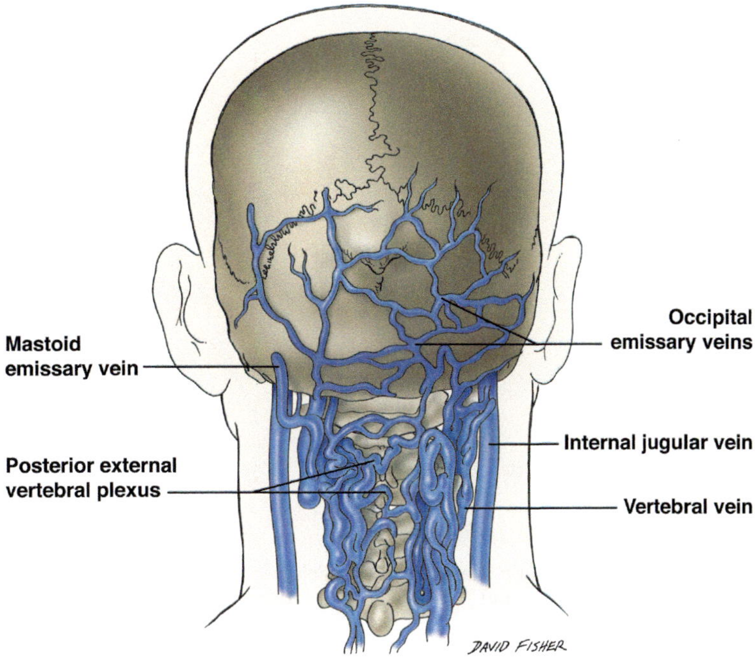

FIG. 20.3 Schematic drawing of the emissary veins of the occiput.

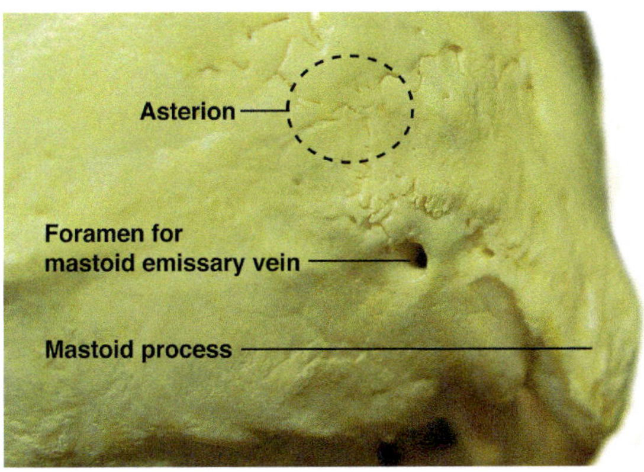

FIG. 20.4 Enlarged right mastoid foramen.

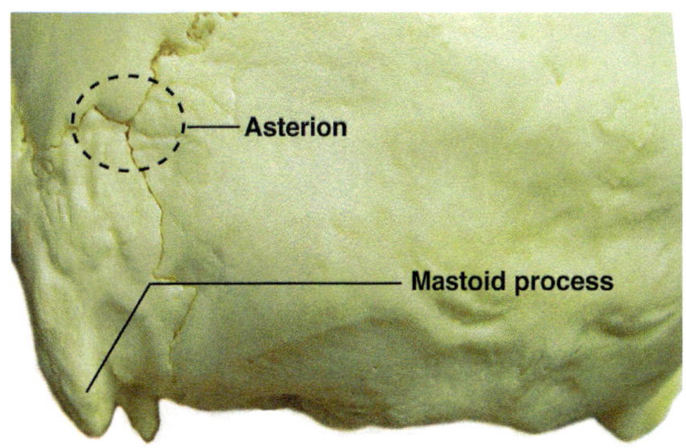

FIG. 20.5 Absence of a left mastoid foramen.

border of the superior rectus muscle. The third segment courses slightly downward, posteromedially, relating to the sloping of the orbit, leaving the muscle cone and enters the anteroinferior portion of the cavernous sinus. Venous tributaries of the SOV are highly variable location and degree to which they join; however, the main venous tributaries include the medial palpebral, superior vortex, anterior ethmoidal, lacrimal, vorticose veins, central retinal, muscular, and the inferior ophthalmic veins.

The inferior ophthalmic vein originates from a venous network that drains the lower lid, inferior rectus and inferior oblique muscles, lacrimal sac, inferior vortex veins, and the inferior conjunctiva. It runs posteriorly along the inferior rectus muscle and drains into the superior ophthalmic vein or the cavernous sinus directly.

The middle ophthalmic vein is present in only 1%–20% of the population, and some refer to it as the second inferior ophthalmic vein as it drains the inferior network. It arises lateral to the medial rectus

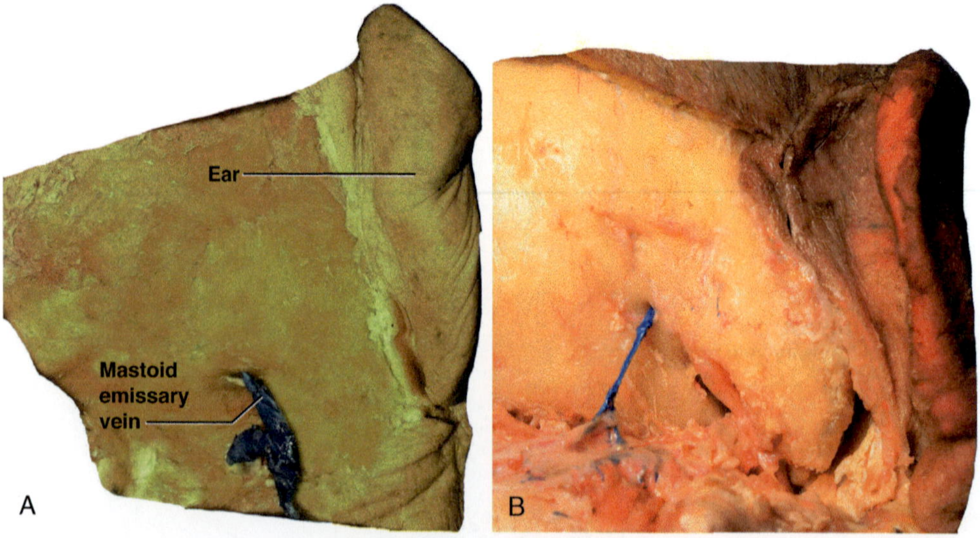

FIG. 20.6 A and B show two cadaveric examples of latex-injected mastoid emissary veins of varying sizes both on right sides and latex injected.

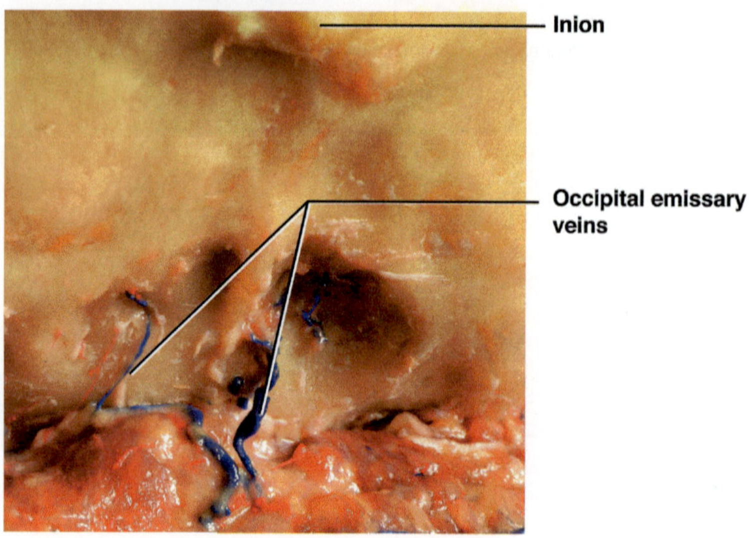

FIG. 20.7 Cadaveric example of latex-injected occipital emissary veins.

and inferior to the lateral rectus muscle and joins the superior ophthalmic vein to drain into the cavernous sinus.

The medial ophthalmic vein is seen in up to 40% of orbital phlebograms. It arises from the inferior root of the first (anterior) segment of the superior ophthalmic vein and runs backward along the orbital roof, near the medial wall, and drains into the cavernous sinus.

Sphenoidal Emissary Vein (Vesalius)

Sphenoidal emissary veins (Vesalian veins) (Fig. 20.12) connect the cavernous sinus with the pterygoid plexus or pharyngeal plexus of veins.[17–19] These veins are not constant and are found in only approximately one in three individuals.[17] When present, the foramen for this vessel is found just medial to the foramen ovale. This emissary vein has been referred to as the accessory sphenoidal emissary vein.

Anterior Condylar Vein

Traveling with the hypoglossal nerve in the hypoglossal canal, the anterior condylar vein (Figs. 20.13 and 20.14) joins the anterior condylar confluent.[20]

Internal Carotid Venous Plexus

The internal carotid plexus of veins (*sinus caroticus*)[21] extends through the carotid canal and connects the cavernous sinus with the internal jugular vein and was first described by Santorini in his *Observationes Anatomicae* published in 1724.[18] This collection of veins is classified by some as emissary veins because it joins the intradural sinuses with extracranial veins.[22] Some have referred to this venous structure as the *vena sodalis carotidis*.

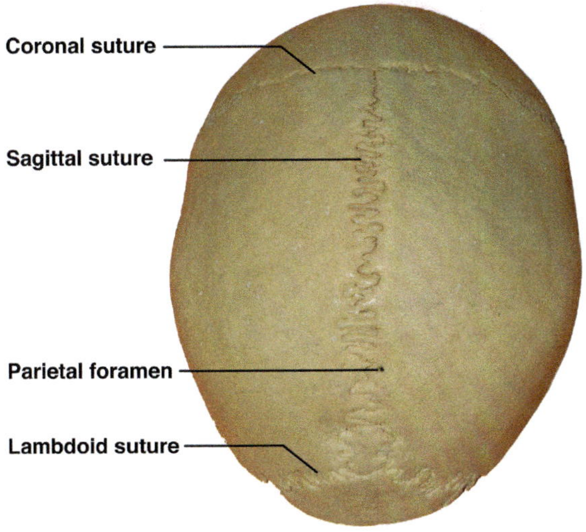

FIG. 20.8 Calvarial illustrating a right parietal foramen.

Emissary Vein of the Foramen Cecum

A vein can travel from the nasal cavity up through the foramen cecum to join the superior sagittal sinus and is known as the emissary vein of the foramen cecum.[18] This vessel is larger at birth than in the adult.

Emissary Veins of the Foramen Lacerum

An inconsistent number of small veins may traverse the cartilage-filled foramen lacerum. Such emissary veins connect the cavernous sinus with the pterygoid plexus of the infratemporal fossa.[17]

Emissary Veins of the Clivus

Some have identified transclival emissary veins[23] (Figs. 20.15 and 20.16). If present, these structures connect the basilar plexus to pharyngeal veins.

Lateral Condylar Vein

First mentioned by Trolard, the lateral condylar vein usually arises from the anterior condylar confluence and drains into the vertebral venous plexus. Matsushima et al.[24] identified this vein in 88.0% of paracondylar areas, with an average diameter of 3.6 mm.

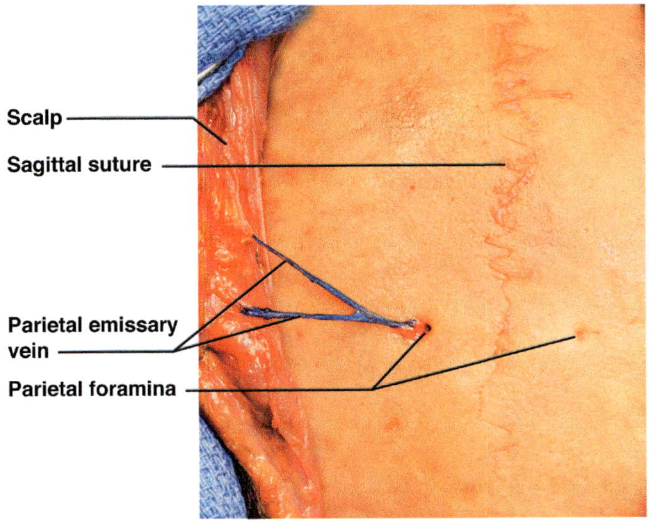

FIG. 20.9 Latex-injected cadaver noting a left-sided parietal emissary vein.

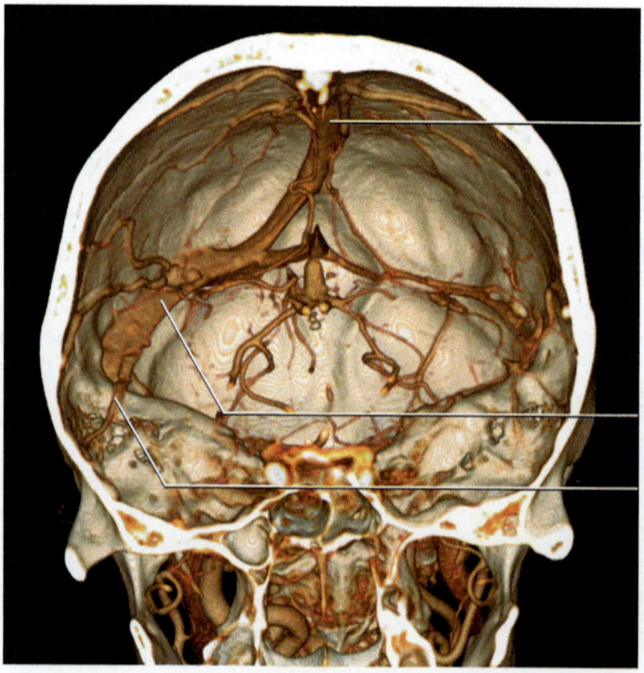

FIG. 20.10 CTA noting a petrosquamous sinus.

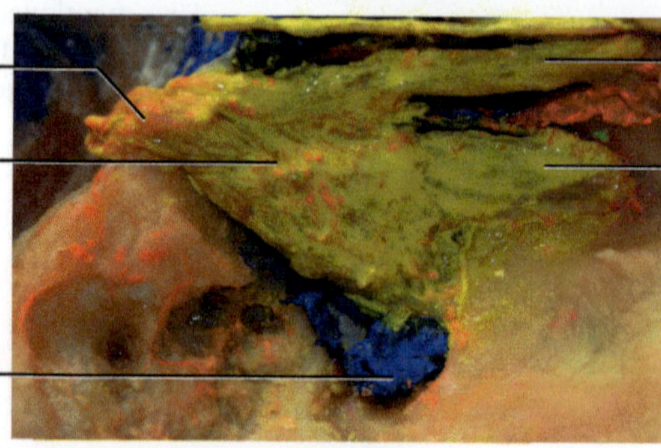

FIG. 20.11 Latex-injected cadaver noting a right-sided parietal emissary vein of the foramen ovale.

In some specimens, it arose from the internal jugular vein, and in some (16.7%) the lateral condylar vein coursed within a small bony canal lateral to the occipital condyle.

Temporal Emissary Vein

This venous structure may connect the remnant of the petrosquamosal sinus (Fig. 20.10) with the deep temporal vein and likely represents the dorsal cerebral vein seen in some mammals.

Superficial Petrosal Emissary Vein

When present, the superficial petrosal emissary vein in the middle cranial fossa to the vein traveling with the facial nerve within the stylomastoid foramen. Such a vein has been considered by some to be a remnant of the embryonic primary head sinus.

CLINICAL CORRELATIONS

Hoshi et al.[25] reported a case of removal of a hypoglossal neurinoma where the condylar emissary veins

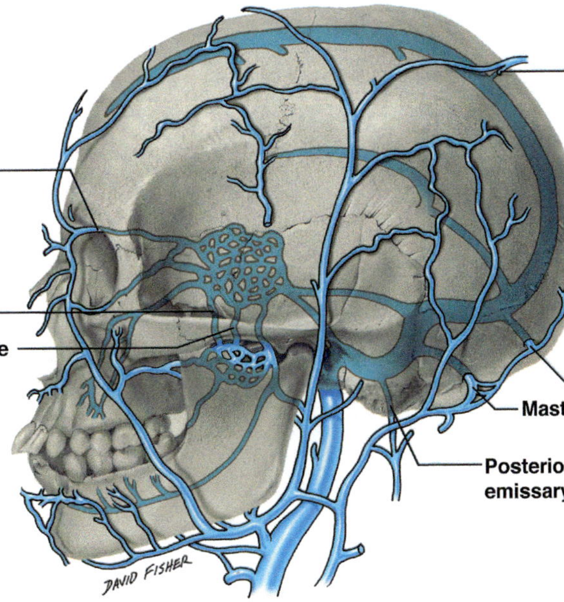

FIG. 20.12 Lateral drawing of additional emissary veins.

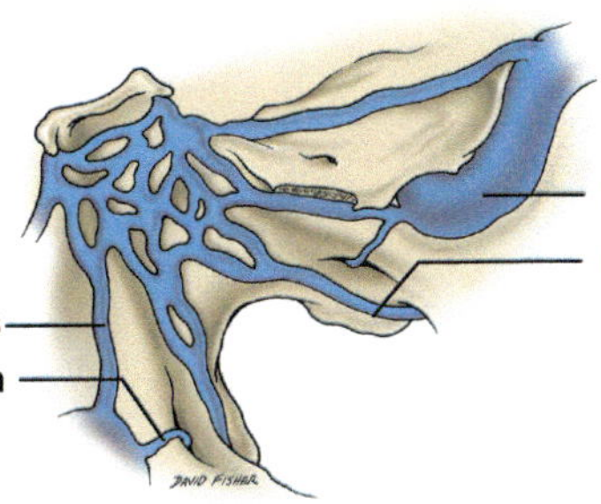

FIG. 20.13 Drawing of the skull base noting the anterior condylar vein and its relationship to regional dural venous sinuses.

were enlarged. Surgical coagulation of these veins caused dural venous sinus thrombosis and infarction of the cerebellum resulting in the death of the patient. Sphenoidal emissary veins and veins of the foramen ovale have been reported to interfere with surgical approaches that are extradural in nature at the base of the skull.

With disease or compression of the internal jugular veins, various emissary veins can increase in size and serve as the primary venous outflow of the brain.[26,27] For example, the main venous outflow of the posterior cranial fossa has been reported to be via the occipital emissary and mastoid emissary veins.[28]

Large posterior condylar veins have been reported to cause tinnitus.[20,29,30] One case of tinnitus was alleviated after decreasing blood flow through the internal jugular vein via direct pressure on the neck, thus altering the flow within the posterior condylar emissary vein.[29] Dural arteriovenous fistulas have been reported to involve the anterior condylar vein. Ernst et al.[22] reported three cases of dural arteriovenous fistula involving the anterior condylar vein within the hypoglossal canal. In a cadaver, Moore et al. identified an

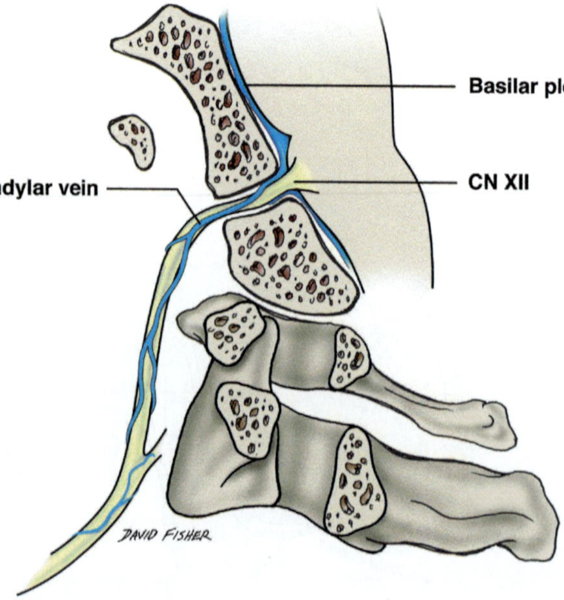

FIG. 20.14 Parasagittal drawing noting the hypoglossal canal and nerve with connections between the basilar venous plexus and anterior condylar vein.

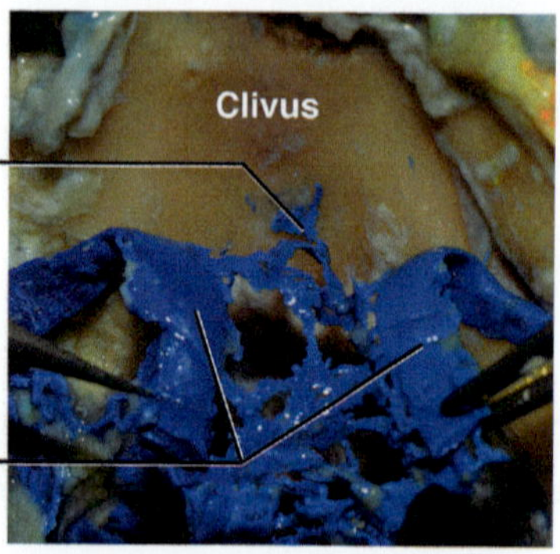

FIG. 20.15 Posterior view of the clivus with the basilar plexus (latex injected) and reflected inferiorly and illustrating a transclival vein.

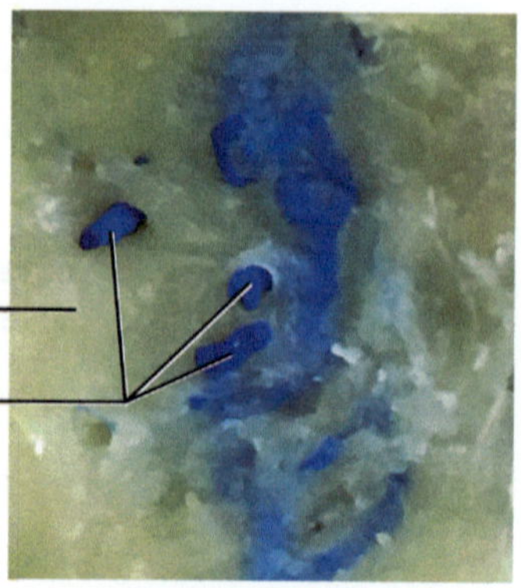

FIG. 20.16 Zoomed in view of latex-injected cadaveric skull base noting transclival veins.

anastomosis between the posterior condylar vein and Batson's plexus.

An enlarged anterior condylar emissary vein was reported to cause compression of the hypoglossal nerve with resultant tongue atrophy.[31] Sinus pericranii is characterized by abnormal communication of pericranial varicosities with the underlying dural sinus.[32,33]

REFERENCES

1. Eckley W. Anatomic and physiological correspondences of child and the adult. *J Am Med Assoc.* 1903;20:1337.
2. Boyd G. The emissary foramina of the cranium in man and the anthropoids. *J Anat.* 1930;65:108–121.
3. Braun JP, Tournade A. Venous drainage in the craniocervical region. *Neuroradiology.* 1977;13:155–158.
4. Williams P, Warwick R, Dyson M, Bannister L. *Gray's Anatomy.* 37th ed. Edinburgh: Churchill Livingstone; 1989.

5. Curé JK, Van Tassel P, Smith MT. Normal and variant anatomy of the dural venous sinuses. *Semin Ultrasound CT MR*. 1994;15:499–519.
6. Louis Jr RG, Loukas M, Wartmann CT, et al. Clinical anatomy of the mastoid and occipital emissary veins in a large series. *Surg Radiol Anat*. 2009;31:139–144.
7. Hacker H. Emissary veins related to the transverse sinus, sigmoid sinus, and torcular herophili. In: Newton THPD, ed. *Radiology of the Skull and Brain*. Vol. 2. St. Louis: C.V. Mosby Company; 1974:1852–1858.
8. Falk D. Evolution of cranial blood drainage in hominids: enlarged occipital/marginal sinuses and emissary foramina. *Am J Phys Anthropol*. 1986;70:311–324.
9. Pearson BW. Microsurgical anatomy of the approach to the base of the skull. *Clin Neurosurg*. 1979;26: 379–390.
10. Irmak MK, Korkmaz A, Erogul O. Selective brain cooling seems to be a mechanism leading to human craniofacial diversity observed in different geographical regions. *Med Hypotheses*. 2004;63:974–979.
11. Lang J. Anatomy of the brainstem and the lower cranial nerves, vessels, and surrounding stuctures. *Am J Otol*. 1985;(suppl).
12. Cheatle A. The mastoid emissary vein and its surgical importance. *Proc R Soc Med*. 1925;18:29–34.
13. Standring S. *Gray's Anatomy*. 39th ed. Elsevier Churchill Livingstone; 2005:1600.
14. Lang Jr J, Samii A. Retrosigmoidal approach to the posterior cranial fossa. An anatomical study. *Acta Neurochir*. 1991;111:147–153.
15. Neuroangio. *Venous Anatomy of the Brain*; 2013. URL http://neuroangio.org/venous-brain-anatomy/.
16. Okudera T, Huang YP, Ohta T, et al. Development of posterior fossa dural sinuses, emissary veins, and jugular bulb: morphological and radiologic study. *Am J Neuroradiol*. 1994;15:1871–1883.
17. Dwight T, Hamann C, McMurrich J, Piersol G. In: Piersol G, ed. *Human Anatomy*. Vol. 1. London: Lippincott Company; 1913:879.
18. Gray H. *Anatomy of the Human Body*. Philadelphia: Lea & Febiger; 1918:1396.
19. Hayashi N, Sato H, Tsuboi Y, Nagai S, Kuwayama N, Endo S. Consequences of preoperative evaluation of patterns of drainage of the cavernous sinus in patients treated using the anterior transpetrosal approach. *Neurol Med Chir*. 2010;50:373–377.
20. Chen Z, Feng H, Zhu G, Wu N, Lin J. Anomalous intracranial venous drainage associated with basal ganglia calcification. *Am J Neuroradiol*. 2007;28:22–24.
21. Rektorzik E. *Ueber das Vorkommen eines Sinus venosus im Canalis caroticus des Menschen. Wien*; 1868.
22. Ernst R, Bulas R, Tomsick T, van Loveren H, Aziz KA. Three cases of dural arteriovenous fistula of the anterior condylar vein within the hypoglossal canal. *Am J Neuroradiol*. 1999;20:2016–2020.
23. Tubbs RS, Kelly DR, Humphrey ER, et al. The tectorial membrane: anatomical, biomechanical, and histological analysis. *Clin Anat*. 2007;20:382–386.
24. Matsushima K, Funaki T, Komune N, Kiyosue H, Kawashima M, Rhoton Jr AL. Microsurgical anatomy of the lateral condylar vein and its clinical significance. *Neurosurgery*. 2015;(suppl 2):135–145.
25. Hoshi M, Yoshida K, Ogawa K, Kawase T. Hypoglossal neurinoma--two case reports. *Neurol Med Chir*. 2000;40:489–493.
26. Ginsberg LE. The posterior condylar canal. *Am J Neuroradiol*. 1994;15:969–972.
27. Marsot-Dupuch K, Gayet-Delacroix M, Elmaleh-Bergès M, Bonneville F, Lasjaunias P. The petrosquamosal sinus: CT and MR findings of a rare emissary vein. *Am J Neuroradiol*. 2001;22:1186–1193.
28. Jeevan DS, Anlsow P, Jayamohan J. Abnormal venous drainage in syndromic craniosynostosis and the role of CT venography. *Childs Nerv Syst*. 2008;24:1413–1420.
29. Lambert PR, Cantrell RW. Objective tinnitus in association with an abnormal posterior condylar emissary vein. *Am J Otol*. 1986;7:204–207.
30. Forte V, Turner A, Liu P. Objective tinnitus associated with abnormal mastoid emissary vein. *J Otolaryngol*. 1989;18:232–235.
31. Shiozawa Z, Koike G, Seguchi K, Shindo K, Sugita K. Unilateral tongue atrophy due to an enlarged emissary vein in the hypoglossal canal. *Surg Neurol*. 1996;45:477–479.
32. Carpenter JS, Rosen CL, Bailes JE, Gailloud P. Sinus pericranii: clinical and imaging findings in two cases of spontaneous partial thrombosis. *Am J Neuroradiol*. 2004;25:121–125.
33. Ota T, Waga S, Handa H, Nishimura S, Mitani T. Sinus pericranii. *J Neurosurg*. 1975;42:704–712.

FURTHER READING

1. Mortazavi MM, Tubbs R, Riech S, et al. Anatomy and pathology of the cranial emissary veins: a review with surgical implicaitons. *Neurosurgery*. 2012;70:1312–1318.

CHAPTER 21

Sinus Pericranii

GRAHAM DUPONT • R. SHANE TUBBS

INTRODUCTION

Stromeyer proposed the name "sinus pericranii" (SP) (Figs. 21.1, 21.2 and 21.3) after lamenting the much longer "varix spurius circumscriptis venae diploicae frontalis" proposed by Hecker, describing what he deemed a strange affliction, wherein he observed a "blood bag" that appeared to make connections with the veins of the diploë and the dural sinuses.[1] Early morphologic descriptions of SP by Stromeyer involved minor trauma in which a recession of bone was palpable, as well as a "blood bag" formed under the skin. Currently, SP is viewed as a rare extradural venous anomaly whereby an abnormal connection is formed between the intracranial dural venous sinuses and the extracranial venous system through an emissary or diploic vein. These abnormal communicating channels redirect venous return to the extracranial periosteum, resulting in swelling of the affected region and on palpation, are soft, compressible, and collapsible masses. Typically, these masses are observed along the midline and frontal regions and involve communication with the superior sagittal sinus (SSS) and present with a bluish discoloration of the skin about the swollen region. Cases that involve off-midline masses have been reported but are scant in comparison with SP observed at the midline.[2–7] Tumorlike in appearance, these nonpulsatile varicosities fluctuate with changes in intracranial pressure, such as during Valsalva maneuvers and Trendelenburg position.[8–10] Often, SP is a finding that occurs in tandem with an array of other congenital defects, such as craniosynostosis, cerebral venous malformations, systemic angiomas, and cavernous hemangiomas.[3,10–12]

Most patients are asymptomatic.[13,14] Although rarely life-threatening, cases of this venous anomaly which have led to complications such as venous infarction, hemorrhage, thrombosis, infection, and emboli have been reported.[4,8,11,15,16] Despite the mechanisms of SP formation being poorly understood, the recognized etiologies of SP are congenital, traumatic, and spontaneously acquired.[8,17]

ANATOMY

SP is characterized by confluence of an extracranial vein with an intracranial dural sinus. The SSS is an important receptacle of venous blood from the meningeal network, flanking venous lacunae, and emissary veins penetrating the fenestrations in the cranial vault.[8,18] In most cases of SP, the SSS is involved in the anastomotic connections to the extracranial venous system via a bony defect, consisting of a single union, or multiple venous intersections that can result in profound diploic erosion, major bypass of usual drainage routes, and venous stasis in the affected regions.[2,5,6,13,19]

Of major connection are the diploic veins and emissary veins that penetrate the cranial vault, serving as a link between the intracranial dural sinuses with the extracranial veins. Although the emissary veins of the calvaria are well understood, the precise anatomy of the diploic venous system is highly variable, and less understood.[20–23] Diploic veins anastomose with themselves, as well as form confluences with microscopic branches of the larger diploic channels, resulting in a venous meshwork that feeds into the penetrating emissary veins of the skull, as well as into the dural venous sinuses.[20,21] The diploic veins are lined by a single endothelial layer and, like the emissary veins, are devoid of valves and thus demonstrate bidirectional flow that can be altered based on changes in intracranial pressure. Because the diploic connections to the dural sinuses are twofold, cases of SP may involve abnormal communications with emissary veins that drain into the SSS, or a direct-to-SSS juncture.

Emissary veins are the primary route of venous efflux when the head is upright, linking the extracranial veins with the intradural sinuses at major regions of the skull. The emissary veins that would appear to be most involved with SP based on their immediate anatomic connections to the SSS are the parietal emissary vein and emissary vein of the foramen cecum.[21,24,25] Other emissary veins have the lowest incidence of SP or none whatsoever.[11,21] Abnormal venous connections as in SP may reroute the typical external-to-internal flow within the emissary veins, further exacerbated by head

Anatomy, Imaging and Surgery of the Intracranial Dural Venous Sinuses. https://doi.org/10.1016/B978-0-323-65377-0.00021-0

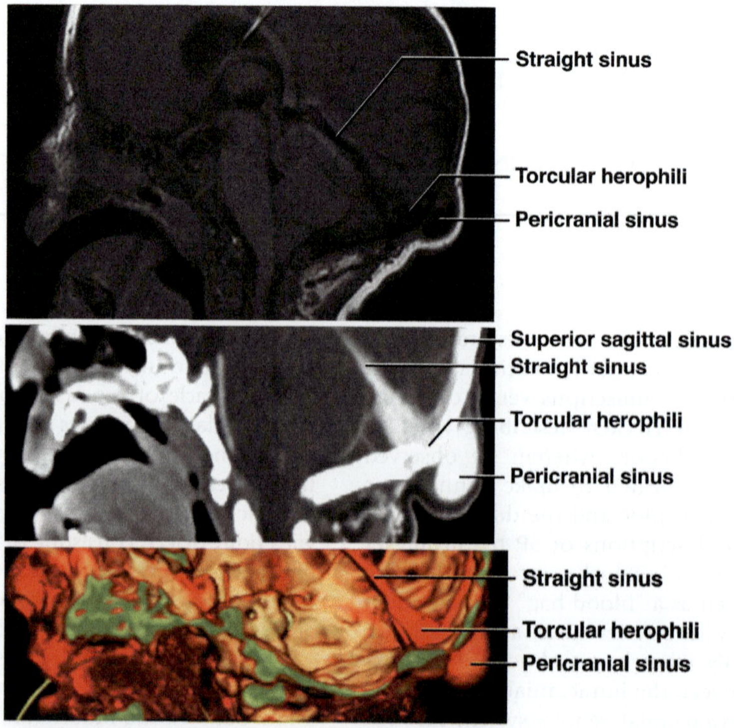

FIGS. 21.1–21.3 (MRI, CT, and CTA) note sinus pericranii connecting internally to the torcular Herophili in a patient with craniosynostosis.

position and intracranial pressure. Interestingly, the emissary veins have been posited to serve as thermoregulatory entities that cool venous blood within the skull.[26,27]

EMBRYOLOGY

Vascularization of the early developing nervous system and skull is an elaborate process involving extensive remodeling and formation of simple endothelial tubes that takes place when the embryo has reached a length of approximately 12–20 mm and continues well on until after birth.[28–30] The process by which the membranes of the brain differentiate alongside developing anastomosing endothelial tubes, wherein cleavage of the cerebrovascular system into external, dural, and cerebral layers is observed, is referred to as the third stage of embryonic development.[28] The embryonic nervous system is encased in a mesodermal (cortical) mantle that is destined for separation into the pia, arachnoid, and dural layers, respectively, each having unique patterns of vascularization. At 5–10 mm, the meningeal venous stalks have emerged from the vena capitis lateralis, with their plexuses located at the anterior (forebrain), middle (midbrain), and posterior (hindbrain) parts of the brain. The plexuses begin to anastomose and at 24–40 mm length, the anterior and middle plexuses begin to recede leaving the tentorial sinus as a major drainage route, and the sagittal plexus and inferior petrosal sinuses appear. As these veins fade, they are replaced by successive caudal vessels, whose medial remnants form the sagittal plexus, and later fuse to form the SSS by the 80-mm stage. The dural venous sinuses thus arise from this developing dural venous network but are not truly considered veins until circulation begins.

Prerequisites of cerebral venous malformations arise from attempts by disappearing pial-dural veins to anastomose to adjoining veins in the pial network; failure to anastomose with an adjoining venous network leads to early stages of cerebral vascular malformation.[29] Vascularization of the cortical mantle proceeds from deep to superficial, wherein the pial surface is impregnated by vasogenic cells that burrow into the ependymal surface, and exit to form a dural anastomosis that is circumferential with the outer surface of the mantle. A cleft is formed within the ependymal venous plexus that directs the majority of the drainage toward the dural venous plexus, and the remaining drainage toward this subependymal venous network. When this occlusion process fails, veins from the dural plexus regress and leave one vessel to drain the entirety of the pial plexus. If further occlusion migrates into the pial network, a "star cluster" is formed, that attempts to send satellites to adjoining veins that will carry it back through to the surface to anastomose with the dural plexus. Propagation of this malformation without vascular remodeling is believed to be how certain cerebral venous malformations arise.[30]

ETIOLOGY AND PATHOLOGY

The pathogenesis of SP is not readily understood, but associations have been put forth that link it with congenital, spontaneous, and traumatic origins.[11,17] In many cases, SP is observed as a symptom complex that most often relates to, and may also be a sign of, abnormal arteriovenous and skull malformations. As a standalone, however, SP seems to be a mostly benign venous anomaly that may resolve itself over time, unless rare complications such as hemorrhage, infection, or emboli are observed that warrant surgical correction.[13]

The congenital origins have been mentioned previously, whereby the venous abnormality may be formed early in embryonic development. Reports mention histologic examination to discriminate between congenital and acquired SP, where it is seen that the endothelial lining of congenital abnormal veins are not comprised of connective tissues such as the acquired types.[14,31] Although congenital cerebral venous malformations form unpredictably, steps have been taken to further categorize the various subtypes and their genetic origins. Sporadic venous malformations comprise 94% of all venous malformation subtypes, with the remaining 6% representing autosomal dominant inheritance—interestingly, a connection was determined between mutation of the TIE2 gene in autosomal dominant inherited venous malformations that also seems to influence the incidence of singly sporadic and multiply sporadic venous malformations.[32,33] These abnormal venous manifestations are a result of the inherited mutation R849W, and the somatic mutation L914F. The vascular endothelial (EC)-specific receptor tyrosine kinase (RTK) TIE2 is critical in angiogenesis and development of the cardiovascular system. Heterozygous substitutions of TIE2 have been found to induce mucocutaneous venous malformations, characterized by bluish cutaneous lesions on the skin and mucosa, as well as common sporadic venous malformations, because of independent hyperphosphorylation of its ligands, the angiopoietins.[32] Nevertheless, inherited venous malformations are very rare and only representative of a small fraction of all cases of venous malformation.

Coexistence of SP with other congenital vascular anomalies seems to explain a trend in venous malformations, specifically that abnormal venous dilatations and vein of Galen aneurysmal malformations redirect venous flow in a way that may instigate abnormal venous connections between the dural sinuses and extracranial venous networks. To further relate the congenital nature of SP, reports have shown the presence of SP with systemic angiomas, persistent trigeminal arteries, facial hemangiomas, solitary venous anomalies, dural sinus malformation, and various cases of craniosynostosis, such as Crouzon's syndrome.[11,19] It has been suggested that intracranial abnormalities as well as absence of calvarial bone or premature suture closure may induce transient intracranial venous hypertension resulting in dilatations of emissary veins and their connections to the dural sinuses.[34] This is further evidenced by observations by Renier and Marchac in which 42% of their cases of craniosynostosis presented with intracranial hypertension.[35] In cases of craniosynostosis, hemangiomas, and aneurysmal malformations, where an asymptomatic extracranial soft mass is observed, SP should be suspect. Albeit, the causal relationship between skull malformations and hypertension suggests a likely association with SP, the etiopathology remains unpredictable and lacking full explanation.

The spontaneous origin of SP has been demonstrated in many cases, wherein sneezing, vomiting, and coughing lead to a varix and erosion of the skull.[10,14] Venous varices occur in the skull as a result of dural sinus occlusion and might exacerbate SP, or via arteriovenous malformations that propagate outward into extracranial venous networks.[11] Cases of spontaneous SP are therefore less clinically complex, simply because of the fact that, compared with its congenital formation, they are not typically an indication of other symptoms. Spontaneous SP may be distinguished from traumatic SP by the incidence of other complications such as ruptures in the dural sinuses or emissary veins through blunt force, leading to brain hemorrhage, thrombosis, and air emboli.[4] These complications may lead to abnormal venous communications because of increased circulation of the diploic and emissary veins.[9,36–38]

PRESENTATION AND SYMPTOMS

The morphologic characteristics of SP make it simple to diagnose; however, most patients are asymptomatic, with occasional headache or vertigo, often leaving SP unappreciated given its rarity. The defining feature of SP is a painless, easily compressible extracranial sac that fluctuates in size based on the position of the patient and during Valsalva maneuvers. This malformation has been reported as a cause of nonspecific chronic headaches.[13]

SP may be found in isolation or in conjunction with other congenital malformations (secondary), such as craniosynostosis, macrocephaly, and other intracranial venous abnormalities.[4,5,12,39,40] It has been reported that the increase in intracranial pressure in utero from craniosynostosis, macrocephaly, tumors, and other coexisting vascular malformations may potentiate venous defects and furthermore redirect venous blood flow through the skull.[12,41]

DIFFERENTIAL DIAGNOSIS

Atretic Cephalocele

For the clinician, it is of great value to understand the distinguishing features of SP, in solitary as well in coexistence with other cranial or cerebral vascular malformations. Often, atretic cephalocele (AC) and SP may be mistaken for one another, because of the similarity in morphologic presentation—small, nonpulsatile subcutaneous/periosteal lesions.[34,42,43] Where a majority of SP cases are asymptomatic, a patient with AC may present with a wide range of neurodevelopmental milestones from no neurologic dysfunction to severe mental retardation due to several cortical and vascular abnormalities.[42] Blue discoloration and overlying hair is typically seen in a patient with SP, whereas AC masses preserve the skin tone and alopecia is observed at the location of the mass.[42,44] Discrimination between AC and SP may be achieved through MRI, whereby the clinician may see a transcalvarial herniation containing neuronal or glial cells, or meninges.[34,42] Other techniques to identify SP include ultrasonography in which a vessel traversing a hyperechoic calvarium may be appreciated. Congenital defects such as AC may also be observed in tandem with other abnormal vascular defects such as persistent falcine sinus.[34,44] The gold standard for identifying SP is angiography with digital subtraction, including angiotomography, and tomography with injected contrast; bony defects and calvarial erosion may be identified with radiography as well as with palpation on recession of the mass.[8,11]

Dermoid Cysts of the Scalp

In continuing with calvarial lesions, the dermoid cyst may also be considered in the differential diagnosis as they can mimic other similar pathologies before being discerned through CT or MRI. Dermoid cysts are benign midline neoplasms that arise during neural tube closure. Dermoid cysts are the most common scalp lesions in children, typically occur at lines of fusion, and are considered congenital in origin if they arise in the head.[45] The defining features of dermoid cysts of the scalp also align with those of SP, nontender, nonpulsatile, with areas of soft and cystic consistency.[45] The main caution with dermoid cysts in the scalp is that they may have an intracranial extension, called "dumbbell dermoid," although incredibly rare.[45,46] It is recommended that all cases of children with midline lesions should be scanned for intracranial extensions of the dermoid cyst. Dermoid cyst may also be confused with meningocele because of similar presentation and may not be identifiable through direct physical examination until X-ray, CT, MRI, or surgery. In relationship to SP, however, the content of dermoid cysts is not homogenous and does not increase or recede on changes in head position. A suspected dermoid cyst should be analyzed histologically as well as undergo imaging before making the proper diagnosis.[46]

Lipomas

Intracranial lipomas are congenital conditions resulting from malformation or persistence of the primitive meninges into lipomatous tissue, most being asymptomatic.[47] Symptomatic patients with lipomas may express seizure, which serves as an important distinguishing feature from SP when considering the differential diagnosis. In rare cases, lipomas may extend extracranially from the interhemispheric fat, appearing as a subcutaneous mass that may mimic SP, dermoid cysts, and meningocele and can thus be misdiagnosed on physical examination.[19,47] Scalp swelling may also be palpable in lipoma cases that make their way through the external table of the skull. Lipomas may also be seen in isolation or in tandem with meningocele and occult spinal dysraphism as part of the signifying cutaneous stigmata.[47,48] Generally, with suspicion of nonpulsatile masses that have intracranial extensions, CT and MRI are the gold standard for determining the direction of diagnosis and treatment.

Meningiomas

Meningiomas are common neoplasms of the nervous system and arise from the cellular elements that form the meninges; these tend to be noncompressive and noninfiltratory, but in rare cases neural tissue may be compressed as a result of tumor encroachment and successive expansion. Of extreme rarity are extracranial meningiomas, known as secondary extracranial meningiomas, that arise from intracranial masses as a result of extension through preformed bony pathways. These tend to appear within the orbit, nasal cavity, and nasopharynx via the cribriform plate. In consideration of its morphologic relation to SP, meningiomas are firm, pink to grayish masses.[49] Meningiomas have been found to compress the SSS, resulting in abnormal venous circuits, so SP is often expressed with meningiomas.[50] Neurologic symptoms may distinguish meningiomas from SP if extracranial masses are observed, as patients may experience cranial neuropathy, facial pain, and paresthesia.[49] There are, however, overlap in aural symptoms in both, as patients may experience vertigo, otherwise there is a very well-defined difference in presentation of meningioma and SP and should, if extracranial masses are present, be properly assessed via CT/MRI.

TREATMENT

Treatment and surgical intervention of SP are highly circumstantial, as there are not precise guidelines and recommendations for managing this medical condition. Indeed, the benign nature of SP results in conservative treatments, most often resulting in surgical correction because of patient cosmetic concerns and fear of trauma. There are also reports documenting the abandonment of plans for surgical correction altogether based on shrinkage of the mass.[40,41] Despite the rarity and lack of precise understanding of the origins and formation of SP, solitary cases have been successfully managed with regular follow-up.[13,41] Digital subtraction angiography is highly versatile and can be used to distinguish SP from other abnormalities that may mimic it and otherwise indicate another method of treatment, as well as reveal abnormal venous circuits draining into the SP. Furthermore, direct visualization of the abnormal venous circuit with cerebral angiography and venography provide precise understanding of the morphologic characteristics of the SP for percutanous excision or endovascular embolization.

Surgical correction of SP involves resection of the extracranial venous mass and ligation of the emissary and diploic veins that communicate with the effected dural sinus, as well as reinforcing the calvarium if there is evidence of erosion.[8,10] Endovascular approaches are also mentioned in various reports; however, it is referred to as a second choice, as it provides less control when traversing the intracranial venous circuits and into the origin of the SP.[5] Endovascular approaches are minimally invasive by nature, so if cosmetics are a concern of the patient and the SP is not a major site of dural venous drainage that could potentially result in hemorrhage, this treatment is viable as primary option. One case mentions the use of ethylene-vinyl alcohol copolymer to assist in obliteration of diploic veins draining into the SP, demonstrating the various methods of obliterating the connections between the SP and dural sinus.[51]

Typically, vascular imaging (CT angiography and CT venography) is used to rule out abnormal vascular formations that may mimic SP, as well as to assess the flow dynamics and drainage pathways of the abnormal venous circuit. Surgical intervention is indicated for the following complications: thrombosis, air embolism, infection, and hemorrhage. Percutaneous alcohol ablations may also be used, but one case report mentions a resulting sixth cranial nerve palsy on a failed treatment of a temporal SP, which was then managed conservatively via warm compress and nonsteroidal medication.[52] Minimally invasive corrections consisting of excision of the extracranial venous mass and successive coagulation and filling of the connecting emissary circuits with bone wax.[4,10,16] In cases in which the bone wax does not adhere to the holes within the skull, methacrylate has been shown to be successful in hemostasis.[3] In cases where craniosynostosis appears to be the cause of the SP, surgical correction will reduce the mass of the extracranial mass once intracranial pressure is attenuated.[5] In cases where the SP is a major outlet (dominant) from the dural venous sinus, treatment should be abandoned to avoid complications involving intracranial venous outflow, such as severe hemorrhage and venous congestion.[5,41,53] Accessory SP, where only a small portion of venous blood exits the sinus and fills the extracranial mass, is treated as mentioned, wherein surgical excision and bone wax are implemented, and is believed to be the most treatable classification of SP.

CONCLUSIONS

The coexistence of SP with many skull and vascular malformations points to an origin needing to be further explored to develop guidelines for treatment. Conditions that have morphologic resemblance to SP should be carefully considered in the differential diagnosis to ensure the proper route of treatment. Currently, surgical correction of SP is amenable as long as it is not a major pathway for dural sinus drainage, otherwise plans for treatment should be delicately considered as the complications may be severe; surgical approaches that mitigate complications such as severe hemorrhage should be investigated.

REFERENCES

1. Stromeyer. About sinus pericranii (translation of original 1850 text). *Surg Neurol*. 1993;40(1):3–4.
2. Nakasu Y, et al. Multiple sinus pericranii with systemic angiomas: case report. *Surg Neurol*. 1993;39(1):41–45.
3. Spektor S, et al. Giant lateral sinus pericranii. Case report. *J Neurosurg*. 1998;88(1):145–147.
4. Ryorin M, et al. Dynamic morphological changes of thrombosed lateral sinus pericranii revealed by serial magnetic resonance images. *Childs Nerv Syst*. 2018;34(1):143–148.
5. Pavanello M, et al. Sinus pericranii: diagnosis and management in 21 pediatric patients. *J Neurosurg Pediatr*. 2015;15(1):60–70.
6. Gandolfo C, et al. Sinus pericranii: diagnostic and therapeutic considerations in 15 patients. *Neuroradiology*. 2007;49(6):505–514.
7. Brisman JL, Niimi Y, Berenstein A. Sinus pericranii involving the torcular sinus in a patient with Hunter's syndrome and trigonocephaly: case report and review of the literature. *Neurosurgery*. 2004;55(2):433.
8. Aburto-Murrieta Y, et al. Sinus pericranii: case report. *Vasc Endovasc Surg*. 2011;45(1):103–105.
9. Güler S, Tatlı B. Rare vascular pathology sinus pericranii; becomes symptomatic with pseudotumor cerebri. *Turk J Pediatr*. 2015;57(6):618–620.
10. Bhutada S, et al. Sinus Pericranii: a case report and review of literature. *Indian J Pediatr*. 2012;79(11):1523–1525.
11. Manjila S, et al. A review of extraaxial developmental venous anomalies of the brain involving dural venous flow or sinuses: persistent embryonic sinuses, sinus pericranii, venous varices or aneurysmal malformations, and enlarged emissary veins. *Neurosurg Focus*. 2018;45(1):E9.
12. Yasuda S, et al. Crouzon disease associated with sinus pericranii: a report on identical twin sisters. *Childs Nerv Syst*. 1993;9(2):119–122.
13. Saba R, et al. Sinus pericranii in a young adult with chronic headache. *BMJ Case Rep*. 2013;2013.
14. Bigot JL, et al. Sinus pericranii: advantages of MR imaging. *Pediatr Radiol*. 2000;30(10):710–712.
15. Zheng JW, et al. Guidelines for the treatment of head and neck venous malformations. *Int J Clin Exp Med*. 2013;6(5):377–389.
16. Crocker M, et al. Symptomatic venous sinus thrombosis following bone wax application to emissary veins. *Br J Neurosurg*. 2008;22(6):798–800.
17. Mastin WM. IV. Venous blood-tumors of cranium communicating with superior longitudinal sinus. *Ann Surg*. 1885;1(4):324–340.
18. Netter FH. *Atlas of Human Anatomy*. 7th ed. Elsevier; 2018.
19. Bollar A, et al. Sinus pericranii: radiological and etiopathological considerations. Case report. *J Neurosurg*. 1992;77(3):469–472.
20. Hershkovitz I, et al. The elusive diploic veins: anthropological and anatomical perspective. *Am J Phys Anthropol*. 1999;108(3):345–358.
21. Mortazavi MM, et al. Anatomy and pathology of the cranial emissary veins: a review with surgical implications. *Neurosurgery*. 2012;70(5):1312–1318; discussion 1318-9.
22. Tubbs R, Shoja M, Loukas M. *Bergman's Comprehensive Encyclopedia of Human Anatomic Variation*. John Wiley & Sons; 2016.
23. García-González U, et al. The diploic venous system: surgical anatomy and neurosurgical implications. *Neurosurg Focus*. 2009;27(5):E2.
24. Bradac G. Applied cerebral angiography. In: *Normal Anatomy and Vascular Pathology*. Springer International Publishing; 2017:163–165.
25. P L, B A, Ter Brugge K. Surgical neuroangiography. In: *Clinical Vascular Anatomy and Variations*. Springer Science & Business Media; 2001:675–678.
26. Louis RG, et al. Clinical anatomy of the mastoid and occipital emissary veins in a large series. *Surg Radiol Anat*. 2009;31(2):139–144.
27. Cabanac M, Brinnel H. Blood flow in the emissary veins of the human head during hyperthermia. *Eur J Appl Physiol Occup Physiol*. 1985;54(2):172–176.
28. Pamir MN, Black P, Falbusch R. Meningiomas: a comprehensive text. In: *Meningeal Anatomy*. Saunders/Elsevier; 2010:11–51.
29. Mullan S, et al. Embryological basis of some aspects of cerebral vascular fistulas and malformations. *J Neurosurg*. 1996;85(1):1–8.
30. Adle-Biassette H, Harding B, Golden J. *Developmental Neuropathology*. John Wiley & Sons; 2018:251–265.
31. Desai K, et al. Sinus pericranii in the frontal region : a case report. *Neurol India*. 2001;49(3):305–307.
32. Limaye N, et al. Somatic mutations in angiopoietin receptor gene TEK cause solitary and multiple sporadic venous malformations. *Nat Genet*. 2009;41(1):118–124.
33. Yadav P, et al. Vascular anomalies of the head and neck: a review of genetics. *Semin Ophthalmol*. 2013;28(5–6):257–266.
34. Weissmann-Brenner A, et al. Soft-tissue mass of fetal scalp with abnormal course of dural sinuses. *Ultrasound Obstet Gynecol*. 2018;52(1):126–127.
35. Renier D, Marchac D. Craniofacial surgery for craniosynostosis: functional and morphological results. *Ann Acad Med Singapore*. 1988;17(3):415–426.
36. Sheu M, et al. Sinus pericranii: dermatologic considerations and literature review. *J Am Acad Dermatol*. 2002;46(6):934–941.

37. Ota T, et al. Sinus pericranii. *J Neurosurg*. 1975;42(6):704–712.
38. Wakisaka S, et al. Sinus pericranii. *Surg Neurol*. 1983;19(3):291–298.
39. Kamble RB, et al. Sinus pericranii presenting with macrocephaly and mental retardation. *J Pediatr Neurosci*. 2010;5(1):39–41.
40. Sanders FH, et al. Extremely large sinus pericranii with involvement of the torcular and associated with Crouzon's syndrome. *Childs Nerv Syst*. 2017;33(9):1445–1449.
41. Goffin J, et al. Sinus pericranii: long-term outcome in a 10-year-old boy with a review of literature. *BMJ Case Rep*. 2018;2018.
42. Wong SL, Law HL, Tan S. Atretic cephalocele - an uncommon cause of cystic scalp mass. *Malays J Med Sci*. 2010;17(3):61–63.
43. Hsu SW, Chaloupka JC. Atretic parietal cephalocele associated with sinus pericranii: embryological consideration. *Brain Dev*. 2012;34(4):325–328.
44. Kim MS, Lee GJ. Two cases with persistent falcine sinus as congenital variation. *J Korean Neurosurg Soc*. 2010;48(1):82–84.
45. Ramnarayan R, Mariappan M. Dermoid cysts of the anterior fontanel in adults. 2018;9:448–449.
46. Crawford R. Dermoid cyst of the scalp: intracranial extension. *J Pediatr Surg*. 1990;25(3):294–295.
47. Aggarwal N, et al. Frontal subcutaneous lipoma associated with interhemispheric lipoma, lipomeningocele, and corpus callosal dysgenesis in a young adult: CT and MRI findings. *Indian J Radiol Imaging*. 2018;28(1):22–26.
48. Schropp C, et al. Cutaneous lesions in occult spinal dysraphism--correlation with intraspinal findings. *Childs Nerv Syst*. 2006;22(2):125–131.
49. Friedman CD, et al. Primary extracranial meningiomas of the head and neck. *Laryngoscope*. 1990;100(1):41–48.
50. Semeraro F, et al. Pseudo-Foster Kennedy syndrome in a young woman with meningioma infiltrating the superior sagittal sinus. *Clin Neurol Neurosurg*. 2012;114(3):272–274.
51. Rangel-Castilla L, et al. Endovascular embolization with Onyx in the management of sinus pericranii: a case report. *Neurosurg Focus*. 2009;27(5):E13.
52. Carpenter JS, et al. Sinus pericranii: clinical and imaging findings in two cases of spontaneous partial thrombosis. *Am J Neuroradiol*. 2004;25(1):121–125.
53. Ellis JA, et al. Determination of sinus pericranii resectability by external compression during angiography: technical note. *J Neurosurg Pediatr*. 2015:1–5.

FURTHER READING

1. Uddin MA, Haq UT, Rafique MZ. Cerebral venous system anatomy. 2006;56:516–518.

CHAPTER 22

The Inferior Petrooccipital Vein

R. SHANE TUBBS

The inferior petrooccipital (Fig. 22.1) vein has infrequently been mentioned in the literature. However, this vessel traveling at the skull base has an important relationship between the venous plexus traveling with the internal carotid artery or cavernous sinus anteriorly to the superior jugular bulb posteriorly. Best described as an emissary vein, the intimate relationship that it shares with the overlying inferior petrosal sinus and as considered a dural venous sinus by some historic authors makes a devoted chapter to its anatomy reasonable.

HISTORY

Kurata et al.[1] stated that Trolard[2] first named the petrooccipital vein and referred to the inferior petrosal sinus as the superior petrooccipital vein.[3] However, in 1743, 147 years earlier, Pietro Tabarrani[4] stated:

> *this new sinus, I believe, has not been hitherto observed by the anatomists on account of the difficult place which it occupies. It is situated on either side between the basilar process and the petrous bone, in the interior of the bone underneath the inferior petrosal sinus; or in order to express myself better, under the groove in which said petrosal sinus pursues its course, exactly there where a certain substance is found which is almost intermediate between cartilage and ligament. There this same sinus pursues its course on the bone of the basilar process; a slight groove, which sometimes is seen imprinted there pointing out the way. The beginning of the said sinus is usually found between the carotid and the sella turcica; but its end is mostly in the foramen jugulare, near its own diverticle, and in connxion with the inferior petrosal sinus.*[4]

In 1863, this structure was rediscovered by Englisch.[5] Interestingly, the inferior petrooccipital vein was once thought to conduct lymph from the pituitary gland.[3]

ANATOMY

The inferior petrooccipital vein travels just inferior to the petrooccipital fissure (suture) and unites the internal carotid artery venous plexus or cavernous sinus anteriorly to the superior jugular bulb posteriorly.[6–8] Trolard[2] found that the inferior petrooccipital vein coursed parallel to the inferior petrosal sinus but external to the skull. Kurata et al.[1] stated that the inferior petrooccipital vein might be incorrectly identified as the inferior petrosal sinus because of their very similar course. This vessel is rarely mentioned in the literature because of both the difficulty in dissecting it and, as alluded to above, because it is superimposed with the more well-known inferior petrosal sinus on angiographic projections. Benndorf[9] suggested that the inferior petroclival vein and inferior petrooccipital sinus might refer to the same structure. Tanoue et al.[10] illustrated the inferior petrooccipital vein and termed it the inferior petroclival vein. However, some have used the former term synonymously for the venous plexus in the carotid canal.[11] Trolard[2] stated that the inferior petrosal sinus might communicate with the inferior petrooccipital vein. Trolard also described the inferior petrooccipital vein as often draining into the anterior condylar confluent.

Tubbs et al. (2014) reported that the inferior petrooccipital vein was identified in 20 of 24 cadaveric sides (83.3%). The vessel had an average length and width of 18 and 1.5 mm, respectively. The range for the length and width was 15–21 mm and 1–1.8 mm, respectively.[13] In general, this vein united the internal carotid venous plexus anteriorly to the superior jugular bulb posteriorly. However, on two sides (10%), the anterior part of this vein communicated directly with the cavernous sinus, and on three sides (15%), the posterior part of the vein drained into the sigmoid sinus. The width was constant on 12 sides (60%), tapered at the vein's last anterior 1–2 cm on 5 sides (25%), and it tapered along its last posterior 1–2 cm on 3 sides (15%). In each of these, the tapering was roughly half of the maximal diameter of the individual veins. The inferior petrooccipital vein was separated from the overlying inferior petrosal sinus by a thin plate of bone on all sides. On eight sides (40%), (three left and five right sides), small venous connections were found between these two venous structures and these perforated the overlying plate of bone. The size of the overlying inferior petrosal sinus was always smaller in diameter when an underlying petrooccipital vein was present ($P < .05$). On four sides (20%) (three left and one right side), the

Anatomy, Imaging and Surgery of the Intracranial Dural Venous Sinuses. https://doi.org/10.1016/B978-0-323-65377-0.00022-2

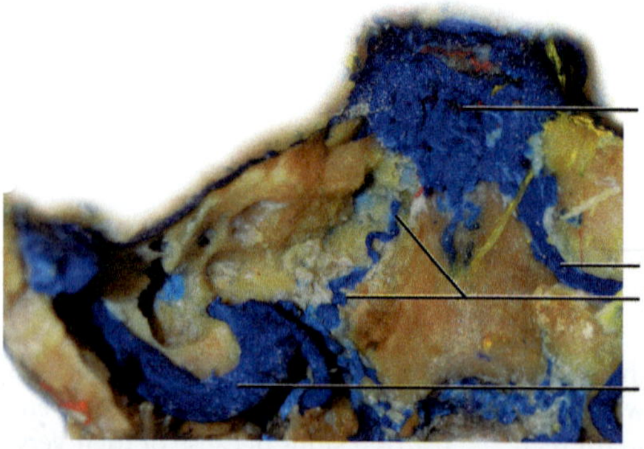

FIG. 22.1 Skull base with latex injection of the internal jugular vein. On the left side, the inferior petrosal sinus has been removed to illustrate the inferior petrooccipital vein. Compare this to the right side where the inferior petrosal sinus is intact.

posterior aspect of the vein communicated with the veins of the hypoglossal canal. On one left and two right sides, diploic veins from the clivus drained into the inferior petrooccipital vein.

CLINICAL APPLICATION

Transvenous approaches for endovascular treatment of carotid-cavernous fistulas or cavernous sinus hormone sampling are often performed via the inferior petrosal sinus. However, this intracranial venous sinus may be unavailable because of pathology or a variant anatomy such as noncommunication with the internal jugular vein. Kurata et al.[1] used the inferior petrooccipital vein as an alternative venous route to the cavernous sinus in four patients. Three of these patients presented with carotid-cavernous fistulas, and the fourth, with Cushing's disease due to a microadenoma in the left pituitary gland. Interestingly, in one of their patients with a carotid-cavernous fistula, the inferior petrooccipital vein was the main venous drainage. Katsuta et al.[12] reported using the inferior petroclival vein, which is usually small, as a useful pathway for introducing catheters for the treatment of dural arteriovenous fistulas. These authors mentioned that the vein, which based on their description is undoubtedly the inferior petrooccipital vein, is usually small, but that the high venous pressures seen with a dural arteriovenous fistula may dilate it significantly, making it a good conduit for approaching such lesions.[12]

REFERENCES

1. Kurata A, Suzuki S, Iwamoto K, et al. A new transvenous approach to the carotid-cavernous sinus via the inferior petrooccipital vein. *J Neurosurg*. 2012;116:581–587.
2. Trolard P. Les veines méningées moyennes. *Rev Sci Biol*. 1890;18:485–499.
3. Swedenborg E. *The Brain Considered Anatomically, Physiologically and Philosophically*. London: James Speirs; 1887.
4. Tabarrani P. *Observationes Anatomicae*. Lucca: Salani e Giuntini; 1743.
5. Speirs J. In: Abtheil i, ed. *Ueber eine constante Verbindung des Sinus cavernosus mit dem hinteren Ende des Sinus petrosus inferior ausserhalb des Schädels Sitzungsberichte der mathematisch-naturwissenschaftlichen Classe der Kaiserlichen Akademie der Wissenschaften Band Xlviii*. Wien: Jahrgaug; 1863.
6. Knott JF. On the cerebral sinuses and their variations. *J Anat*. 1882;16:27–42.
7. San Millan Ruiz D. *Systèmes Veineux De La Base Du Crâne Et De La Jonction Cranio-Cervicale : Anatomie Macroscopique Et Radiologique Et Implications Cliniques*. Thèse de doctorat. Genève, Univ. Genève, no. Méd. 10493; 2006.
8. San Millan Ruiz D, Gailloud P, Rufenacht DA, Delavelle J, Henry F, Fasel JH. The craniocervical venous system in relation to cerebral venous drainage. *AJNR Am J Neuroradiol*. 2002;23:1500–1508.
9. Benndorf G. *Dural Cavernous Sinus Fistulas*. New York: Springer; 2009.
10. Tanoue S, Kiyosue H, Sagara Y, et al. Venous structures at the craniocervical junction: anatomical variations evaluated by multidetector row CT. *Br J Radiol*. 2010;83:831–840.
11. van Loveren HR, Aziz KMA, Sanan A, Chicoine MR, Tew JM. In: Pensak ML, ed. *Jugular Foramen Tumors Controversies in Otolaryngology*. New York: Thieme; 2001.
12. Katsuta T, Matsushima T, Uda K. Surgical anatomy of the skullbase venous system: petroclival region. *Noshinkeigeka*. 2008;17:738–744.
13. Tubbs RS, Watanabe K, Loukas M, Cohen-Gadol AA. Anatomy of the inferior petro-occipital vein and its relation to the base of the skull: application to surgical and endovascular procedures of the skull base. *Clin Anat*. 2014;27(5):698–701.

CHAPTER 23

Dural Venous Sinus Connections to the Vertebral Venous Plexus

R. SHANE TUBBS

HISTORY

In 1819, Breschet was the first to give a detailed description of the vertebral venous plexus[1] (Figs. 23.1–23.3). Over a century later, in 1940, Batson[2] highlighted the functional importance of this primarily longitudinal collection of veins running the length of the vertebral canal and having connections with the intracranial dural venous sinuses. This group of veins, which acts as a bypass system to the caval system, is collectively referred to as *Batson's plexus*. This latter term is collectively used to describe both the external and internal plexuses of vertebral veins.[3]

Only vague statements regarding the cranial confluence of the vertebral venous system are found in the literature. For example, Groen et al.[4] stated that the vertebral venous plexus finds "a cranial terminus in the dural sinuses," and Falk[5] mentioned that distally, the marginal sinus drains freely into the vertebral venous plexus (Fig. 23.1). Even studies dedicated to evaluating the spinal venous plexus[5] and sinuses near the foramen magnum have not commented on the specific anatomy of the intracranial connections.[6–10]

Embryology and Evolutionary Considerations

The formation of the dural venous sinuses of the posterior cranial fossa is directly related to fetal brain growth.[11] By the sixth fetal month at the foramen magnum, the occipital (plexiform at this point) and marginal sinuses form as a result of the inferior growth of the cerebrum over the midbrain and cerebellum.[11] Falk[5] studied ancient hominid bipeds and found that many had enlarged occipital and marginal sinuses. This author hypothesized that selection for bipedalism may have resulted from epigenetic adaptations for pathways to bring blood to the vertebral venous plexus but as bipedalism became established, alternative routes for delivering blood to the vertebral plexus became established possibly because of the development of larger crania.

Anatomy

The vertebral venous plexuses extend from the coccyx to the skull base. Traditionally, the vertebral venous plexus has been described as consisting of four parts, an anterior external (outside the spinal canal) and internal (inside the spinal canal, epidural) components and a posterior external and internal (epidural) component[3] (Fig. 23.1). The internal plexuses are formed by veins in a column-like configuration, and dorsal to the spinal cord, these travel as two vertebral venous channels on either side of the midline. Ventral to the spinal cord, the anterior internal plexus, traveling between the layers of the posterior longitudinal ligament, collects the basivertebral vein and laterally, as the left and right longitudinal sinuses, communicates with the segmental veins (e.g., posterior intercostal, lumbar veins) via the veins of the intervertebral foramina[12]. The posterior external vertebral venous plexus ramifies over the posterior parts of the spinous and transverse processes and laminae and articular facets to then connect to the posterior internal vertebral venous plexus. The anterior vertebral venous plexus spans out over the anterolateral aspects of the vertebral bodies and connects primarily with the segmental veins. Stringer et al.[13] studied the internal and external vertebral venous plexuses. These authors found bicuspid valves in 34% of veins sampled from the external vertebral venous plexus. The direction of flow was always found to be toward the internal vertebral venous plexus. The flow of venous flow at the craniocervical junction depends on such things as posture, anatomic variation, and pathology. Based on the study by Stringer et al.,[13] longitudinal channels with transverse interconnections were characteristics of the internal vertebral venous plexus. Interestingly, these authors identified trabeculae within the internal vertebral venous plexus that were similar to the anatomy seen within the dural venous sinuses. They concluded that such trabeculae might inhibit venous overdistension or collapse of the vein, maintain unidirectional flow and velocity of venous blood flow, or are possibly

Anatomy, Imaging and Surgery of the Intracranial Dural Venous Sinuses. https://doi.org/10.1016/B978-0-323-65377-0.00023-4

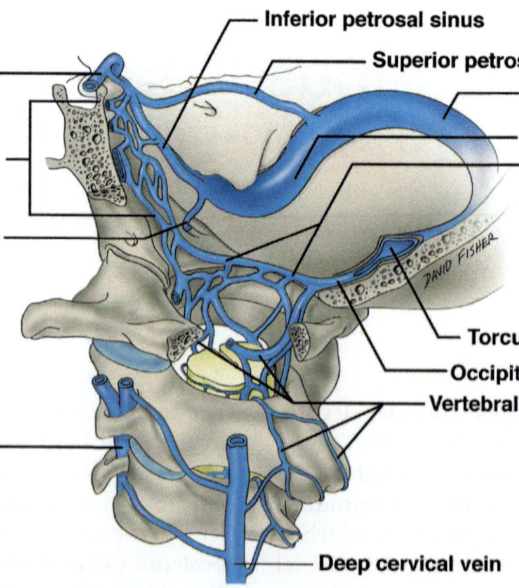

FIG. 23.1 Schematic drawing of the vertebral venous plexus of the upper cervical spine and its confluence with the dural venous sinuses at the skull base, for example, marginal sinus.

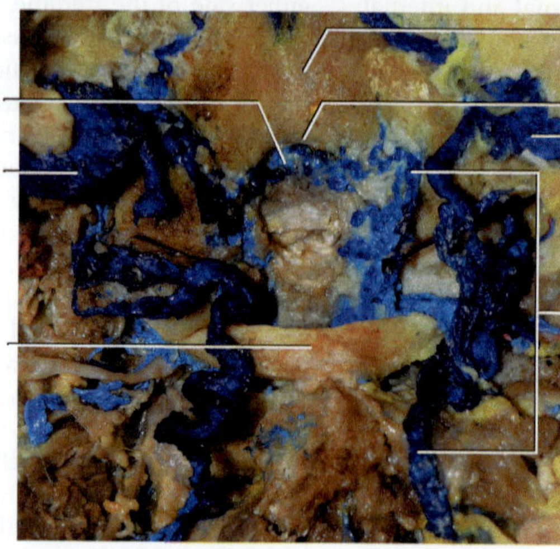

FIG. 23.2 Latex-injected cadaveric specimen noting the dural venous sinuses of the skull base and connections to the vertebral venous plexus.

involved in heat regulation.[13] Others have also hypothesized that the vertebral venous plexus may be involved in thermoregulatory regulation and "cooling" of the spinal cord.[14]

Communication between the intradural and extradural spinal venous compartments is of clinical and surgical importance. Connections between the intradural and extradural parts of the spinal venous sinuses can occur transdurally, but more commonly, this is via the exiting radicular (medullary) veins at or near the dural nerve sheath. These radiculomedullary veins merge and receive drainage from the spinal nerve roots via superficial nerve root veins. Within the nerve root, longitudinal veins receive blood from the venules surrounding the nerves and empty into draining branch veins that then exit the dural nerve sheath and subsequently empty into the superficial nerve root veins.[15] This system of venous drainage of the spinal nerve root

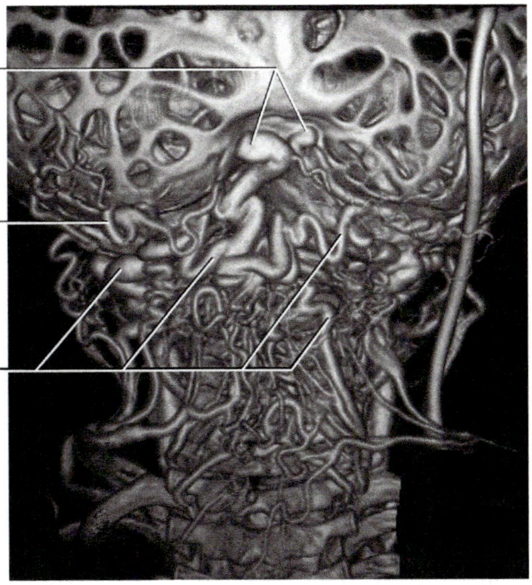

FIG. 23.3 Patient with craniosynostosis and enlarged vertebral venous plexus.

contains transverse coils in the venules, longitudinal veins, and draining branch veins that potentially allow for compensation of extra blood volume. The radiculomedullary veins drain into the extradural vertebral venous plexus via the spinal nerve venous pathways.[16]

Because some investigators[17] have found that the vertebral venous plexus is the main intracranial venous outflow in the upright position and is a secondary pathway of intracranial egress during Valsalva maneuvers or with compromised internal jugular veins, a study aimed at better quantitating this anatomy seemed reasonable. Moreover, recently, the vertebral venous plexus has been used for transvenous embolization of dural arteriovenous fistulas (AVFs) involving the marginal sinus.[18]

Tubbs and Cohen-Gadol[19] found vertebral venous plexuses in all specimens at the craniocervical junction. These were always composed of multiple interwoven vessels concentrated anteriorly (i.e., anterior vertebral plexuses), posteriorly (i.e., posterior vertebral venous plexuses) and laterally (i.e., lateral vertebral venous plexuses). More often than not, these were concentrated anteriorly and within the vertebral canal (e.g., anterior internal vertebral venous plexus). The veins making up the plexus tended to be largest for the anterior internal vertebral venous plexus. The mean diameter of the veins making up the anterior external, anterior internal, lateral internal, posterior internal, and posterior external venous plexuses was 1.7 mm (range 1.0–2.0 mm), 2.3 mm (range 1.8–2.7 mm), 0.9 mm (range 0.5–1.2 mm), 1.2 mm (range 0.8–1.6 mm), and 1.0 mm (range 0.8–1.3 mm), respectively. These authors[19] also found a previously unnamed lateral internal vertebral venous plexus was identified on 10 sides (33%) (6 left and 4 right sides). The lateral internal vertebral venous plexus, when present, connected to the lateral marginal sinus on all sides. The anterior external vertebral venous plexus connected to the basilar venous plexus via transclival emissary veins in two cadavers (13%). The remaining anterior vertebral venous plexus veins either connected intracranially via very small perforating branches through the anterior atlantooccipital membrane (33%) or had no direct gross connections inside the cranium (53%). The anterior internal vertebral plexus, which traveled between the layers of the posterior longitudinal ligament at the skull base (i.e., the tectorial membrane), connected to the anterior half of the marginal sinus in 10 cadavers (33%) and on three sides into the anterolateral parts of the marginal sinus (20%). In two specimens (13.3%), no intracranial connection was identified. The posterior internal venous plexus connected to the posterior aspect of the marginal sinus on 80% of sides and directly into the occipital sinus on two sides (13.3%). No obvious intracranial connection was found on one cadaver (6.7%).

The posterior external venous plexus connected to the veins of the hypoglossal canal in three cadavers (20%) and into the posterior aspect of the marginal sinus on two cadavers (13.3%) via connections through the posterior atlantooccipital membrane. However, this venous plexus connected primarily to the suboccipital venous plexus and had little connectivity to the intracranial venous sinuses[19].

Pathology

Lv et al.[20] reported dural AVFs with spinal perimedullary venous drainage at the craniocervical junction in four patients. Asakawa et al.[21] reported cervical myelopathy resulting from intracranial dural AVF in a patient who presented with progressive myelopathy and respiratory insufficiency. Angiography identified an AVF at the skull base, which drained to the internal vertebral venous plexus. Imaging found enlarged spinal veins and edema of the spinal cord.[22] The progressive myelopathy in this patient was abated following a combined embolization and surgical procedures where the fistula was coagulated via suboccipital craniotomy.

Kinouchi et al.[23] reviewed their patients with dural AVF of the spine and reported that seven of these patients had presented with subarachnoid hemorrhage and a single patient had presented with quadriparesis. Imaging also found that for craniocervical AVF, arterial feeders were derived from radicular branches of the vertebral artery. In one patient with myelopathy, the venous outflow was inferior into the spine. However, in the patients with subarachnoid hemorrhage, the venous outflow was cranial into the venous sinuses.

Yoshida et al.[24] reported a patient with motor and sensory loss due to a craniocervical dural AVF, who also had signal change in the adjacent spinal cord. The AVF was positioned at the point where the vertebral artery pierced the posterior atlantooccipital membrane and underlying dura mater. Ligation of the venous outflow resulted in improvement of the patient's symptoms. Yousry et al.[25] studied patients with postural headache and found that the majority of patients, 17 of 20 (85%), had enlargement of their anterior internal vertebral venous plexus. The authors hypothesized that imaging indicative of dilatation of the anterior internal vertebral venous plexus could lead to the diagnosis of intracranial hypotension in such patients.

Sato et al.[26] reviewed nine cases of dural AVFs and perimedullary AVFs. Each of these fistulas shared perimedullary veins (anterior spinal vein, seven cases; anterolateral spinal vein, two cases), which were enlarged and acted as the main drainage, and this drainage was rostrally directed in most cases.

SURGICAL CONSIDERATIONS

Most often, veins of the upper cervical region both of the vertebral venous plexus and other tributaries, for example, deep cervical vein, are easily controlled during surgical approaches. However, diseases (e.g., craniosynostosis or achondroplasia) that impede venous outflow from the cranium can result in enlarged veins in this area that if injured, may result in significant hemorrhage that is difficult to control. Additionally, some cases have been reported where the majority of venous outflow from the skull is via the vertebral venous plexus and not the internal jugular vein.[27] These cases can be because of venous sinus thrombosis or because of congenital defects, for example, craniosynostosis. Additionally, as mentioned above, AVF in this region and normal variants necessitate a greater appreciation for the anatomy of the veins of the upper spine connecting intracranially. Preoperative Magnetic Resonance Venography (MRV), such as before occipitocervical fusion, could assist in identifying such veins and help guide the surgical procedure, especially when enlarged due to pathology.

REFERENCES

1. Nathoo N, Caris EC, Wiener JA, Mendel E. History of the vertebral venous plexus and the significant contributions of Breschet and Batson. *Neurosurgery*. 2011;69:1007–1014.
2. Batson OV. The function of the vertebral veins and their role in the spread of metastases. 1940;*Clin Orthop Mar*. 1995: 4–9.
3. Griessenauer CJ, Raborn J, Foreman P, Shoja MM, Loukas M, Tubbs RS. Venous drainage of the spine and spinal cord: a comprehensive review of its history, embryology, anatomy, physiology, and pathology. *Clin Anat*. 2015;28:75–87.
4. Groen RJ, Grobbelaar M, Muller CJ, et al. Morphology of the human internal vertebral venous plexus: a cadaver study after latex injection in the 21-25-week fetus. *Clin Anat*. 2005;18:397–403.
5. Falk D. Evolution of cranial blood drainage in hominids: enlarged occipital/marginal sinuses and emissary foramina. *Am J Phys Anthropol*. 1986;70:311–324.
6. Woodhall B. Variations of the cranial venous sinuses in the region of the torcular herophili. *Arch Surg*. 1936;33. 397–314.
7. Browder J, Kaplan HA. *Cerebral Dural Sinuses and Their Tributaries*. Springfield: Royal Society of Medicine Press; 1976.
8. Dora F, Zileli T. Common variations of the lateral and occipital sinuses at the confluens sinuum. *Neuroradiology*. 1980;20:23–27.
9. Kimbel WH. Variation in the pattern of cranial venous sinuses and hominid phylogeny. *Am J Phys Anthropol*. 1984;63:243–263.
10. Caruso RD, Rosenbaum AE, Chang JK, Joy SE. Craniocervical junction venous anatomy on enhanced MR images: the suboccipital cavernous sinus. *Am J Neuroradiol*. 1999;20:1127–1131.
11. Okudera T, Huang YP, Ohta T, et al. Development of posterior fossa dural sinuses, emissary veins, and jugular bulb: morphological and radiologic study. *Am J Neuroradiol*. 1994;15:1871–1883.

12. Schaeffer JP, ed. *Morris' Human Anatomy*. 11th ed. New York: The Blakiston Company; 1953.
13. Stringer MD, Restieaux M, Fisher AL, Crosado B. The vertebral venous plexuses: the internal veins are muscular and external veins have valves. *Clin Anat*. 2012;25:609–618.
14. Hoogland PV, Wessels Q, Vorster W, Groen RJ, Greyling LM, Kotzé SH. The posterior intercostal vein: a thermoregulatory gateway to the internal vertebral venous plexus. *Clin Anat*. 2013;26:735–740.
15. Jinkins J. Spinal vasculature. In: John J, Brown B, Seigafuse S, Palumbo R, eds. *Atlas of Neuroradiologic Embryology, Anatomy, and Variants*. Philadelphia: Lippincott Williams & Wilkins; 2000:563–578.
16. Lasjaunias P, Berenstein A. Spinal and spinal cord arteries and veins. In: John J, Brown B, Seigafuse S, Palumbo R, eds. *Atlas of Neuroradiologic Embryology, Anatomy, and Variants*. New York: Springer-Verlag; 1990.
17. Epstein HM, Linde HW, Crampton AR, Ciric IS, Eckenhoff JE. The vertebral venous plexus as a major cerebral venous outflow tract. *Anesthesiology*. 1970;32:332–337.
18. Choi HS, Kim DI, Kim BM, Kim DJ, Ahn SS. Endovascular treatment of dural arteriovenous fistula involving marginal sinus with emphasis on the routes of transvenous embolization. *Neuroradiology*. 2012;54:163–169.
19. Tubbs RS, Cohen-Gadol AA, Demerdash A, et al.Intracranial connections of the vertebral venous plexus: anatomical study with application to neurosurgical and endovascular procedures at the craniocervical junction. *Oper Neurosurg (Hagerstown)*. 2018;14:51–57.
20. Lv X, Yang X, Li Y, Jiang C, Wu Z. Dural arteriovenous fistula with spinal perimedullary venous drainage. *Neurol India*. 2011;59:899–902.
21. Asakawa H, Yanaka K, Fujita K, Marushima A, Anno I, Nose T. Intracranial dural arteriovenous fistula showing diffuse MR enhancement of the spinal cord: case report and review of the literature. *Surg Neurol*. 2002;58:251–257.
22. Hendrix P, Griessenauer CJ, Cohen-Adad J, et al. Spinal diffusion tensor imaging: a comprehensive review with emphasis on spinal cord anatomy and clinical applications. *Clin Anat*. 2015;28:88–95.
23. Kinouchi H, Mizoi K, Takahashi A, Nagamine Y, Koshu K, Yoshimoto T. Dural arteriovenous shunts at the craniocervical junction. *J Neurosurg*. 1998;89:755–761.
24. Yoshida S, Oda Y, Kawakami Y, Sato S. Progressive myelopathy caused by dural arteriovenous fistula at the craniocervical junction--case report. *Neurol Med Chir*. 1999;39:376–379.
25. Yousry I, Forderreuther S, Moriggl B, et al. Cervical MR imaging in postural headache: MR signs and pathophysiological implications. *Am J Neuroradiol*. 2001;22:1239–1250.
26. Sato K, Endo T, Niizuma K, et al. Concurrent dural and perimedullary arteriovenous fistulas at the craniocervical junction: case series with special reference to angioarchitecture. *J Neurosurg*. 2013;118:451–459.
27. Choudhary AK, Dias MS, Iantosca M. Intracranial venous drainage through spinal veins. *Del Med J*. 2014;86:181–184.

CHAPTER 24

Diploic Veins

SATOSHI TSUTSUMI

INTRODUCTION

The calvarial diploic veins (DVs) are intraosseously formed, distinct venous networks that were first described in 1928.[5] Neurosurgeons and plastic surgeons can encountered bleeds from the DVs during surgery at any cranial site. Although cranial emissary veins have been well investigated,[8,10] we lack systematic knowledge about the DVs. The DVs have received little attention because of their peculiar location beneath the hard compact bones, which makes extensive investigations difficult, and because bleeding is often not profuse and is controlled with ease.[3] Furthermore, the DVs are inconsistently visualized with conventional neuroimaging techniques and they have been infrequently documented in association with pathologic conditions such as dural arteriovenous fistulas,[1,2,13] tumors,[9,15] and sinus pericranii.[11] Investigations have attempted to reveal the distribution of DVs with radiography,[4] corrosion cast models[7,12] cadaver dissection,[3,20] magnetic resonance imaging (MRI),[6] and in experimental study[14]; however, detailed morphology of the DVs and their distributions are not well understood. To our knowledge, there has been only an infusion study that has demonstrated the direct communications between the DVs and superior sagittal sinus (SSS).[7] Recently, we reported peculiar morphologies and distribution of the DVs and their potential function as cerebrospinal fluid (CSF) pathways.[16–19]

In the present chapter, morphology and distribution of the DVs are characterized based on our investigations with MRI, cadaver dissection, and laboratory examination with a brief review of the literature concerning the DVs.

Major DV Pathways

Examinations with thin-sliced, contrast MRI involving the whole cranial vault, were performed for a total of 100 outpatients, and the DVs with irregular contours and peculiar branching patterns were well delineated. Furthermore, the DVs could be classified into four major pathways: pteriofrontoparietal (PFP), frontoorbital (FO), occipitoparietal (OP), and occipitocervical (OC) route depending on the topological differences in the calvarium. The PFP connected the lateral edge of the sphenoparietal sinus to the SSS in the parietal region and was the most prominent type. The PFP route showed a near-vertical, superoinferior course: the single trunk from the pterional region to the level of the frontal eminence changed direction posteriorly and divided into several branches, which coursed toward the parietal SSS. These branches showed racemose pattern in patients with well-developed DVs. The FO route consisted of two major parts, the orbital and pterional parts. The PFP and FO parts fused proximally with the sphenoparietal sinus and descended as the middle meningeal vein, which coursed inferomedially along the middle cranial fossa, passed downward through the floor adjacent to the foramen ovale, and finally drained into the pterygoid plexus. The OP route coursed in the superoinferior direction as a single trunk and connected the junction part of the transverse-sigmoid sinus to the SSS. This route arose as several tributaries from the parietal SSS converged in a single trunk at the level of the parietal eminence, coursed inferiorly, and finally drained into the transverse-sigmoid sinus junctional region. The OC route was delineated as a unique, unpaired pathway. It occurred as a single major channel coursing in the superoinferior direction in the median occipital bone, drained extracranially passing through the lower part of the occipital bone, and finally joined the suboccipital venous channels. In the cephalad, the OC connected to the parietooccipital SSS in 42% of cases. The OC communicated with the confluence of the sinuses (torcular Herophili) via various sizes of channels. In summary, the calvarial diploic system was found to communicate with the intracranial dural sinuses at the lateral edge of the sphenoparietal sinus, frontoparietal region of the SSS, torcular Herophili, and at the region of the transverse sinus-sigmoid sinus junction (Fig. 24.1). Degrees of development of the PFP, FO, OP, and OC showed considerable interindividual diversity in addition to common asymmetry in the same subject.[16]

Anatomy, Imaging and Surgery of the Intracranial Dural Venous Sinuses. https://doi.org/10.1016/B978-0-323-65377-0.00024-6

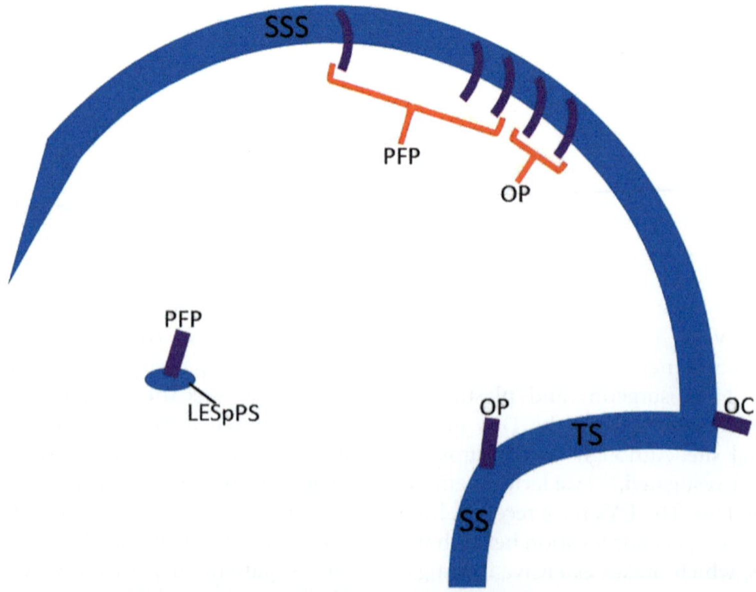

FIG. 24.1 Schematic drawing of the major communicating sites between the calvarial diploic veins and intracranial dural sinuses. *LESpPS*, lateral edge of the sphenoparietal sinus; *OC*, occipitocervical route; *OP*, occipitoparietal route; *PFP*, pteriofrontoparietal route; *SS*, sigmoid sinus; *SSS*, superior sagittal sinus; *TS*, transverse sinus.

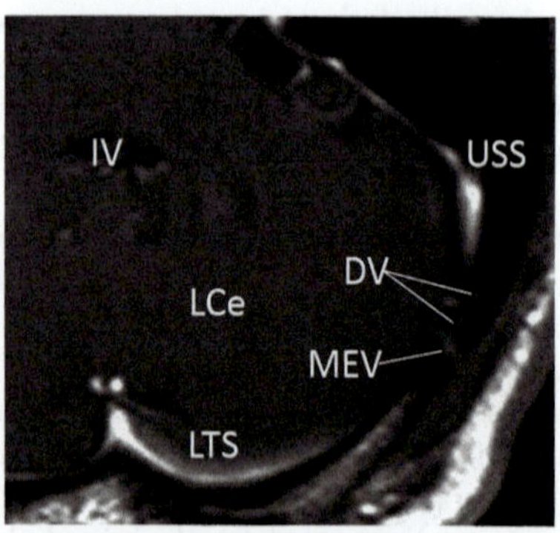

FIG. 24.2 Postcontrast T1-weighted axial magnetic resonance image sectioned at the level of the transverse sinus-sigmoid sinus junction showing a mastoid emissary vein on the left communicating with a diploic vein. *DV*, diploic vein; *IV*, fourth ventricle; *LCe*: left cerebellar hemisphere; *LTS*, lower margin of the transverse sinus; *MEV*, mastoid emissary vein; *USS*, upper margin of the sigmoid sinus.

Diploic Veins Communicating With the Mastoid Emissary Vein

In another study, with thin-sliced, contrast MRI that was performed for a total of 96 outpatients,[19] 5.6% of the mastoid emissary veins were identified to communicate with the DVs distributing in the region (Fig. 24.2).

Diploic Veins Anastomosing With the Supraorbital Subcutaneous Vein

Our recent investigation with thin-sliced, contrast MRI that was performed for a total of 90 outpatients suggested that 6.6% of the supraorbital DVs had anastomotic channels with the subcutaneous veins through the anterior wall of the supraorbital rim, 9.4% through the inferior wall of it, and 7.2% through the supraorbital foramen (Fig. 24.3, unpublished data).

Diploic Veins and Contiguous Arachnoid Protruding Upward Into the Skull

A total of 150 patients who underwent thin-sliced, coronal T2-weighted MRI found a peculiar, pairing structure formed by the DVs and contiguous arachnoid protruding upward into the skull (AP) (Fig. 24.4). On T2-weighted images, the DVs appeared to have a homogenous hyperintensity similar to the intensity of the CSF. Furthermore, morphology of the DVs delineated on T2-weighted sequence was in accordance with that on the contrast images. In 150 patients, the total number of AP-DV pairings identified in the cerebral convexity was 489 on the right and 498 on the left. When the cerebral convexity was divided into three parts–anterior (A), middle (M), and posterior (P) third,–55% were found in M, 27% in P, and 18% in A. The total number of

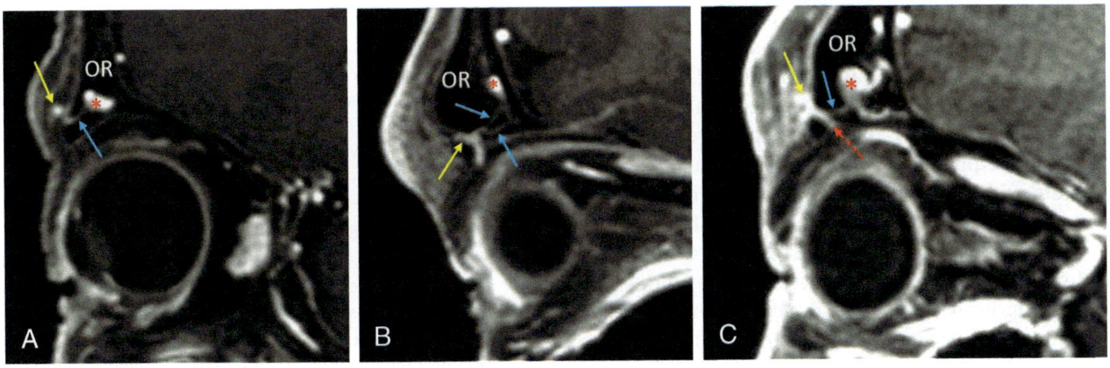

FIG. 24.3 Postcontrast T1-weighted sagittal magnetic resonance images of different patients showing variable morphologies of the diploic veins distributing in the supraorbital rim and their anastomotic channels with the subcutaneous veins through the anterior wall **(A)**, through the inferior wall **(B)**, and through the supraorbital foramen **(C)**. OR: supraorbital rim; asterisk: diploic vein of the supraorbital rim; blue arrow: anastomotic channel; yellow arrow: subcutaneous vein; dotted red arrow in **C**: supraorbital foramen.

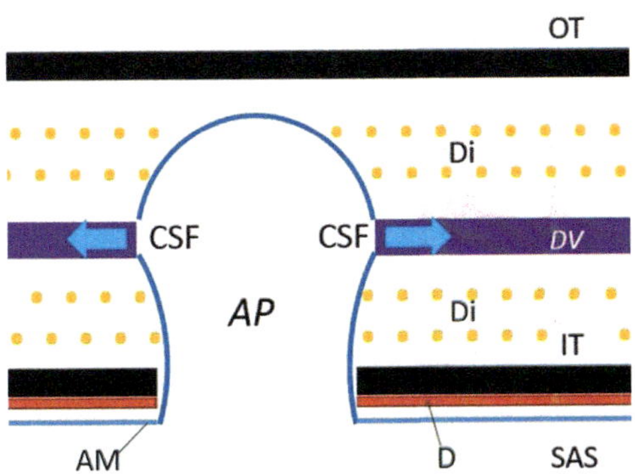

FIG. 24.4 Schematic drawing of a pairing structure formed by the diploic veins and contiguous arachnoid protruding upward into the skull that is assumed to function as cerebrospinal fluid pathway. *AM*, arachnoid membrane; *AP*, arachnoid protrusion; *CSF*, cerebrospinal fluid; *D*, dura mater; *Di*, diploe; *DV*, diploic vein; *IT*, inner table; *OT*, outer table; *SAS*, subarachnoid space; arrow: permeation of cerebrospinal fluid.

AP-DV pairings identified in the skull base was 375, 159 on the right, and 216 on the left. In the skull base, 53% of these pairings were located in the middle fossa and 47% in the posterior fossa. Neither APs nor DVs were found in the anterior fossa.[17]

Cadaver Dissection

Observations on three cadaver heads (six sides) found that the FO and PFP are the most predominant among the four major DV pathways and are distributed disparately over the skull. In all of the six sides, the FO and PFP were interrupted at a conventional frontotemporal craniotomy.[17]

Laboratory Investigation

For a total of 41 patients who underwent craniotomy surgeries in various cranial regions, levels of prostaglandin D synthase (PGDS) and cystatin C (CysC) proteins with low molecular weights, known as CSF-specific biomarkers, were measured in the diploic and peripheral venous bloods. In these patients, the DV/peripheral vein ratios were significantly elevated for PGDS in the frontal, temporal, parietal regions, and the skull base ($P<.05$), and did not reach a statistical significance for CysC.[18]

COMMENTS

In our investigations with contrast MRI, morphology of the DVs and their distributions over the calvaria were well delineated. Depending on the topographic differences, the calvarial DVs could be classified into four major pathways. On cadaver specimens, the FO and PFP were most predominant and consistently interrupted at a frontotemporal craniotomy.[16] In another study with contrast MRI, 5.6% of the mastoid emissary veins were found to communicate with the DV.[19] In addition, our recent investigation suggested that at least a part of the DVs distributing in the supraorbital bone had anastomotic channels with the adjacent subcutaneous veins. Furthermore, examination with contrast and noncontrast, T2-weighted MRI delineated pairing structures were formed by the DVs and contiguous arachnoid. They were identified most frequently over the middle third of the cerebral hemisphere, roughly corresponding to the parietal region of the skull.[17] In addition, laboratory investigation showed that the DV/

peripheral vein ratios were significantly elevated for PGDS in most of the calvarial regions.[18]

The functional implications of the DVs remain elusive. In our investigations, the pterional, parasagittal parietal, asterional, and suboccipital regions were thought to be pivotal for the DVs where the DVs communicate with the dural sinuses.[16] In addition, it was suggested that the supraorbital region may be an essential center of the calvarial DV system functioning as a conduit connecting to the subcutaneous venous system. Furthermore, laboratory investigation suggested that some CSF-specific biomarkers could dissolve into DVs through the contiguous arachnoids.[18] This means that at least a part of the intracranial CSF may permeate into the DVs. In other words, the DVs may function not only as venous networks distributing over the calvaria but also as draining pathways of the intracranial CSF. These speculations may be a clue for approaching the precise anatomic knowledge and functional implications of the DVs, but have to be verified in a systematic manner in future studies.

CONCLUSIONS

The DVs appear to be relatively consistent venous networks distributing over the calvaria that connect with the intracranial dura sinuses, suboccipital venous channels, subcutaneous veins in the supraorbital region, and possibly, with the mastoid emissary veins. At least a part of the DVs are contiguous with the arachnoids protruding into the skull. Based on the appearance on MRI and outcomes of laboratory investigation, the DVs seems to function as draining pathways of the intracranial CSF.

REFERENCES

1. Benndorf G, Lehmann TN. Bilateral diploic arteriovenous fistula causing scalp hematoma. *J Neurosurg*. 2004;100:950–955.
2. Burger IM, Tamargo RJ, Broussard J, Gailloud P. Combined surgical and endovascular treatment of a spontaneous diploic arteriovenous fistula. Case report. *J Neurosurg*. 2005;103:179–181.
3. García-González U, Cavalcanti DD, Agrawal A, et al. The diploic venous system: surgical anatomy and neurosurgical implications. *Neurosurg Focus*. 2009;27:E2.
4. Hershkovitz I, Greenwald C, Rothschild BM, et al. The elusive diploic veins: anthropological and anatomical perspective. *Am J Phys Anthropol*. 1999;108:345–358.
5. Jefferson G, Stewart D. On the veins of the diplö. *Br J Surg*. 1928;16:70–88.
6. Jivraj K, Bhagava R, Aronyk K, Quateen A, Walji A. Diploic anatomy studied in-vivo by MRI. *Clin Anat*. 2009;22:296–301.
7. Johnston KD, Walji AH, Fox RJ, Pugh JA, Aronyk KE. Access to cerebrospinal fluid absorption sites by infusion into vascular channels of the skull diplö. *J Neurosurg*. 2007;107:841–843.
8. Mortazavi MM, Tubbs RS, Riech S, et al. Anatomy and pathology of the cranial emissary veins: a review with surgical implications. *Neurosurgery*. 2012;70:1312–1319.
9. Ohigashi Y, Tanabe A. A huge frontal meningioma associated with intraoperative massive bleeding and severe brain swelling--case report. *J Clin Neurosci*. 2001;8(suppl 1):54–58.
10. Reis CV, Deshmukh V, Zabramski JM, et al. Anatomy of the mastoid emissary vein and venous system of the posterior neck region: neurosurgical implications. *Neurosurgery*. 2007;61:193–201.
11. Rizvi M, Behari S, Singh RK, et al. Sinus pericranii with unusual features: multiplicity, associated dural venous lakes and venous anomaly, and a lateral location. *Acta Neurochir*. 2010;152:2197–2204.
12. San Millán Ruíz D, Fasel JH, Rüfenacht DA, Gailloud P. The sphenoparietal sinus of breschet: does it exist? An anatomic study. *AJNR Am J Neuroradiol*. 2004;25:112–120.
13. Shim JH, Yoon SM, Shim JJ, Kim RS. A case of intraosseous dural arteriovenous fistulas involving diploic vein treated with transarterial onyx embolization. *J Korean Neurosurg Soc*. 2011;50:260–263.
14. Toriumi H, Shimizu T, Shibata M, et al. Developmental and circulatory profile of the diploic veins. *Microvasc Res*. 2011;81:97–102.
15. Tsutsumi S, Yasumoto Y, Ito M. Case of calvarial fibrous dysplasia presenting with cyst degeneration [Japanese]. *Noshinkeigeka*. 2011;39:163–168.
16. Tsutsumi S, Nakamura M, Tabuchi T, Yasumoto Y, Ito M. Calvarial diploic venous channels: an anatomic study using high-resolution magnetic resonance imaging. *Surg Radiol Anat*. 2013;35:935–941.
17. Tsutsumi S, Ogino I, Miyajima M, et al. Cranial arachnoid protrusions and contiguous diploic veins in CSF drainage. *AJNR Am J Neuroradiol*. 2014;35:1735–1739.
18. Tsutsumi S, Ogino I, Miyajima M, Ito M, Arai H, Yasumoto Y. Cerebrospinal fluid drainage through the diploic and spinal epidural veins. *J Anat*. 2015;227:297–301.
19. Tsutsumi S, Ono H, Yasumoto Y. The mastoid emissary vein: an anatomical study with magnetic resonance imaging. *Surg Radiol Anat*. 2017;39:351–356.
20. Tubbs RS, Salter EG, Wellons 3rd JC, Blount JP, Oakes WJ. The sphenoparietal sinus. *Neurosurgery*. 2007;60(2 suppl 1):ONS9–12.

CHAPTER 25

Variations of the Intracranial Dural Venous Sinuses

SHAMFA C. JOSEPH • ELIAS RIZK • R. SHANE TUBBS

The dural venous sinuses develop from a widespread venous network, which allows for multiple variations.[1] Insufficient knowledge on these variations can lead to misdiagnosis and can complicate interventional neurosurgical procedures. It is therefore important to understand not just the anatomy of the most consistent presentation of the dural sinuses but also the variant anatomy.

SUPERIOR SAGITTAL SINUS

The diameter of the superior sagittal sinus varies from 3.0 to 4.5 mm.[2] Its length varied from 24 to 27 cm in one study.[3] In one study of 100 patients, 7% had hypoplasia of the rostral superior sagittal sinus.[4] Browder and Kaplan[5] found that the length of rostral sinus atresia ranged from 1 to 9 cm. There have also been reports of complete absence of the superior sagittal sinus.[6,7,8]

Duplication of the superior sagittal sinus is uncommon.[9–11] Woodhall[12] reported two cases where it was doubled, and Knott[6] and Malacarne[13] described early bifurcation of the sinus into the transverse sinuses. In a study of 50 children with developmental delays, Widjaja and Griffiths[14] observed "high splitting" of the superior sagittal sinus. In another patient, they also observed a shortened superior sagittal sinus, which was drained anteriorly by two prominent cortical veins. Bisaria[2,15] found splitting of the superior sagittal sinus into two and three channels with and without partition. The superior sagittal sinus can drain into the torcular Herophili, superior jugular bulb, or left or right transverse sinuses.

INFERIOR SAGITTAL SINUS

Knott[6] noted an inferior sagittal sinus that terminated in the superior sagittal sinus instead of passing through the straight sinus. This sinus can also be absent.[5] Saxena et al.[16] reported absence of the inferior sagittal sinus in 1 of 76 cases.

TORCULAR HEROPHILI

Labbé[17] quoted Hallet's first description of an absence of the torcular Herophili. Woodhall[12] described five types of torcular Herophili and added one type to the classification by Edwards.[18]

1. The plexiform type (56%): This type consisted of several channels that provided communication between the sides.
2. The ipsilateral type (31%): The superior sagittal sinus ran toward one side and the straight sinus ran to the opposite side.
3. The common pool type (9%): The straight and superior sagittal sinuses merged and both transverse sinuses drained this junction.
4. The unilateral type (4%): Both the superior sagittal and straight sinuses entered the same transverse sinus with absence of the contralateral transverse sinus.
5. The occipital type: This is characterized by the persistence of a large single sinus, or of a paired occipital sinus with a large marginal sinus.

Woodhall[12] suggested different draining patterns of the transverse sinus with resultant forms of the torcular. In the plexiform type, the sagittal and straight sinuses can drain equally into both sides of the transverse sinus, or one draining solely into one side of the transverse sinus and the other draining into the other transverse sinus.

Browning et al.[19] described four patterns:

1. Type I (36%): The superior sagittal and straight sinuses form a confluence from which the two transverse sinuses arise.
2. Type II (24%): both the superior and the straight sinuses bifurcate with union of their right and left branches to form the corresponding transverse sinus.
3. Type III (24%): The superior sagittal sinus deviates to the right of the left transverse sinus, whereas the straight sinus bifurcates into two branches. One branch joins the superior sagittal sinus, whereas the other branch becomes the opposite transverse sinus.

Anatomy, Imaging and Surgery of the Intracranial Dural Venous Sinuses. https://doi.org/10.1016/B978-0-323-65377-0.00025-8

4. Type IV (16%): This is similar to type III; however, the drainage of the straight and sagittal sinuses is reversed.

Bisaria[2,15] described three types of variations of the torcular Herophili:

1. Type 1 (24.5%): The superior sagittal sinus drains into one transverse sinus and the straight sinus into the other.
2. Type 2 (9.1%): The superior sagittal sinus and the straight sinus fork into the transverse sinuses.
3. Type 3 (57.3%): The torcular Herophili is present with varying degrees of partitioning.

Bisaria[2,15] also observed other rare variations including (1) doubled straight sinuses uniting to form one sinus and then becoming continuous with the left transverse sinus; (2) the transverse sinus originating from a tentorial vein; (3) a circular defect in the roof of a transverse sinus; and (4) the drainage of the tentorial vein into the torcular Herophili.

Fukusumi et al.[20] noted several different configurations of the torcular Herophili with other venous sinuses. There were four different patterns of drainage of the superior sagittal sinus into the transverse sinus.

1. Type I (20%): The superior sagittal sinus drained into the torcular Herophili, which bifurcated into two transverse sinuses.
2. Type II (26.7%): There were two superior sagittal sinus (right and left limbs) that both drained into the same side of the transverse sinus.
3. Type III (44.2%): The superior sagittal sinus drained completely into the right transverse sinus.
4. Type IV (9.2%): The superior sagittal sinus drained completely into the left transverse sinus.

Singh et al.[21] described the following four patterns of flow through the dural sinuses:

1. Confluence type (35%): The superior sagittal sinus drained into a common pool of venous sinuses.
2. Bifurcation type (14%): The superior sagittal sinus divided into bilateral transverse sinuses.
3. Right dominant type (41%): The superior sagittal sinus drained only into the right transverse sinus.
4. Left dominant type (10%): The superior sagittal sinus drained only into the left transverse sinus.

Kobayashi et al.[22] described the following different patterns of the torcular Herophili:

1. Type I (32.7%): The superior sagittal sinus, straight sinus, and transverse sinus merged.
2. Type II: The superior sagittal sinus bifurcated into the left and right transverse sinuses:
   a. The superior sagittal sinus drained into the right transverse sinus (31.5%).
   b. The superior sagittal sinus drained into the left transverse sinus (6.2%).
3. Type III: The superior sagittal sinus and the straight sinus branch into the bilateral transverse sinus (18.9%).
4. Type IV: The straight sinus branches into the left and right transverse sinuses.
   a. The straight sinus drained into the right transverse sinus (3.1%).
   b. The straight sinus drained into the left transverse sinus (4.4%).
5. Type V:
   a. The straight sinus drained into the occipital sinus (0.5%).
   b. The straight sinus communicated with veins other than the occipital sinus (0.4%).
6. Type VI:
   a. The left transverse sinus was aplastic (0.4%).
   b. The right transverse was aplastic (0.9%).
7. Type VII: The straight sinus branched into bilateral transverse sinuses and the superior sagittal sinus drained into the straight and left transverse sinuses (0.2%).
8. Type VIII: The superior sagittal sinus branched into the left and right transverse sinuses, and the straight sinus branched into the superior sagittal and left transverse sinuses (0.4%).
9. Type IX: The superior sagittal sinus branched into the right transverse sinus and occipital sinus. The straight sinus drains into the left transverse sinus and occipital sinus, and the superior sagittal sinus communicated with the straight sinus via the small anastomotic veins (0.4%).

Surendrababu et al.[23] found that 39% of the superior sagittal sinus drained into the right transverse sinus, 15% drained into the left transverse sinus, and the remainder drained into the torcular Herophili. Another variation was noted by Curé et al.[24] where the basal vein of Rosenthal drained near the torcular Herophili. Browder and Kaplan[5] noted triangular, figure of eight, and circular configurations of the torcular Herophili.

TRANSVERSE SINUS

Hollinshead[25] reported hypoplasia or absence of a transverse sinus. Knott[6] mentioned that Lower was the first to describe the right transverse sinus being larger than the left transverse sinus.[6] The right transverse sinus is reported to be larger in four times more cases than the left side.[20] However, the left transverse sinus can be longer than the right side.[23,26] Browder and Kaplan[5] found that 33% of specimens had right-side transverse sinus dominance; 16% showed equal dominance; 8% showed left side dominance; and the remainder had a variety of developmental aberrations. They also observed that in cases where there was doubling of the distal 1–3 cm of the superior sagittal sinus, the smaller channel was the origin of a small transverse sinus. They also found that in some cases, the lumen of the transverse sinus was also narrowed by the presence of a vascular mesh. Another variation found by Browder and Kaplan[5] was the presence of numerous connections joining the torcular Herophili to the transverse sinus.

Aplasia and hypoplasia of one transverse sinus might be seen, with the latter being more prevalent.[27] They are mainly noticed on the left side but may also be seen in the right transverse sinus. In total aplasia, both the superior sagittal sinus and straight sinus drain into the contralateral transverse sinus.[28] Rarely, one or both sinuses can be absent.[29]

Developmental abnormalities of the proximal transverse sinus were observed in 13 of 422 specimens studied by Browder and Kaplan.[5] There was narrowing on the right side in five cases; on the left side in seven cases; and on both sides in one specimen. In the case with narrowing on both sides, it was observed that the superior sagittal sinus continued as a large occipital sinus that joined the marginal sinus. Browder and Kaplan[5] reported atresia of the transverse sinus in 11 of the 422 specimens and doubling of a part of it in 14 specimens. Barkow,[30] Hoople,[31] Knott,[6] Laff,[32] and Malacarne[13] described the transverse sinus exiting the skull via the mastoid foramen. Hoople[31] reported a similar case. Barkow's[30] also had absence of the sigmoid sinus. Hahn[33] and Streit[34] observed cases where the transverse sinus was separated by a fibrous septum or a bony ridge.

SIGMOID SINUS

Williams[35] and others[28,36,37] reported unilateral absence of the sigmoid sinus. Rutting[38] described a diverticulum of the sigmoid sinus. Furstenberg[39] described a sigmoid sinus ending in a blind pouch and draining through a large mastoid foramen.

Hypoplasia or total aplasia of the sigmoid sinus is usually seen on the left side. In cases of total absence or hypoplasia of both the transverse sinus and sigmoid sinus, the superior petrosal sinus may pass directly through the mastoid foramen, and a large inferior petrosal sinus may be present.[28,35] Surendrababu et al.[23] reported a hypoplastic sigmoid sinus on the right in 6 patients and on the left in 19 patients. Sarmiento and Eslait[40] classified the sigmoid sinus into three types and how this changed the size of Trautmann's triangle:

- Type 1 (22.3%): Posterior placed sigmoid sinus increasing the size of the Trautmann's triangle.
- Type 2 (57.5%): Anterior placed sigmoid sinus reducing the area of the Trautmann's triangle.
- Type 3 (20.2%): Medially placed sigmoid sinus reducing the area of the Trautmann's triangle.

Tomura et al.[41] found that 1.6% of cases had an anteriorly located sigmoid sinus.

Dai et al.[42] found that the sigmoid sinus in males tends to be situated more laterally and posteriorly when compared with females. Compared with the left sinus, the right side tends to protrude more deeply with greater cross-sectional area and situated more laterally. This might be related to the right-side dominance of venous sinus drainage. Duplication of the sigmoid sinus is less frequent than the transverse sinus, and the two channels can be separated by a bony or fibrous septum.[28] On rare occasions, the sigmoid sinus may have an unusual anterior course reaching up to the posterior wall of the external auditory canal.[43]

STRAIGHT SINUS

Saxena et al.[44] examined the straight sinus in 43 cadavers and found that 13.85% were doubled with 9.3% in the median position and 4.65% in the paramedian position. Magden[45] found the straight sinus in 26.7% of cadavers to be doubled. In two cases (3.5%), the sinus was triple, being either median or paramedian.

The length of the straight sinus ranges between 4 and 7 cm.[16] In cases of absent inferior sagittal sinus, the straight sinus is formed by the continuation of the great cerebral vein. It may also communicate with the occipital sinus, the cavernous sinus through tentorial veins, and the right transverse sinus.[16,46]

Hasegawa et al.[47] examined the anatomic variations of the straight sinus in 108 control cases and 5 cases with a pineal region tumor. In 108 cases, the length of the straight sinus was 51±5.2. The angle of the straight sinus to the nasion-tuberculum sellae line was 51 ± 6.7°; the angle to the tuberculum sellae-inion line was 44 ± 5.0°; and the angle the nasion-inion line was 47 ± 5.0°. The straight sinus coursed posteriorly at 1.4 ± 4.5° to the bregma-inion line. The straight sinus was placed into three groups based on the relationship with the corpus callosum. They included the following:

- Type 1 (63%): The extended line of the slope of the straight sinus is tangential to the upper aspect of the splenium of the corpus callosum.
- Type 2 (26%) (high angle type): The extended line was far above the tangent line.

- Type 3 (11%) (low angle type): The extended line was far below the tangent line.

The straight sinus can also be completely or partially absent. Van den Bergh et al.[48] described a case of congenital absence of the straight sinus in a patient with Aarskog syndrome (x-linked recessive syndrome). Knott[6] also described one instance in which the sinus was completely absent. However, Hsu and Chalopka[49] reported a case of a 16-year-old male with a midline persistent falcine sinus (connecting the vein of Galen and the posterior 1/3 of the superior sagittal sinus) with the absence of only the proximal end of the straight sinus. The distal end of the straight sinus drained the cortical veins of the occipital lobe and the superior cerebellum. Kim and Lee[50] reported two cases of persistent falcine sinus with the complete absence of the straight sinus in a 60-year-old woman and an 11-year-old girl. Ryu[51] examined the CTA of 586 patients and found that 12 patients had a falcine sinus with 1 associated with a dysplastic tentorium. Three patients had an absent straight sinus, eight patients had a rudimentary straight sinus, and four patients had a normal sinus.

SUPERIOR PETROSAL SINUS

The superior petrosal sinus can be completely absent or enlarged, passing into the mastoid foramen to compensate for a small or absent transverse sinus.[6,28,35] A communication between the ophthalmic vein and the superior petrosal sinus has been described.[6,52] Theile also noted an aberrant termination of the superior petrosal sinus into the foramen spinosum of the middle cranial fossa.[34] On rare occasions, the vein of Labbé may drain into the superior petrosal sinus, which can make surgical approaches at the skull base extremely difficult or impossible.[53] Seven percent of the 14 fixed cadaver heads examined by Avci et al.[53] showed the vein of Labbé draining directly into the superior petrosal vein. The superior petrosal sinus may be absent.[6,54]

Tubbs et al.[55–57] observed different arrangements of the superior petrosal sinus from studying the relationship between the superior petrosal sinus and the porus trigeminus. In the 25 (50 sides) cadaver heads, 68% of the superior petrosal sinuses were superior to the opening of Meckel's cave; 18% were inferior; and 16% surrounded the opening of Meckel's cave. It was also observed that the superior petrosal sinuses that coursed inferiorly to the porus trigeminus were generally smaller than those that coursed superiorly or around the opening of Meckel's cave.[55–57]

Coates[58] examined 31 cadavers (63 sinuses identified) to determine the relationship of the superior petrosal sinus to the trigeminal nerve. In eight specimens, both right and left sinuses passed over the cranial surface of the trigeminal nerve root. Both right and left sinuses passed under the trigeminal nerve root in three cases. The sinus divided on both sides in three cases with some portions passing under the trigeminal root and others passing over the trigeminal nerve root.

On rare occasions, the basal vein of Rosenthal may drain into the superior petrosal sinus.[24]

Occasionally, the superior petrosal sinus may communicate with the superior ophthalmic veins through an aberrant vein termed the ophthalmopetrosal sinus in up to 9% of the cases, according to Knott.[8] The foramen of the ophthalmopetrosal sinus of Hyrtl is rarely seen in humans. The foramen may vary in size and may be found on one or both sides.[59]

Tanoue et al.[60] have classified the proximal communication of the superior petrosal sinus into three types. In type A, most common, the superior petrosal sinus runs along the lesser sphenoid wing and connects with the anterior aspect of the cavernous sinus. In type B, the superior petrosal sinus runs along the lesser sphenoid wing and connects with the foramen ovale venous plexus or the pterygoid venous plexus, in addition to the anterior aspect of the cavernous sinus. In type C, a hypoplastic superior petrosal sinus connects with the anterior aspect of the cavernous sinus.[60] In other occasions, the superior petrosal sinus communicates via an aberrant vein with the superior ophthalmic vein.[8] The superior petrosal sinus can be absent.[28]

INFERIOR PETROSAL SINUS

Major variations in the inferior petrosal sinus are extremely rare. Theile described drainage of this sinus into the superior thyroid vein.[34] Rubinstein et al.[61] examined the anatomic variations in the course of the inferior petrosal sinus in relation to the glossopharyngeal nerve and found that in 22 of the 25 specimens, the inferior petrosal sinus entered the foramen by passing inferior to the horizontally positioned and laterally coursing glossopharyngeal nerve. In the other three cases, the inferior petrosal sinus entered the foramen more inferiorly, heading inferiorly anteromedial or medial to the glossopharyngeal nerve as it descended into the foramen. In the jugular foramen of 16 of 20 specimens, the inferior petrosal sinus coursed inferiorly and laterally running between the descending portion of the glossopharyngeal nerve anteriorly, and the vagus and the accessory nerves posteriorly. In three specimens, the sinus remained medial to the nerves but passed medial to, and then posterior to all three nerves in 1 specimen. The junction of the inferior petrosal sinus to the jugular venous system was also varied. In four of the cases, the junction was within the jugular foramen. In eight cases, it was found in the extracranial opening of the jugular foramen. In 15 cases, it was found below the skull base. In evaluating the anatomy and the normal variations of the craniocervical veins, Tanoue et al.[62] reported two variations in the draining patterns of the inferior petrosal sinus, including the following:

- Type A (92%): The inferior petrosal sinus originated from the posterosuperior aspect of the cavernous sinus, coursed along the petroclival fissure, and drained into the medial portion of the jugular through the anterior edge of the jugular foramen.
- Type B (8%): The inferior petrosal sinus coursed along the petroclival fissure, penetrated the midportion of the petroclival fissure, and drained into the medial aspect of the jugular bulb

Knott[6] examined 11 skulls (22 sinuses) and found that the inferior petrosal sinus terminated near the lower margin of the jugular foramen in eight sinuses; slightly above the jugular foramen in nine sinuses; and a little below in the remaining five sinuses. In two sinuses, it ended 3/8th of an inch below the skull.

Variations at the junction of the inferior petrosal sinus and the internal jugular vein (internal jugular vein) have been classified into four types. In type I, the inferior petrosal sinus drains directly into the superior jugular bulb. In type II, the inferior petrosal sinus drains into a communicating vein that links the superior jugular bulb to the deep cervical plexus. In type III, the poorly formed inferior petrosal sinus is represented by a plexus of veins. In type IV, the inferior petrosal sinus drains directly into the deep cervical venous plexus. An incomplete type IV in which an extremely small channel links the internal jugular vein to the point of junction between the inferior petrosal sinus and the vertebral venous plexus was described. Inferior petrosal sinus communication with the vertebral venous plexus is via the anterior condylar vein (anterior condylar vein, mostly), lateral condylar vein, or both.[63–68]

As mentioned above, the inferior petrosal sinus can extend below the skull. Unilateral and bilateral extracranial extension of the inferior petrosal sinus may represent the most common type of inferior petrosal sinus termination. In these cases the inferior petrosal sinus courses parallel to the internal jugular vein, separated by variable distance, up to 100 mm (the longest reported) below the jugular foramen before joining it, reaching up to the level of C5. In other conditions, the extracranial inferior petrosal sinus may divide into two branches draining into the internal jugular vein at different levels before or after the confluence with the anterior condylar vein. One of these branches may also subdivide and join at different level. A second division of the subdivided branches may also be seen. In the jugular foramen, the inferior petrosal sinus and the jugular bulb may be close enough to establish a small anastomosis en passant by direct contact of their walls.[65–67,69] The inferior petrosal sinus may also be valvular at this level.

Absence of the inferior petrosal sinus has been described but is not uncommon.[67] Mitsuhashi et al.[67] classified the inferior petrosal sinus-internal jugular vein junction. In type A, the inferior petrosal sinus drains into the superior jugular bulb; in type B, the inferior petrosal sinus drains into the internal jugular vein at the level of the extracranial opening of the hypoglossal canal; in type C, the inferior petrosal sinus drains into internal jugular vein at a lower extracranial level, either as a single route (C1) or with another upper venous route (C2); in type D, the inferior petrosal sinus forms a plexus and has multiple junctions to the internal jugular vein around the jugular foramen; in type E, the inferior petrosal sinus drains directly into the vertebral venous plexus with no connection to the internal jugular vein; in type F, the inferior petrosal sinus is absent.[67] Types D and E are corresponded to types III and IV, respectively, of the classifications of Shiu et al. and Miller et al.

Zhang et al.[68] have subdivided the classification of Mitsuhashi et al. by adding the patterns of inferior petrosal sinus anastomosis with sigmoid sinus, anterior condylar vein, lateral condylar vein, and vertebral venous plexus. Type A is divided into A1: inferior petrosal sinus directly draining into superior jugular bulb, and A2: inferior petrosal sinus having two branches after leaving the cranium to communicate with sigmoid sinus and superior jugular bulb. Type B is divided into B1: inferior petrosal sinus draining into internal jugular vein at the level of hypoglossal canal, and B2: inferior petrosal sinus draining into internal jugular vein at the level of hypoglossal canal and having a communicating branch with sigmoid sinus. To type C, they added C3: inferior petrosal sinus drains into internal jugular vein at a lower extracranial level either alone or with other higher branch but having a communicating branch with sigmoid sinus. Type D was divided into D1: plexuslike inferior petrosal sinus draining into internal jugular vein near the jugular foramen, and D2: plexuslike inferior petrosal sinus draining into internal jugular vein near the jugular foramen and having a communicating branch with sigmoid sinus. In this study, a communicating branch between sigmoid sinus and inferior petrosal sinus was seen in 19% of the cases, especially in type B2.[68]

The diameter of the inferior petrosal sinus at its confluence with the internal jugular vein ranged between 0.8 and 5.7 mm and is usually larger on the right side.[68,69]

In a rare case, the inferior petrosal sinus drained into the superior thyroid vein.[28]

TENTORIAL SINUSES

The first observation of cerebellar tentorial sinuses was described in a study on the torcular Herophili and lateral sinuses by Gibbs and Gibbs,[2,5,15,70–74] all commented on its presence in anatomic or radiographic studies. Duval et al.[75] looked at 23 skulls and recorded the presence of the tentorial sinus in more than half of the cases. Matsushima et al.[76] studied 26 sides of the cerebellar tentorium from 13 specimens and classified the tentorial sinuses into the following four groups:

1. Group I (69.2%): The sinuses receive venous blood from the cerebral hemisphere through bridging veins.
2. Group II (88.5%): The sinuses are drained and formed by the terminal portions of the cerebellar hemispheric or vermian veins.
3. Group III (42.3%): Many small veins originating in the tentorium join to form a small sinus.
4. Group IV (7.6%): The sinus is formed by a bridging vein from the cerebral hemisphere or brain stem to the tentorial free edge.

Group II was further classified into five different subgroups.

The variable position of the tentorial sinus may be explained during development. As the temporal lobe and the cranial fossae expand cranioventrally, the tentorial sinus is pulled into the dural mesenchyme. This process may be responsible for the difference in position of the tentorial sinus from a medial to lateral position on the middle cranial fossa floor.[77]

Muthukumar and Palaniappan[78] studied the anatomy of the tentorial venous sinuses in 80 cadavers and found that 86% had these sinuses. They observed three types of tentorial sinuses.

- Type I (25%): This type was the largest and was often found in the medial 1/3 of the tentorium cerebelli. They often had a branching staghorn appearance and usually drained into the straight sinus, the torcular Herophili, and the medial 1/3 of the transverse sinus.
- Type II (25%): This type was the smallest of the three types and was usually found in the lateral 1/3 of the tentorium cerebelli. They usually drained into the junction of the transverse sinus and the superior petrosal sinus and into the lateral 1/3 of the transverse sinus.
- Type III (50%): The size of type III ranged from small to medium. They had a tendency to drain into the straight sinus, torcular Herophili, and the medial 1/3 of the transverse sinus.

The tentorial sinus, located on each half of the tentorium, is divided into medial and lateral groups.[79–82]

Miabi et al.[79] reported variations in the lateral tentorial sinus in 104 of 110 lobes and classified them into three types:

- Type I (candelabra): found in 30 (28.8%)
- Type II (independent veins): found in 22 (21.1%)
- Type III (venous lakes): found in 37 (35.55)

The lateral tentorial sinus was indeterminate in 15 (14.4%) cases. Instead of draining into the vein of Galen, the basal vein of Rosenthal may drain into the tentorial sinus.[24] The tentorial sinus may be absent. It can also have the occipital sinus and an accessory common internal cerebral vein as abnormal tributaries.[8] Occasionally, the tentorial sinuses are absent.[8]

FALCINE VENOUS PLEXUS/SINUS

A falcine sinus is a normal anatomic structure that usually involutes after birth. It is located within the falx cerebri and is mostly seen posteriorly connecting the posterior part of the superior sagittal sinus with the straight sinus or the posterior part of the inferior sagittal sinus. Crosby et al.[83] stated that the inferior sagittal sinus "begins in about the middle of the border of the falx with the convergence of the facial plexus of veins." Kaplan et al.[84] also acknowledged finding these channels in the falx. This venous plexus can communicate with the superior sagittal sinus. Rhoton[85] noted that this connection could be large enough that the superior sagittal sinus will drain primarily into the straight and inferior sagittal sinus. Tubbs et al.[86,87] studied 27 adult specimens and found an extensive network of small tributaries within the falx cerebri in all the specimens. These channels were most prominent in the posterior 1/3 and within the inferior 2/3 of the falx cerebri. All the venous channels communicated with the inferior sagittal sinus. The authors further classified the venous channels based on their communication with the superior sagittal sinus.

1. Type I (37%): No communication with the superior sagittal sinus.
2. Type II (26%): Limited communication with the superior sagittal sinus.
3. Type III (37%): Extensive communication with the superior sagittal sinus.

According to Curé et al.[24] a falcine sinus may be seen in cases where there is an absent, small, or stenotic straight sinus. Falcine sinuses are often seen in patients who have vein of Galen malformations. It has also been suggested by Yokota et al.[88] that the falcine sinus may actually be an "accessory straight sinus" seen in fetal specimens at 5 months, running upward within the falx between the vein of Galen and the superior sagittal sinus.

Hsu and Chalopka[49] noted the presence of a midline persistent falcine sinus connecting the vein of Galen and the posterior 1/3 of the superior sagittal sinus in a 16-year-old male. Kim and Lee[50] reported observing two cases of persistent falcine sinus in a 60-year-old woman and an 11-year-old girl. An anterior falcine sinus draining the paramedian cortical veins of the frontal lobes into inferior sagittal sinus has also been reported in a patient with agenesis of the anterior 1/3 of the superior sagittal sinus.[89] The falcine sinus is mostly seen in those with a congenitally absent straight sinus, which has the same embryonic origin with the falcine sinus, and is almost always associated with other anomalies, including bifid cranium, vein of Galen malformation, arteriovenous malformation, agenesis of the corpus callosum, Apert syndrome, osteogenesis imperfecta, Chiari malformation type II, occipital encephalocele, acrocephalosyndactyly, absent tentorium cerebelli, and bilateral giant parietal foramina. Acquired lesions in association with persistent falcine sinus are uncommon and include venous sinus thrombosis or obstruction of the straight sinus by a mass lesion. A persistent falcine sinus with no associated anomalies is thought to be rare.[90,91] However, Ryu[51] has reported this finding in 2.1% of 610 consecutive patients on computed tomography angiography.

OCCIPITAL SINUS

The occipital sinus, the smallest of all venous sinuses, usually lies in the midline near the posterior attachment of the falx cerebelli. It starts caudally at the level of the foramen magnum where it communicates with the marginal sinus (when present) anteriorly and the vertebral venous plexus inferiorly, and ends cranially at the confluence of sinuses.[92] The length of the occipital sinus ranges between 1.5 and 7 cm, and its width ranges between 1 and 19 mm near its termination,[27] and it is relatively wider in neonates.[14,93] Sometimes, the occipital sinus is quite large and may even replace one of the sigmoid sinuses. This is especially true in cases of an absent transverse sinus. In such cases, the occipital sinus functions as the main drainage canal, and the marginal sinus would also be large.[13,25,93]

In most cases, a single occipital sinus is observed, but double occipital sinus and total absence of the sinus are not uncommon.[27,93,94] In other studies, however, absent occipital sinus, rather than its presence, was the most common variation.[14,95] Triple occipital sinus is rare,[96] and in some conditions, the OC is composed of a mesh of venous collaterals.[97] A single occipital sinus may be midline in position, right-sided, or left-sided. The median occipital sinus may occasionally divide into two or more divisions, either caudally or cranially.[27,92,93]

An age-related regression in the occipital sinuses may occur. In the MRV study by Rollins et al., the occipital sinus was found in 13% of patients who were 25 months of age but in only 2% of children older than 5 years.[97]

This occipital sinus appears to be present with high frequency in anatomic studies.[6,12,19,70,98–101] Knott[6] detected its presence in 42 of 44 specimens. Thirty-three specimens had a single occipital sinus. Eighteen of these originated above the torcular Herophili; seven opened into the left lateral sinus; five opened into the right lateral sinus; and three connected with the straight sinus ¼ inch in front of the torcular Herophili. A bilateral sinus was found in the nine other specimens. In one of the nine cases, the occipital sinus was found lying beneath the dura mater on both sides of the internal occipital crest. Three cases had very small occipital sinuses that ended below the anastomosing network at the posterior lip of the margin of the foramen magnum. The left occipital sinus in 2 cases, continued on to form the marginal sinus to join the lateral sinus at the jugular foramen. A connection was made with the veins of the spinal canal. Browder and Kaplan[5] noted the presence of a single occipital sinus in 75%, paired occipital sinuses in 8%, and absent in 15% of the specimens studied. In 2% of cases, the sinus served as a major draining pathway.[5] Das and Hasan[27] looked at 200 adult cadavers and found the occipital sinus to be present in 129 specimens. He also noted a single midline occipital sinus in 35% of the specimens, a double sinus in 22.5% of the specimens, a single left-sided sinus in 4% of specimens, and a single right-sided sinus in 3% of specimens.

The size of the occipital sinus varies significantly. This can potentially cause great difficulty in posterior fossa surgical approaches.[25] Hollinshead[25] reported that sometimes the occipital sinus can be so large that it replaces the sigmoid sinus. The course of the occipital sinus may also deviate from the common presentation. Instead of passing in the midline, sometimes it deviates to one side and merges with the sigmoid sinus as it passes through the jugular foramen.[25]

Tubbs et al.[102,103] reported a larger than usual occipital sinus (1.5 × 6 cm) that drained directly into the jugular foramen and subsequently into the internal jugular vein instead of its normal drainage into the marginal sinus. An occipital sinus draining into the sigmoid sinus has been termed an oblique occipital sinus.[96] This is referred to as the oblique occipital sinus.[104,105] Another variation of the occipital sinus is where it drains directly into the bulb of the left lateral sinus with no drainage into the right lateral sinus.[104,105]

The occipital sinus may be duplicated or absent. Variations of the ipsilateral lateral sinus have been observed when the occipital sinus was absent or drained into the jugular bulb. When the lateral sinus is rudimentary, the occipital sinus functions as the main drainage.[104,105]

Baker[106] described a huge occipital sinus receiving drainage form the straight and superior sagittal sinuses in 2% of cases. He also reported that in 25%–30% of cases, the occipital sinus may be doubled or even absent in up to 3% of cases. D'Costa et al.[94] studied the variations in the falx cerebelli in 52 cadavers of South Indian origin and found in 8 (15.4%) of cases; there was a duplicated falx cerebelli with duplicated occipital venous sinuses. No marginal sinus was found. Each of the falx cerebelli had a distinct occipital venous sinus attached to its border.

Shoja et al.[107] described a rare variation of the occipital sinus, which they termed a "lateral occipital sinus" in a young male cadaver. The specimen examined had a duplicated falx cerebelli (right and left) and an accessory falx cerebelli attached to the underside of the tentorium cerebella 3.4 mm lateral to the base of the right falx cerebelli. There was an occipital sinus measuring 2.5 mm, which was found near the right posterolateral rim of the foramen magnum. No marginal sinus was observed. Embedded within the dura mater and posterolateral to the foramen magnum at the right floor, an additional venous sinus was discovered, which they referred to as a "lateral occipital sinus." The lateral occipital sinus traveled superiorly and posteromedially and divided into a medial and two lateral branches. The medial branch connected the right sigmoid sinus to the occipital sinus and the two lateral branches connected the right transverse sinuses.

Tanoue et al.[62] used contrast-enhanced CT with a multidetector scanner to study the anatomic variations of the veins at the craniocervical junction in 50 patients. The occipital sinus was seen on 18 cases. Four cases were the "prominent type" occipital sinuses that originated from the torcular Herophili, coursed along the internal occipital crest and drained into the right sigmoid sinus. Seven of the other types of the occipital sinus drained into the marginal sinus and three drained into the sigmoid sinus.

TERMINATION OF THE SUPERIOR SAGITTAL, STRAIGHT, TRANSVERSE, AND OCCIPITAL SINUSES

Termination of the superior sagittal sinus into the transverse sinus is the most common anatomic variation of the sinus. It ends into the right transverse sinus in most cases (right dominance) but may also end into the left transverse sinus (left dominance) and the confluence of sinuses (codominance). This pattern of dominance varies with patient age and is more similar to the adult pattern after 5 years of age. In children less than 2 years, the codominance pattern was reported to be the highest.[97] This termination usually occurs at the level of internal occipital protuberance but may also occur above this level. In other cases, the superior sagittal sinus may fork and join with a forked straight sinus and then becomes continuous with the transverse sinus. A partition of the dura mater may also be seen in the terminal portion of the sinus, dividing this part of the sinus into unequal channels. This dural partition may also extend and divide the confluence of sinuses, the straight sinus, or the transverse sinus. In rare occasions, the superior sagittal sinus may be divided into three channels with variant terminations. In one case, this termination included a superficial threadlike transverse sinus overlying a deeper transverse sinus.

Fukusumi et al.[20] have classified the drainage pattern of the superior sagittal sinus into the transverse sinus into four types. Type I: The superior sagittal sinus reaches a centrally located confluence and then divides into the bilateral transverse sinus. Type II: The superior sagittal sinus bifurcates into right and left limbs, draining into the same side transverse sinus. Type III (most common): The superior sagittal sinus drains predominantly into the right transverse sinus. Type IV: The superior sagittal sinus drains predominantly into the left side.[20] Same classification was also applied by Singh et al. based on the occipital bone impressions for dural venous sinuses around the confluence. They also added that type I was seen more commonly in females, whereas male mostly showed type III termination.[21]

Similarly, the straight sinus may reach a centrally located confluence before dividing into bilateral transverse sinus (type I), prematurely bifurcate into right and left channels before joining the corresponding transverse sinus (type II), drain predominantly into the right transverse sinus (type III), or predominantly into the left transverse sinus (type VI).[16,20] The first two types are most commonly observed, and draining into the left transverse sinus is more than the right.[23]

In most cases, the occipital sinus terminates in the confluence of sinuses but may also terminate into transverse sinus, superior sagittal sinus, or straight sinus.[27] In the latter condition, the occipital sinus is termed the oblique occipital sinus and functions as the main drainage canal when the transverse sinus is rudimentary.[104,105] A more developed oblique occipital sinus was reported by Shoja et al.[107] in association with other dural variations. In this case, the sinus was found posterolateral to the foramen magnum coursing superiorly and posteromedially and connecting the terminal portion of the right sigmoid sinus to the occipital and right transverse sinuses via one medial and two lateral branches, respectively.[107] On rare occasions, the occipital sinus may drain into the superior bulb of the internal jugular vein, in association with either normal, hypoplastic, or absent transverse sinus and sigmoid sinus.[108]

Based on their findings, Kopuz et al.[93] have classified the venous sinuses termination in the region of the confluence of sinuses in neonates into six types. In type I, the superior sagittal sinus was continuous with the right transverse sinus, and two occipital sinuses were opened to the confluence. In type II, the superior sagittal sinus was also continuous with the right transverse sinus, but more than two occipital sinuses were seen opening into the confluence. Types III and IV are similar to types I and II, respectively, except that the superior sagittal sinus is continuous with the left transverse sinus. In type V, the superior sagittal sinus is draining into the confluence, to which both transverse sinus and two occipital sinuses are connected. In type VI, the superior sagittal sinus bifurcates before joining the transverse sinus.[93]

MARGINAL SINUS

The marginal sinus is an inconstant remnant of the embryonic posterior venous plexus. When present, it encircles the internal aspect of the foramen magnum and has a diameter ranging between 7 and 15 mm, which tapers to 3–5 mm anteriorly and posteriorly. The marginal sinus connects anteriorly with the basilar venous plexus on the superior surface of the inferior clivus and with the occipital sinus posteriorly at the junction of the left and right posterior parts of the marginal sinus. However, the marginal sinus and occipital sinus may not be connected. Extracranially, it communicates with the internal vertebral venous plexus, paravertebral or deep cervical veins in the suboccipital region. Moreover, it may join the distal portions of the sigmoid sinus via small connections that pass across the intracranial surface of, and communicate with, the veins of the hypoglossal canal.

Knott[6] described this sinus in two of the specimens studied. Similarly, Woodhall and Seeds[101] and Browning[19] also described them as large venous lakes at the foramen magnum region. Caruso et al.[109] also detected this sinus on MR imaging of the craniocervical junction. Tubbs et al.[110,111] examined the marginal sinus in 15 cadaveric specimens and found that 93% demonstrated drainage into the hypoglossal canal. Seventy-three percent (11 specimens) were pierced by the hypoglossal nerve root. Eighty percent (12 specimens) communicated with the basilar venous plexus, and 100% communicated with the occipital venous sinus. All specimens had communication with the sigmoid sinus. In all left sides, the vertebral artery coursed through the marginal sinus as it pierced the posterior atlantooccipital membrane. Eighty-seven percent ran through the marginal sinus on the right side. Browder and Kaplan[5] and Hollinshead[25] found that large occipital sinuses usually corresponded to large marginal sinuses.

CAVERNOUS SINUS

This sinus might be completely absent.[8,112] Knott[6] noted a smaller than usual size of the cavernous sinus. The structures within the cavernous sinus also vary. According to Knott[6] and Bergman et al.[8] the cavernous sinus can receive a vein via the foramen rotundum.

Tanoue et al.[60] evaluated 37 patients using 3D fast gradient echo MR imaging and discovered four different patterns of communication between the cavernous sinus and the superficial middle cerebral vein:

1. Type A: The superficial middle cerebral vein connects with the proximal sphenoparietal sinus and flows into the frontal aspect of the cavernous sinus.
2. Type B: The superficial middle cerebral vein connects with the lateral aspect of the cavernous sinus independently.
3. Type C: The superficial middle cerebral vein turns downward and connects with the pterygoid venous plexus through the middle cranial fossa.

4. Type D: The superficial middle cerebral vein runs across the pyramidal ridge and connects with the superior petrosal sinus or transverse sinus via the tentorial sinus.

Takahashi et al.[113] classified the termination of the superficial middle cerebral vein into four groups:

1. Cavernous type (35.4%): The superficial middle cerebral vein entered the anterolateral aspect of the cavernous sinus.
2. Paracavernous type (10.4%): The superficial middle cerebral vein coursed outside of the cavernous sinus and entered the foramen ovale or the superior petrosal sinus.
3. Laterocavernous type (16.7%): The superficial middle cerebral vein ran between the two layers of the lateral wall of the cavernous sinus and entered the pterygoid venous plexus. The diameter of the superficial middle cerebral vein was smaller within the lateral wall.
4. Absent superficial middle cerebral vein (35.4%).

Controversy has arisen in literature regarding the structure of the medial wall of the cavernous sinus, which at the same time forms the lateral part of the pituitary capsule. This is especially important in identifying the route of pituitary tumor extension. In a systematic review by Gonçalves et al., they found that four studies concluded that the medial wall of the cavernous sinus is composed of a loose, fibrous structure that might have small histologic defects representing important sites of adenoma extension. On the other hand, 10 studies presumed that the medial wall is formed by a single, thin layer of dura that may allow direct extension.[114] Special attention should be given to the study of Diao et al., which has shown that the medial wall of the cavernous sinus consists of both the meningeal dura and weblike loose fibrous network, which are located at the anterosuperior and posteroinferior aspects of the sinus, respectively.[115]

SPHENOPARIETAL SINUS

Tanoue et al.[60] evaluated 37 patients and noted three variations of the sphenoparietal sinus:

1. Type a (72%): The sphenoparietal sinus coursed along the lesser sphenoid wing and connected with the anterior aspect of the cavernous sinus.
2. Type b (4%): The sphenoparietal sinus coursed along the lesser sphenoid wing and connected with the foramen ovale venous plexus or the pterygoid venous plexus.
3. Type c (14%): A hypoplastic sphenoparietal sinus entered the cavernous sinus.

Tubbs et al.[86,87] studied the sphenoparietal sinus of 15 cadavers and found that most sinuses began at the lateral tip of the lesser wing of the sphenoid bone and ended in the cavernous sinus near the passage of the ophthalmic nerve. The sinus had a connection with the Sylvian vein in all except one specimen. They also observed that one sinus drained into the foramen rotundum rather than the cavernous sinus. Ten specimens had temporal veins from the anterior temporal tip that drained into the sphenoparietal sinus.

Suzuki and Matsumoto[116] studied 500 superficial middle cerebral veins in 250 patients and found that the superficial middle cerebral vein was present in 456 sides and 62% drained into the sphenoparietal sinus or the cavernous sinus and 12% joined an emissary vein.

Knott[6] noticed that when the sphenoparietal sinus was inadequately represented, small veins were found. Cruveilhier[117] described this venous sinus as draining diploic and meningeal veins and coursing between the middle and anterior parts of the base of the skull, occupying a transversally oriented gutter, and ending in the cavernous sinus.

Hédon[118] added that the superficial middle cerebral vein ends in this sinus under the lesser wing of sphenoid bone or that it constitutes the sphenoparietal sinus. Later, authors also supported these findings and added that the superficial middle cerebral vein could either join the sphenoparietal sinus or drain directly into the cavernous sinus.[15,80,119,120]

BASILAR PLEXUS

Tubbs et al.[86,87] examined 20 cadavers and found a basilar plexus in all of them. They observed that in 35%, the basilar venous plexus communicated with veins draining into the hypoglossal canal. In 60%, the basilar plexus communicated with the marginal sinus. In two specimens, a connection between the internal vertebral plexus and the basilar plexus was observed. They also noted that the concentration of the venous channels in the basilar plexus decreased as the structure descended inferiorly to a plane between the right and left jugular tubercles.

Aquini et al.[121] studied 32 basilar plexuses. In 23 (71.8%) specimens, the basilar plexus was the widest intercavernous connection. The pattern of distribution varied. At the level of the dorsum sellae, the basilar plexus appeared as transverse, irregular vascular channels. In 24 cases, it did not have a well-defined vascular pattern.

PETROSQUAMOUS SINUS

This sinus communicates with the deep temporal and middle meningeal veins and courses along the angle between the petrous and squamous portion of the temporal bone until it terminates in the transverse sinus or the posterior portion of the superior petrosal sinus.[25] The petrosquamous sinus usually disappears during fetal development and is variably present in adults. It might be found unilaterally or bilaterally and is more common on the left side.[122,123] It has been reported more commonly in women and in patients with severe, congenital inner ear anomalies, including aplasia of the semicircular canals, patients with hypoplasia of the internal jugular vein, and patients with other craniovertebral anomalies, including sigmoid sinus hypoplasia/aplasia, facial nerve dehiscence, and craniostenosis.[123–125] A persistent petrosquamous sinus functions as an emissary vein that connects the intra- and extracranial venous networks. Nevertheless, it is often described as part of the dural venous sinuses. It arises from the dorsolateral portion of the transverse sinus at the junction with the sigmoid sinus and before the confluence with the transverse sinus with the superior petrosal sinus.[123] It may also arise from the sigmoid sinus,[124] and in a rare occasion, the origin was reported from a dilated mastoid emissary vein.[126] It then courses along the junction of the squamous and petrous parts of temporal bone (the petrosquamosal suture), where it marks a groove that sometimes becomes a canal (canal of Vergi). It has two emptying pathways: one anteroinferiorly into the retromandibular vein via the retroarticular foramen and one anteromedially into the pterygoid venous plexus via the foramen ovale or foramen spinosum, and ultimately drains into the external jugular vein (EJV), which marks the main drainage pathway of this sinus.[92,108,123,127] San Millan Ruiz et al.[108] reported one case in which the anterior portion of the petrosquamous sinus gave rise to two branches, the medial branch reaching the foramen ovale and the lateral branch connected extracranially with a deep temporal vein.[108] The petrosquamous sinus receives tributaries from the middle and superficial temporal veins, the masseteric veins, and the internal maxillary vein. It may also drain the posterior temporal diploic vein and the emissary veins of the cranial fossa. The diameter of the petrosquamous sinus is usually as small as that of a silk thread but might reach a diameter of 2–4 mm, and it may have an irregular contour and tortuous course in the manner of a diploic vein.[108,123] Rarely, when the sigmoid sinus is absent or severely hypoplastic, the petrosquamous sinus may represent the major or the only drainage pathway of the transverse sinus, directing the venous blood to the EJV system. In such occasions, the EJV system becomes the major encephalic outflow pathway in the affected side.[108]

Knott[6] found this sinus present bilaterally in 7 of 44 specimens and unilaterally in 19 specimens. Similarly, Vernieuwe[128] found this sinus in 12 of 60 specimens. Streit,[34] Laff,[32] Zuckerkandl et al. (1873),[129] and Cheatle[130] all noted such a variation. Stewart[131] reported the there was some association between the petrosquamous and the passage of infection from the middle ear to the brain. Small veins from the middle ear may drain through the petrosquamous fissure into this sinus.[25] Cheatle[130] described two cases where infection passed through the petrosquamous from the veins of the middle ear and entered the lateral sinus.

San Millan Ruiz et al.[108] observed 13 cranial venous systems and found that a petrosquamous sinus was found in 5 of the 26 corrosion casts. In two of the five cases, a connection with the emissary veins of the foramen ovale was observed. The anterior portion of petrosquamous sinus in 1 of the cases divided into two branches: a medial and a lateral branch, which connected extracranially to the deep temporal vein. The petrosquamous sinus had an irregular contour and a tortuous course in three cases. The other two cases had a smooth contour and were less tortuous. When the sigmoid sinus is absent or underdeveloped, the petrosquamous sinus may serve as the main outflow pathway of the transverse sinus.[108] San Millan Ruiz et al.[108] also described a large petrosquamous sinus found in a 7-year-old girl. On the left side, the petrosquamous sinus drained the transverse sinus. It had an anterior-lateral and anterior-medial branch that connected it to the external jugular vein. The anterior lateral branch communicated with the deep temporal veins and the anterior-medial branch communicated with the emissary veins of the middle cranial fossa. The anterior-lateral branch left the skull through the postglenoid foramen located in the temporal squama. The sigmoid sinus and the internal jugular vein were absent. According to San Millan Ruiz et al.,[108] only the connection of the petrosquamous sinus with the middle meningeal vein and the transverse sinus persists in humans. The lateral connection with the deep temporal vein usually disappears.[108]

Knott[6] observed that this sinus was present on both sides in 7 of 44 cases. It was found only on one side in 19 cases. Of these 19 cases, 11 were found on the left side and 8 were found on the right side.

OPHTHALMOPETROUS/ OPHTHALMOPETROSAL/SINUS OF HYRTL

From the superior orbital fissure, this sinus travels over the great wing of the sphenoid and the anterior surface of the temporal bone and ends in the transverse sinus.[25] Knott[6] was able to locate this sinus in 4 of 44 specimens. This sinus passes backward from the superior orbital fissure over the greater wing of the sphenoid and petrous portion of the temporal bone and terminates in the transverse sinus.[6,86,87] This sinus can also terminate by exiting through the middle meningeal vein[25] or anteriorly through the foramen ovale.[25,86,87] San Millan Ruiz[132] suggested that an orbital vein, which was one of the branches observed feeding the middle and the lateral 1/3 of the sinus of the lesser wing in a dissected specimen, could have been an ophthalmomeningeal vein of Hyrtl.

ACCESSORY SINUS OF KELCH

Becker described this sinus in 23 of 31 specimens. Of the 23 skulls, 16 showed it on both sides and the remainder showed it only on the left side.[131] Knott[6] observed this sinus in three cases. The sinuses of Hyrtl, Kelch, and Verga may all represent the same structure.

ACCESSORY SINUS OF VERGA

This sinus communicates between the cavernous sinus or the ophthalmic vein anteriorly and the transverse sinus posteriorly.[6,25,52] The sinuses of Hyrtl, Kelch, and Verga may all represent the same structure.

ANTERIOR AND POSTERIOR INTERCAVERNOUS SINUSES/CIRCULAR SINUS

Browder and Kaplan[5] found these to be present in all their specimens. Knott,[6] on the other hand, found this to be absent in 26 of 44 specimens studied. Renn and Rhoton[133] found that 76% had an anterior intercavernous sinus and 32% had a posterior intercavernous sinus. They also noted that the anterior intercavernous sinuses were usually larger than the posterior intercavernous sinuses; however, either one or both can be absent. Tubbs et al.[55-57] studied the morphology of the anterior and posterior intercavernous sinuses in 35 cadavers and classified them into four types:

- Type I (80%): Had both an anterior and posterior intercavernous sinus.
- Type II (25% of type I): Had a circular connection between the anterior and posterior intercavernous sinuses.
- Type III (17%): Only an anterior intercavernous sinus.
- Type IV (2.9%): Only a posterior intercavernous sinus.

Tubbs et al.[55-57] also found that in 80% of specimens, the anterior intercavernous sinus was larger than the posterior intercavernous sinus. In five specimens, the anterior intercavernous sinus occupied the entire anterior wall of the sella turcica. Six specimens had an inferior intercavernous sinus, which was much smaller than the other intercavernous sinuses.

Aquini et al.[121] studied the intercavernous sinuses and all had an anterior intercavernous sinus. It was the broadest intercavernous connection in three cases and occupied the entire sella turcica in 17 cases. In 22 cases, it had a curvilinear shape. A posterior intercavernous sinus was the widest interconnection in one case and was also found in all specimens.

INFERIOR INTERCAVERNOUS SINUS

First described by Winslow, this sinus is located at the inferior surface of the pituitary body. Knott[6] described this sinus in 6 of 44 specimens. In 12 cases, instead of the circular sinus, Knott[6] found a single intercavernous vein beneath the pituitary body. Eighty percent of the 35 cadaveric heads examined by Tubbs et al.[55-57] had both anterior and posterior intercavernous sinuses. Twenty-five percent of these cases had a circular connection between them. Aquini et al.[121] observed the inferior intercavernous sinus in 96.9% by serial section and 75% in X-ray studies. Five specimens had the largest intercavernous connections. The inferior intercavernous sinus presented in three different ways on the floor of the sella turcica. They were the plexuslike type, the venous lake, and the mixed type.

REFERENCES

1. Streeter GL. The development of the venous sinuses of the dura mater in the human embryo. *Am J Anat.* 1915;18:145.
2. Bisaria KK. Anatomic variations of venous sinuses in the region of the torcular Herophili. *J Neurosurg.* 1985;62:90–95.
3. Brockmann C, Kunze SC, Schmiedek P, Groden C, Scharf J. Variations of the superior sagittal sinus and bridging veins in human dissections and computed tomography venography. *Clin Imag.* 2012;36:85–89.
4. San Millan Ruiz D, Fasel JHD, Gailloud P. Unilateral hypoplasia of the rostral end of the superior sagittal sinus. *AJNR Am J Neuroradiol.* 2012;33:286–291.

5. Browder J, Kaplan H. *Cerebral Dural Sinuses and Their Tributaries*. Illinois: Thomas C; 1976.
6. Knott JF. On the cerebral sinuses and their variations. *J Anat Physiol*. 1881;16:27–42.
7. Portal. *Cours d'anatomie med Cit nach Labbé*. 1803.
8. Bergman R, Thompson SA, Afifi AK, Saadeh FA. Cardiovascular system. In: Bergman R, ed. *Compendium of Human Anatomic Variation*. Baltimore-Munich: Urban & Schwarzenberg; 1988:93.
9. Otsubo Y, Sato H, Sato N, Ito H. Cephaloceles and abnormal venous drainage. *Childs Nerv Syst*. 1999;15:329–332.
10. Tubbs RS, Loukas M. Duplication of the superior sagittal sinus. *Clin Anat*. 2006;19:728.
11. Neumann JO, Herweh C, Halatsch ME. Congenital duplication of the superior sagittal sinus and parietal encephalocele after vacuum extraction delivery. *Acta Neurochir*. 2010;152:713–716.
12. Woodhall B. Variations of the cranial venous sinuses in the region of the torcular Herophili. *Arch Surg*. 1936;33:297.
13. Malacarne MV. In: Briolo G, ed. *Encefalotomia nuova universale*. Torino; 1780.
14. Widjaja E, Griffiths PD. Intracranial MR venography in children: normal anatomy and variations. *AJNR Am J Neuroradiol*. 2004;25:1557–1562.
15. Bisaria KK. The superficial sylvian vein in humans: with special reference to its termination. *Anat Rec*. 1985;212:319–325.
16. Saxena RC, Beg MA, Das AC. The straight sinus. *J Neurosurg*. 1974;41:724–727.
17. Labbé C. Anomalies des sinus de la dure-mère. Dévelopment de ces sinus. Considérations sur la suppléance reciproque de ces canaux veineaux dans les cas d'absence de l'un d'eux description de quelque sinus peu connus. *Archives de physiologie normale et pathologique*. 1883;3:1–27.
18. Edwards EA. Anatomic variations of the cranial venous sinuses. Their relation to the effect of jugular compression in lumbar manometric test. *Arch Neurol Psychiatr*. 1931;26:801–814.
19. Browning H. The confluence of dural venous sinuses. *Am J Anat*. 1953;92:307–329.
20. Fukusumi A, Okudera T, Takahashi S, et al. Anatomical evaluation of the dural sinuses in the region of the torcular herophili using three dimensional CT venography. *Acad Radiol*. 2010;17:1103–1111.
21. Singh M, Nagashima M, Inoue Y. Anatomical variations of occipital bone impressions for dural venous sinuses around the torcular Herophili, with special reference to the consideration of clinical significance. *Surg Radiol Anat*. 2004;26:480–487.
22. Kobayashi K, Matsui O, Suzuki M, Ueda F. Anatomical study of the confluence of the sinuses with contrast-enhanced magnetic resonance venography. *Neuroradiology*. 2006;48:307–311.
23. Surendrababu N, Subathira, Livingstone RS. Variations in the cerebral venous anatomy and pitfalls in the diagnosis of cerebral venous sinus thrombosis: low field MR experience. *Indian J Med Sci*. 2006;60:135–142.
24. Curé JK, Tassel PV, Smith MT. Normal and variant anatomy of the dural venous sinuses. *Sminars in Ultrasouns, CT and MRI*. 1994;15:499–519.
25. Hollinshead WH. 2nd ed. *Anatomy for Surgeons*. Vol. 1. Maryland: Harper & Row; 1968:12–22, 83–85.
26. Srijit D, Shipra P. Unusual venous sinuses. *Bratisl Lek Listy*. 2007;108:104–106.
27. Das AC, Hasan M. The occipital sinus. *J Neurosurg*. 1970;33:307–311.
28. Waltner J. Anatomic variations of the lateral and sigmoid sinuses. *Arch Otolaryngol Head Neck Surg*. 1944;39:307–312.
29. Hamnett NT, Ogungbo B, Nahser H, Javadpour M. Anomalous cerebral venous sinus drainage. *Br J Neurosurg*. 2010;24:497–498.
30. Barkow JCL. *Anatomische Abhandlungen*. F Hirt Breslau; 1851:1.
31. Hoople GD. Anormaly of the lateral sinus: report of a case. *Ann Otol Rhinol Laryngol*. 1936;45:1019.
32. Laff HJ. Unilateral absence of sigmoid sinus. *Arch Otolaryngol*. 1930;11:151.
33. Hahn R. *Arch ital di otol*. 1914;25:203.
34. Streit H. Ueber otologisch wichtige anormalien der hirnsinus, uber accessorische sinus und bedeutendere venenverbindungen. *Arch f Ohneuheilk*. 1903;58(85):161.
35. Williams HL. Apparent unilateral absence of sigmoid sinus noted at operation. *Arch Otolaryngol*. 1930;12:339–341.
36. Kiritsi O, Noussios G, Tsitas K, Chouridis P, Lappas D, Natsis K. Anatomical variants of the emissary veins: unilateral aplasia of both the sigmoid sinus and the internal jugular vein and development of the petrosquamosal sinus. A rare case report. *Folia Morphol*. 2011;70:305–308.
37. Deeb ZL, Rotenberg D, Black FO. Aplasia of sigmoid sinus with high-lying jugular bulb. *AJNR Am J Neuroradiol*. 1981;2:187–188.
38. Ruttin E. Kloaken und blindsackbildung am sinus sigmoideus. *Acta Otolaryngol*. 1926;9:217–220.
39. Furstenberg AC. Septic thrombophlebitis of the sigmoid sinus. *Trans Am Acad Ophtal*. 1937;42:424.
40. Sarmiento PB, Eslait FG. Surgical classification of variations in the anatomy of the sigmoid sinus. *Otolaryngol Head Neck Surg*. 2004;131:192–199.
41. Tomura N, Sashi R, Kobayashi M, Hirano H, Hashimoto M, Watari J. Normal variations of the temporal bone on high-resolution CT: their incidence and clinical significance. *Clin Radiol*. 1995;50:144–148.
42. Dai PD, Zhang HQ, Wang ZM, Sha Y, Wang KQ, Zhang TY. Morphological and positional relationships between the sigmoid sinus and the jugular bulb. *Surg Radiol Anat*. 2007;29:643–651.
43. Gangopadhyay K, McArthur PD, Larsson SG. Unusual anterior course of the sigmoid sinus: report of a case and review of the literature. *J Laryngol Otol*. 1996;110:984–986.

44. Saxena RC, Beg MA, Das AC. Double straight sinus-report of six cases. *J Neurosurg*. 1973;39:540–542.
45. Magden AO. Triple straight sinus-report of 2 cases. *Anat Anzeiger*. 1991;173:17–22.
46. Browder J, Kaplan HA, Krieger AJ. Anatomical features of the straight sinus and its tributaries. *J Neurosurg*. 1976;44:55–61.
47. Hasegawa M, Yamashita J, Yamashima T. Anatomical variations of the straight sinus on magnetic resonance imaging in the infratentorial supracerebellar approach to pineal region tumors. *Surg Neurol*. 1991;36:354–359.
48. Van den Bergh P, Fryns JP, Wilms G, Piot R, Dralands G, Van den Bergh R. Anomalous cerebral venous drainage in Aarskog syndrome. *Clin Genet*. 1984;25:288–294.
49. Hsu S, Chaloupka JC. Atretic parietal cephalocele associated with sinus pericranii: embryological consideration. *Brain Dev*. 2012;34:325–328.
50. Kim MS, Lee GH. Two cases with persistent falcine sinus as congenital variation. *J Korean Neurosurg Soc*. 2010;48:82–84.
51. Ryu CW. Persistent falcine sinus: is it really rare? *AJNR Am J Neuroradiol*. 2010;31:367–369.
52. Verga. *Ann Univers di Medicina*. 1856:175.
53. Avci E, Dagtekin A, Akture E, Uluc K, Baskaya MK. Microsurgical anatomy of the vein of Labbe. *Surg Radiol Anat*. 2011;33:569–573.
54. Hyrtl. Der sinus opththalmo-petrosus. *Wien Med Wochenschr*. 1862;12:290–291.
55. Tubbs RS, Griessenauer C, Loukas M, Cohen-Gadol AA. The circular sinus: an anatomic study with neurosurgical and neurointerventional applications. *World Neurosurg*. 2013;12:1341–1343.
56. Tubbs RS, Mortazavi MM, Krisnamurthy S, Verma K, Griessenauer CJ, Cohen-Gadol AA. The relationship between the superior petrosal sinus and the porus trigeminus: an anatomical study/laboratory investigation. *J Neurosurg*. 2013. https://doi.org/10.3171/2013.4.JNS122062.
57. Tubbs RS, Watanabe K, Loukas M, Cohen-Gadol AA. Anatomy of the inferior petro-occipital vein and its relation to the base of the skull: application to surgical and endovascular procedures of the skull base. *Clin Anat*. 2013. https://doi.org/10.1002/ca.22268.
58. Coates AE. A note on the superior petrosal sinus and its relation to the sensory root of the trigeminal nerve. *J Anat*. 1934;68:428.
59. Shapiro R, Robinson F. The foramina of the middle cranial fossa: a phylogenetic, anatomic and pathologic study. *Am J Roentgenol Radium Ther Nucl Med*. 1967;101:779–794.
60. Tanoue S, Kiyosue H, Okahara M, et al. Para-cavernous sinus venous structures: anatomic variations and pathologic conditions evaluated on fat-suppressed 3D fast gradient-echo MR images. *AJNR Am J Neuroradiol*. 2006;27:1083–1089.
61. Rubinstein D, Burton B, Walker A. The anatomy of the inferior petrosal sinus, glossopharyngeal nerve, vagus nerve, and accessory nerve in the jugular foramen. *AJNR Am J Neuroradiol*. 1995;16:185–194.
62. Tanoue S, Kiyosue H, Sagara Y, et al. Venous structures at the craniocervical junction: anatomical variations evaluated by multidetector row CT. *Br J Radiol*. 2010;83:831–840.
63. Shiu PC, Hanafee WN, Wilson GH, Rand RW. Cavernous sinus venography. *Am J Roentgenol Radium Ther Nucl Med*. 1968;104:57–62.
64. Miller DL, Doppman JL, Chang R. Anatomy of the junction of the inferior petrosal sinus and the internal jugular vein. *AJNR Am J Neuroradiol*. 1993;14:1075–1083.
65. Ayeni SA, Ohata K, Tanaka K, Hakuba A. The microsurgical anatomy of the jugular foramen. *J Neurosurg*. 1995;83:903–909.
66. Gailloud P, Fasel JH, Muster M, Desarzens F, Ruefenacht DA. Termination of the inferior petrosal sinus: an anatomical variant. *Clin Anat*. 1997;10:92–96.
67. Mitsuhashi Y, Nishio A, Kawahara S, et al. Morphologic evaluation of the caudal end of the inferior petrosal sinus using 3D rotational venography. *AJNR Am J Neuroradiol*. 2007;28:1179–1184.
68. Zhang W, Ye Y, Chen J, et al. Study on inferior petrosal sinus and its confluence pattern with relevant veins by MSCT. *Surg Radiol Anat*. 2010a;32:563–572.
69. Zhang WG, Ye YY, Chen JH, Chen R, Kuang LQ, Li X. Imaging study of the long extracranial extension of the inferior petrosal sinus with MSCT. *Clin Anat*. 2010b;23:160–167.
70. Gibbs E, Gibbs F. The cross section areas of the vessels that form the torcular and the manner in which flow is distributed to the right and to the left lateral sinus. *Anat Rec*. 1934;59:419–426.
71. Babin E, Megret M. Variations in the drainage of the basal vein. *Neuroradiology*. 1973;6:154–161.
72. Chung JI, Weon YC. Anatomic variations of the deep cerebral veins,tributaries of basal vein of Rosenthal: embryologic aspects of the regressed embryonic tentorial sinus. *Intervent Neuroradiol*. 2005;11:123–130.
73. Huang Y, Wolf B. Veins of the posterior fossa. In: Newton T, Ports D, eds. *Radiology of the Skull and Brain*. Vol. II. St Louis: Mosby; 1974.
74. Huang YP, Wolf BS, Okudera T. Angiographic anatomy of the inferior vermian vein of the cerebellum. *Acta Radiol Diagn*. 1969;9:327–344.
75. Duval JM, Latouche X, MOndine P, Robillard D. Sinus of the cerebellar tentorium. *Bull Assoc Anat*. 1975;59:855–862.
76. Matsushima T, Suzuki SO, Fukui M, Rhoton Jr AL, de Oliveira E, Ono M. Microsurgical anatomy of the tentorial sinuses. *J Neurosurg*. 1989;71:923–928.
77. Dolenc VV, Rogers LA. *Venous Anatomy of the Lateral Sella Compartment. Cavernous Sinus: Developments and Future Perspectives*; 2009. Retrieved from: http://books.google.com/books?id=A3b_GBvxBDUC&pg=PA40&dq=tentorial+sinus&hl=en&sa=X&ei=a2TDUdbRLYeG9gSt1oHoDw&ved=0CDwQ6AEwAQ#v=onepage&q=tentorial%20sinus&f=false.

78. Muthukumar N, Palaniappan P. Tentorial venous sinuses: an anatomic study. *Neurosurgery*. 1998;42:363–371.
79. Miabi Z, Midia R, Rohrer SE, et al. Delineation of lateral tentorial sinus with contrast-enhanced MR Imaging and its surgical implications. *AJNR Am J Neuroradiol*. 2004;25:1181–1188.
80. Oka K, Rhoton Jr AL, Barry M, Rodriguez R. Microsurgical anatomy of the superficial veins of the cerebrum. *Neurosurgery*. 1985;17:711–748.
81. Sakata K, Al-Mefty O, Yamamoto I. Venous consideration in petrosal approach: microsurgical anatomy of the temporal bridging vein. *Neurosurgery*. 2000;47:153–161.
82. Rhoton AL. The cerebral veins [suppl]. *Neurosurgery*. 2002;51:159–205.
83. Crosby E, Humphrey T, Lauer E. *Correlative Anatomy of the Nervous System*. New York: The Macmillan Company; 1962.
84. Kaplan HA, Browder J, Krieger AJ. Venous channels within the intracranial dural partitions. *Radiology*. 1975;115:641–645.
85. Rhoton A. Rhoton's cranial anatomy and surgical approaches. In: Rhoton A, ed. *Schaumburg: Congress of Neurological Surgeons*. 2003.
86. Tubbs RS, Hansasuta A, Loukas M, et al. The basilar venous plexus. *Clin Anat*. 2007;20:755–759.
87. Tubbs RS, Loukas M, Shoja MM, Oakes WJ. Accessory venous sinus of Hyrtl. *Folia Morphol*. 2007d;66:198–199.
88. Yokota A, Oota T, Matsukado Y, Matsukado Y, Okudera T. Structures and development of the venous system in congenital malformations of the brain. *Neuroradiology*. 1978;16:26–30.
89. Matouk CC, Mandell DM, Krings T, Willinsky RA, Ter Brugge KG. Persistant anterior falcine sinus: demonstration by CT angiography. *Can J Neurol Sci*. 2011;38:760–761.
90. Tubbs RS, Loukas M, Louis Jr RG, et al. Anatomy of the falcine venous plexus. *J Neurosurg*. 2007a;107:155–157.
91. Cai CQ, Zhang QJ, Yang WD, Wang CX, Shen CH. Neuroimages of persistent falcine sinus in children. *World J Pediatr*. 2009;5:63–64.
92. Adeeb N, Mortazavi MM, Tubbs RS, Cohen-Gadol AA. *Childs Nerv Syst*. 2012;28(6):827–837.
93. Kopuz C, Aydin ME, Kale A, Demir MT, Corumlu U, Kaya AH. The termination of superior sagittal sinus and drainage patterns of the lateral, occipital at confluens sinuum in newborns: clinical and embryological implications. *Surg Radiol Anat*. 2010;32:827–833.
94. D'costa S, Krishnamurthy A, Nayak SR, et al. Duplication of falx cerebelli, occipital sinus, and internal occipital crest. *Rom J Morphol Embryol*. 2009;50:107–110.
95. San Millan Ruiz D, Gailloud P, Rufenacht DA, Delavelle J, Henry F, Fasel JH. The craniocervical venous system in relation to cerebral venous drainage. *AJNR Am J Neuroradiol*. 2002;23:1500–1508.
96. Lang J. *Clinical Anatomy of the Posterior Cranial Fossa and its Foramina*. New York: Thieme; 1991.
97. Rollins N, Ison C, Booth T, Chia J. MR venography in the pediatric patient. *AJNR Am J Neuroradiol*. 2005;26:50–55.
98. Balo J. The dural venous sinuses. *Anat Rec*. 1950;106:319–324.
99. Padget DH. The cranial venous system in man in reference to development, adult configuration and relation to the arteries. *Am J Anat*. 1956;98:307–355.
100. Woodhall B. Anatomy of cranial blood sinuses with particular reference to the lateral sinuses. *Laryngoscope*. 1939;49:966–1010.
101. Woodhall B, Seeds AE. Cranial venous sinuses, correlation between skull markings and roentgenograms of the occipital bone. *Arch Surg*. 1936;33:867–875.
102. Tubbs RS, Loukas M, Shoja MM, Apaydin N, Ardalan MR, Oakes JW. Lateral lakes of Trolard: anatomy, quantitation and surgical landmarks. *J Neurosurg*. 2008;108:1005–1009.
103. Tubbs RS, Shoja MM, Loukas M. An unusual finding of the posterior cranial fossa: one case report. *Ital J Anat Embryol*. 2008;113:83–86.
104. Tubbs RS, Bosmia AN, Shoja MM, Loukas M, Curé JK, Cohen-Gadol. The oblique occipital sinus: a review of anatomy and imaging characteristics. *Surg Radiol Anat*. 2011;33:747–749.
105. Tubbs RS, Denardo AJ, Cohen-Gadol AA. Intercavernous connection between the internal carotid arteries. *J Neurosurg Pediatr*. 2011;8:625–627.
106. Baker AB. *Clinical Neurology*. Vol. 3. New York: Hoeber-Harper; 1955:1686.
107. Shoja MM, Tubbs RS, Loukas M, Shokouhi G, Oakes WJ. A complex dural-venous variation in the posterior cranial fossa: a triplicate falx cerebelli and an aberrant venous sinus. *Folia Morphol*. 2007;66:148–151.
108. San Millan Ruiz D, Gailoud P, Yilmaz H, et al. The petrosquamosal sinus in humans. *J Anat*. 2006;209:711–720.
109. Caruso RD, Rosenbaum AE, Chang JK, Joy SE. Craniocervical junction venous anatomy on enhanced MR images: the suboccipital cavernous sinus. *AJNR Am J Neuroradiol*. 1999;20:1127–1131.
110. Tubbs RS, Ammar K, Liechty P, et al. The marginal sinus. *J Neurosurg*. 2006;104:429–431.
111. Tubbs RS, Kelly DR, Lott R, Salter EG, Oakes WJ. Complete ossification of the human falx cerebri. *Clin Anat*. 2006;19:147–150.
112. Santorini. *Obs Anat*. 1714;3:25.
113. Takahashi S, Sakuma I, Otani T, et al. Venous anatomy of the sphenoparietal sinus: evaluation by MR Imaging. *Intervent Neuroradiol*. 2007;13:84–89.
114. Goncalves MB, de Oliveira JG, Williams HA, Alvarenga RM, Landeiro JA. Cavernous sinus medial wall: dural or fibrous layer? Systematic review of the literature. *Neurosurg Rev*. 2012;35:147–153; discussion 153–144.
115. Diao Y, Liang L, Yu C, Zhang M. Is there an identifiable intact medial wall of the cavernous sinus? Macro-microscopic anatomical study using sheet plastination. *Neurosurgery*. 2013;73:106–109.
116. Suzuki Y, Matsumoto K. Variations of the superficial middle cerebral vein: classification using three-dimensional CT angiography. *AJNR Am J Neuroradiol*. 2000;21:932–938.

117. Cruveilhier J. *Traité D'anatomie Descriptive: Angéologie. Book Traité D'anatomie Descriptive: Angéologie. 3.* Paris: Labbé; 1852.
118. Hédon C. *Etude anatomique sur la circulation veineuse de l'encéphale.* 1888.
119. Wolf BS, Huang YP, Newman CM. The superficial sylvian venous drainage system. *Am J Roentgenol Radium Ther Nucl Med.* 1963;89:398–410.
120. Hacker H. Normal supratentorial veins and dural sinuses. Radiology of the skull and brain: angiography. In: Newton T, Potts D, eds. St Louis: Mosby; 1974:1851–1862.
121. Aquini MG, Marrone ACH, Schneider FL. Intercavernous venous communications in the human skull base. *Skull Base Surg.* 1994;4:145–150.
122. Conroy GC. The emissary foramina: their value in platyrrhine systematics. *Am J Phys Anthropol.* 1982;57:7–12.
123. Marsot-Dupuch K, Gayet-Delacroix M, Elmaleh-Berges M, Bonneville F, Lasjaunias P. The petrosquamosal sinus: CT and MR findings of a rare emissary vein. *AJNR Am J Neuroradiol.* 2001;22:1186–1193.
124. An YH, Wee JH, Han KH, Kim YH. Two cases of petrosquamosal sinus in the temporal bone presented as perioperative finding. *Laryngoscope.* 2011;121:381–384.
125. Giesemann AM, Goetz GF, Neuburger J, Lenarz T, Lanfermann H. Persistent petrosquamosal sinus: high incidence in cases of complete aplasia of the semicircular canals. *Radiology.* 2011;259:825–833.
126. Chauhan NS, Sharma YP, Bhagra T, Sud B. Persistence of multiple emissary veins of posterior fossa with unusual origin of left petrosquamosal sinus from mastoid emissary. *Surg Radiol Anat.* 2011;33:827–831.
127. Wysocki J. Morphology of the temporal canal and postglenoid foramen with reference to the size of the jugular foramen in man and selected species of animals. *Folia Morphol.* 2002;61:199–208.
128. Vernieuwe S. *Rev Laryngol.* 1921;53:207.
129. Zuckerkandl E. *Monatsschrift Ohrenh.* 1873;7:102.
130. Cheatle A. *Trans Int Congr Oto.* 1899;6:160.
131. Stewart JP. The persistence of fetal blood sinuses and their relation to the middle ear spaces. *Arch Otolaryngol Head Neck Surg.* 1929;10:266–275.
132. San Millan Ruiz D, Fasel JHD, Ru¨fenacht DA, Gailloud P. The sphenoparietal sinus of Breschet: does It exist? An anatomic study. *AJNR Am J Neuroradiol.* 2004;25:112–120.
133. Renn W, Rhoton A. Microsurgical anatomy of the sellar region. *J Neurosurg.* 1975;43:288–298.

CHAPTER 26

Imaging Techniques for the Dural Venous Sinuses

MATTHEW PROTAS • AMIT SINGLA

INTRODUCTION

The dural venous sinuses (DVSs) are endothelial-lined sinuses, which lie between the two layers of dura (meningeal and endosteal layers). They collect venous blood from the brain, meninges, and calvaria and deliver it to the internal jugular veins at the skull base. There are two groups of DVS. The superior group drains the majority of the brain and skull and includes the superior and inferior sagittal sinuses and the straight, occipital, transverse, and sigmoid sinuses (Fig. 26.1). These sinuses converge at the torcular Herophili and drain the blood into the internal jugular veins. The inferior group (Fig. 26.2) drains the Sylvian veins, the basal and medial parts of the undersurface of the brain, and the orbits. This system collects the blood at the cavernous sinuses and then drains either into the pterygoid plexus or via the inferior petrosal sinuses, basilar plexus into the internal jugular vein.

Many imaging modalities can be used to visualize the DVS. These imaging modalities include computed tomography venography (CTV), magnetic resonance imaging (MRI), magnetic resonance venography (MRV) with time-of-flight imaging (TOF-MRV), contrast-enhanced MRV, and digital subtraction angiography (DSA). The imaging modality of choice can vary with the pathology suspected. The common pathologies related to DVS include dural venous sinus thrombosis (DVST), vein of Galen malformation (VOGM),

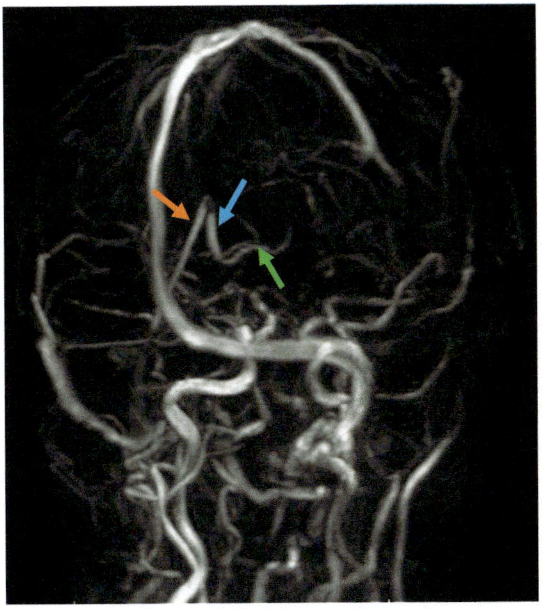

FIG. 26.1 Magnetic resonance venography noting the straight sinus (*orange arrow*), vein of Galen (*blue arrow*), and internal cerebral veins (*green arrow*). The sagittal, transverse, and sigmoid sinuses are also shown.

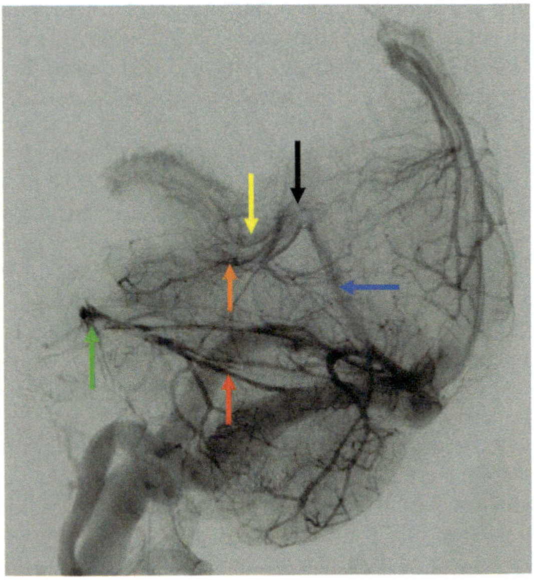

FIG. 26.2 Angiogram (venous phase) noting the cavernous sinus (*green arrow*), superior petrosal sinus (*red arrow*), basal vein (*orange arrow*), internal cerebral vein (*yellow*), vein of Galen (*black arrow*), and straight sinus (*blue arrow*).

Anatomy, Imaging and Surgery of the Intracranial Dural Venous Sinuses. https://doi.org/10.1016/B978-0-323-65377-0.00026-X

dural arteriovenous fistula (dAVF). In adults, DSA is the modality of choice for the diagnosis of dAVF. Ultrasonography (USG) is usually sufficient for the diagnosis of VOGM. Noninvasive techniques, such as MRI with contrast-enhanced MRV, have gradually replaced DSA as the imaging modality of choice for DVST.

COMPUTED TOMOGRAPHY TECHNIQUES

Before MRI, unenhanced and contrast-enhanced CT imaging were used to make the diagnosis of the some of the pathologies of DVST. Different radiologic signs were noted to be helpful for the diagnosis of DVST, such as empty delta sign, cord sign, and dense vein sign. These signs, however, were not reliable rendering the patients to DSA, which was the gold standard test for the diagnosis of DVST pathologies. With the advent of helical CT scans, data acquisition during optimal vascular contrast enhancement became possible, which was the main limitation with the conventional CT scanners before. This resulted in a technique called CTV, the term initially coined by Casey in 1996.[1]

CTV can be defined as a fast thin-section volumetric helical CT examination performed with a time-optimized bolus of contrast medium to enhance the cerebral venous system. Ozsvath et al.[2] reported that the imaging protocol with helical CT scanner provided high-resolution images of the intracranial vasculature and also allowed reformatting of the images in any desired plane as well as 3D projection images. They reported CTV to be superior to MRV because of less acquisition time of 1 min in comparison with several minutes for 2D phase contrast (PC) MRV and up to 8–10 min with 2D TOF-MRV, which makes CTV more suitable for uncooperative/unstable patient.[2] CTV was proved to be a reliable method to investigate the structure of the cerebral veins, with a reported sensitivity of 95% with multiplanar reformatted (MPR) images compared with DSA as the standard of reference. MPR images from CTV were superior to DSA images in showing the cavernous sinus, inferior sagittal sinus, and basal vein of Rosenthal.[3]

One major drawback of CTV over MRV is the use of ionizing radiation and iodinated contrast material, which makes MRV a less-invasive examination. Other drawbacks of CTV include that it requires complex post-processing (in particular, the removal of bony structures from the reconstructed images) and provides limited visualization of skull base structures. The 3D visualization of the cerebral venous system with conventional CTV can be difficult because of close proximity to the bony structures, which necessitates bone subtraction for better visualization of the venous structures.[4]

Bone subtraction techniques described include conventional bone subtraction technique[5] and dual energy bone subtraction technique.[6] Dual energy bone subtraction technique exploits the differences in attenuation of iodine and calcium at different X-ray energies because of their different atomic numbers differentiating vessels filled with contrast medium from bones or calcified plaques. It also allows simultaneous acquisition of low- and high-energy data in one examination and thus allows simultaneous imaging without interscan motion and with the use of only a small additional radiation dose in contrast to conventional bone subtraction technique.[6] To improve on these bone subtraction techniques which are semiautomatic and operator-dependent, matched mask bone elimination was another technique described for bone removal because of its user-independent and fully automatic nature.[7,8]

Magnetic Resonance Imaging

With the recent advancements in the MRI, DVS can be visualized with as good a correlation as with DSA.[9] Imaging of the cerebral venous system using MRI can be achieved by using either nonenhanced or contrast-enhanced methods.

NONENHANCED CEREBRAL VENOGRAPHY TECHNIQUES

Two-Dimensional Time-of-Flight Magnetic Resonance Venography

TOF-MRV relies on the difference in magnetization between the nuclei in the flowing blood and the stationary tissue. High-signal intensity of the inflowing fully magnetized blood contrasts against the low-signal intensity of stationary tissue. The typical characteristics of TOF-MRV include a conventional gradient echo (GRE), short TR, intermediate or high flip angle, and short TE. Advantages include sensitivity to slow flow, short acquisition time (5–8 min), and no requirement for an injection. Limitations include artifactual intravascular signal loss due to insensitivity to in-plane flow or due to tortuosity and turbulent flow, high signal from background substances with short T1 values and patient motion causing vessel misregistration.[10]

Phase Contrast Magnetic Resonance Venography (3D and 2D PC MRV)

PC MRV is based on the shift in the phase of magnetization when the material moves in the presence of magnetic field gradient. The typical characteristics of

PC MRV include a conventional GRE sequence, bipolar gradients along one or more axis, and a velocity-encoding variable that adjusts the bipolar gradient strength to produce a phase shift of 180 degrees. Advantages include the ability to quantify flow and determine the direction of flow and greater suppression of the background tissues. Disadvantages include the need to predict VENC and long acquisition times.[10]

CONTRAST-ENHANCED CEREBRAL MAGNETIC RESONANCE VENOGRAPHY TECHNIQUES

Gadolinium-Enhanced Three-Dimensional Magnetic Resonance Venography

Gadolinium-enhanced 3D MRV gained popularity because of the flow-related limitations of nonenhanced cerebral MRV techniques. Moreover, paramagnetic effects of the contrast agent shorten the intravascular T1 relaxation time resulting in increased signal intensity of the blood without saturation effects. The typical characteristics of Gd-enhanced 3D MRV include a GRE sequence with modified ordering of k-space acquisition, keeping TR and TE as short as possible and using an intermediate flip angle. Advantages include enhanced visualization of the vasculature, faster acquisition times, suppression of the background tissues, and avoidance of the in-plane saturation effects. Disadvantages include contrast cost, patient discomfort, and risk of allergic reactions.[11,12]

Fluoro/Auto-Triggered Gadolinium-Enhanced Three-Dimensional Magnetic Resonance Venography

This auto-triggered elliptic centric-ordered 3D MRV is based on the empirically determined 8-s delay before initiation of the centric filling of the k-space. This is to ensure sufficient contrast material perfusing the intracranial venous system after moving through the cerebral circuit.[11] Advantages include the shorter repetition time, better suppression of the background tissue signal, and higher spatial resolution images.[12]

Time-Resolved Gd-Enhanced MR Venography

In this technique, multiple 3D image sets are acquired during passage of the contrast agent, increasing the possibility of obtaining the 3D image set showing only arteries or only veins. It also provides information on the bolus transit time indicating the blood flow rate. Time-resolved 3D MR angiographic technique is one such technique, which gives dynamic information of flow and can be helpful where the timing of venous drainage within the normal cerebral perfusion cycle is of interest, such as dAVFs. The images are repeatedly obtained every 1–4 s over a 1–3 min period and retrospectively analyzed for arterial, capillary, and venous phases (Du et al., 1996)[13]. The main disadvantage is low spatial resolution compared with the other contrast-enhanced sequences.

DIGITAL SUBTRACTION ANGIOGRAPHY

DSA, when used by a skilled radiologist, is the gold standard for imaging the DVS. Lately, however, this technique is being replaced by newer less-invasive techniques. When examining pathology, DSA is typically not the first-line imaging modality used, as it is invasive and diagnosis can be achieved with the combined usage of other less-invasive imaging techniques.[14] However, when ambiguity arises, DSA provides the highest quality imaging and reconstruction of the DVS.

Although it is one of the gold standards for investigation of the DVS, DSA can be prone to error in assessing the sinus stenosis because of the high collateral flow from anastomosing veins entering the sinuses, which can result in decreased opacification of the sinus thus adding an artifact to the image. Poor positioning of the catheter tip, such as that located in the collateral vessel, can also result in false-negative interpretation of the sinus dimensions making it look stenosed.[14] 3D rotational venography with associated cross-sectional reconstruction is a newer technique that provides a novel view of the cerebral venous vasculature. Although this technique is invasive and expensive, it is a good adjunct to 2D DSA and recommended when previous imaging is equivocal. Its images are comparable with cone-based CT images. Some limitations are that the quality of the subtracted 3D images and MPR images are dependent on windowing and have a high potential for human error.[15]

ULTRASOUND

Ultrasound (US) is limited in its ability to evaluate DVS in adults; its most effective use is in the fetus. It is a good imaging modality for assessment of venous sinuses in neonates because of the open sutures and fontanelles in this population; moreover, it does not require sedation or anesthesia.[16] A sagittal view of the brain is imperative for viewing the midline sinuses and seeing abnormalities, such as a falcine sinus.[17,18] For the sagittal view, the anterior fontanelle, or the metopic suture, is used as an acoustic window.[17,19,20] Axial and slightly oblique planes can be used to demonstrate the veins from the middle of the brain toward the straight sinus and torcular as well as the vessels at the base of the skull. One also can use transvaginal US to appreciate the intracerebral arterial and venous systems. Sensitive high-definition color Doppler is imperative for viewing the venous sinuses because of slow flow of the blood in the sinuses. The spatial course of the vasculature can be appreciated using 3D color Doppler reconstruction of the vascular region using so-called "glass-body mode tool."[17] The superior sagittal sinus, internal cerebral veins, great vein of Galen, straight sinus, and the torcular all can be visualized in a fetus as young as 11–13 weeks. The inferior sagittal sinus is visible in the third trimester. The transverse sinus is visualized in the transcerebellar plane, whereas using a more caudal view can visualize the sigmoid sinuses. Visualization of the superficial venous system is difficult through US but can be achieved through tracking its anastomosis with larger vessels.[17]

IMAGING OF DURAL ARTERIOVENOUS MALFORMATIONS

DSA is the gold standard in the diagnosis and characterization of these vascular malformations, but advances in both MRI and CT have helped in further characterizing these lesions and also evaluating the surrounding brain structures that may be affected.

Noncontrast CT imaging techniques are limited in the diagnosis of dAVF except in the volumetric measurement of the distribution of hematoma or edema secondary to venous congestion. When cortical venous reflux is present, a curvilinear pattern of calcification can be seen at the corticomedullary junction adjacent to the bottom of the cerebral sulci on plain CT.[21] Nodular structures adjacent to the sinus wall and the former curvilinear pattern with calcification when imaged on high-intensity MRI and CT are highly sensitive and specific findings of dAVF. These findings indicate meningeal branch-feeding arteries that correspond to secondary increased flow via arteriovenous malformation.[22] Low densities on noncontrast CT and high-intensity areas on T2-weighted MRI can indicate brain edema in the subcortical areas of patients with venous congestion caused by dAVF.[22]

MRI can also demonstrate engorged dilated tortuous vessels or abnormal vascular enhancement apart from the changes secondary to venous hypertension (De Marco, 1990).[23] Dynamic susceptibility contrast-MR perfusion imaging was described to be a sensitive marker for the evaluation of impaired venous drainage in the setting of cerebral dAVF and permits for the quantitative evaluation of mean transit time, cerebral blood volume (CBV), and cerebral blood flow. In patients with cerebral dAVF with retrograde cortical venous drainage, there are increased CBV values involving the affected cerebral hemisphere secondary to impaired venous drainage.[24]

Unenhanced 3D TOF magnetic resonance angiography (MRA) is a noninvasive technique that does not require contrast material, which can be useful in the diagnosis of dAVFs. However, it is limited in the evaluation of dAVFs because of the lack of hemodynamic information but can suggest the presence of a lesion by abnormal flow enhancement, such as dilated meningeal branches and shunted veins. These findings can also be seen in healthy patients limiting the specificity of TOF-MRA in the diagnosis of dAVF.[25]

DSA remains the gold standard investigation for diagnosis of dAVF, as it is the most sensitive and specific diagnostic tool for evaluating the existence of abnormal shunting blood flow.[22] Comparison studies indicated that gross characterization of intracranial dAVF can be similar for both unenhanced 3T 3D TOF-MRA and DSA, but unenhanced MRA cannot replace DSA.[26,27] In certain locations such as cavernous sinus, cone beam CT has been reported to more effective than traditional imaging modalities, such as DSA and 3D rotational angiography, at imaging-feeding arteries and shunt points of the cavernous sinus in patients with dAVFs.[28]

VEIN OF GALEN MALFORMATION

US examination is the study of choice in case of vein of Galen aneurysmal malformations (VGAMs) because of its noninvasive character, safety, and low cost. Aneurysms in the vein of Galen appear as hypoechoic cystlike or tubular mass midline masses posterior to the roof of the third ventricle and superior to the thalamus representing the dilated median prosencephalic vein.[17,29] This malformation typically is diagnosed in the late second and early third trimesters as sufficient dilatation of the vein does not occur till that time. Dilated pericallosal arteries, when they appear on US, also indicate VOGMs. Doppler imaging will further delineate this mass from other cystic and solid tumors, such as pineal meningiomas, by showing turbulent flow through the cystic structure instead of a masslike structure.[17] USG is also imperative in postnatal follow-up after endovascularly treated VGAM as well as for antenatal diagnosis of a VGAM. This importance is because of its usefulness in accurately measuring the volume and shape of the lesion.[30]

VGAM can be identified on plain CT as a round masslike lesion with isodensities or with slightly higher density compared with the surrounding brain parenchyma. Its appearance is especially noticeable in the pineal region. Contrast CT, when used with these patients, is also effective at imaging dilated collateral veins [31]

The gold standard for diagnosis of a VGAM is MRI (Figs. 26.3 and 26.4) because of its accurate visualization of soft tissue as well as its ability to differentiate VGAM from dAVF that drain into the vein of Galen. Imaging of major arterial vessels is also more sensitive and specific with MRI imaging than with contrast CT.[32] MRI imaging will also demonstrate large, rounded masslike lesions in the posterior pineal region with varying intensities, depending on the flow velocity and turbulence.[31,32] DSA rarely is required in the diagnosis of VGAM, as the combination of MRI with T1, T2, fluid-attenuated inversion recovery (FLAIR), and venography is sufficient.[32] However, DSA is the only available modality that provides a detailed evaluation of the VGAM angioarchitecture and hemodynamics necessary for treatment purposes.

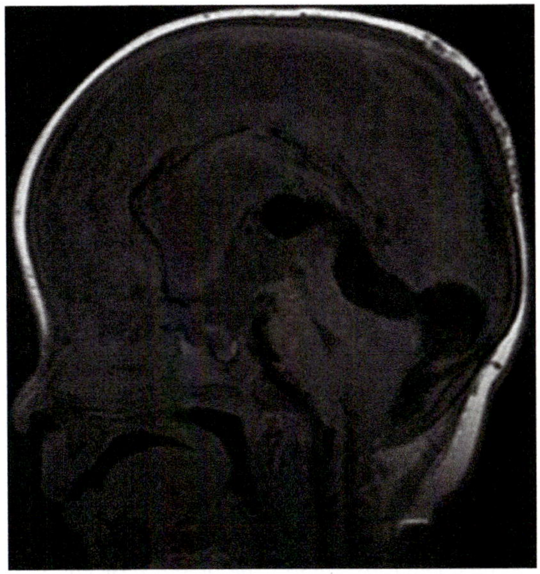

FIG. 3 Sagittal T1-weighted MRI without contrast: Dilation of vein of Galen, straight sinus, and the torcular Herophili is seen.

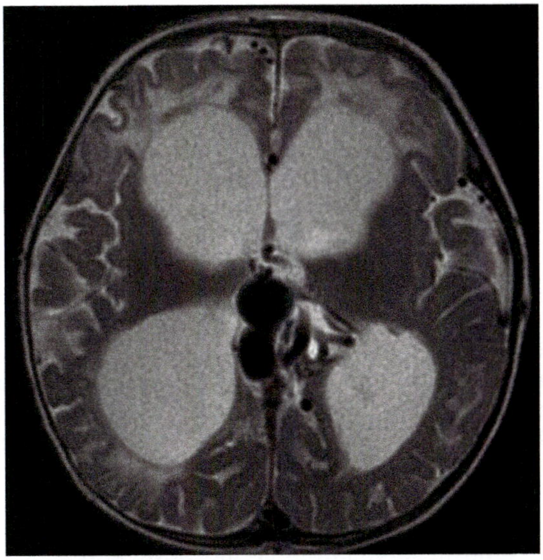

FIG. 4 T2-weighted MRI: Enlarged vein of Galen with fistulous vessels mainly fed by posterior cerebral artery branches. In addition, note the hydrocephalus.

DURAL VENOUS SINUS THROMBOSIS

Computed Tomography and Magnetic Resonance Imaging

CT is often the first imaging modality obtained for the patients in emergency setting presenting with nonspecific symptoms such as headache, nausea, or focal neurologic deficits, which are often the symptoms of the patients with DVST. A typical imaging finding in patients with DVST is direct visualization of a hyperattenuating thrombus (the dense or filled delta sign) in the occluded sinus or in the cortical vein (cord sign). However, less than one-third of DVST cases present with direct visualization of thrombus, as it depends on the attenuation of the clot.[33,34] Using modern multidetector row CT scanner, sensitivity of the direct signs for DVST has been reported to be as high as 64.6%. In the first 2 weeks, thrombotic blood is usually hyperdense on an unenhanced CT scan compared with the brain parenchyma; therefore, these signs are usually present only during the first 2 weeks. Other indirect signs of DVST include infarcts due to venous backpressure, which are often hemorrhagic, subarachnoid/subdural hemorrhages and diffuse cerebral edema. Avsenik et al. reported the sensitivity of the noncontrast CT to be close to 100% with 83% specificity for diagnosing DVST making it a valuable tool in the emergency setting.[35] However, the spontaneous hyperdensity of the sinuses is not very specific and can be seen in a range of other conditions such as young patients with high hematocrit, dehydrated patients in which the sinuses may demonstrate a bright signal on the CT.

On CT head with contrast, a triangular filling defect due to nonopacification of the clot with opacification of the sinuses and collateral veins is seen. This sign called "empty delta sign" is the most commonly seen direct finding on CT imaging in patients with DVST. This can also be seen on the MRI with contrast. An empty delta sign on contrast-enhanced MRI and CT is highly suggestive of DVST.[33,36] Indirect findings of DVST on postcontrast CT head include parenchymal enhancement because of luxury perfusion in the areas of ischemia and tentorial enhancement secondary to venous stasis or hyperemia of the dura mater.

MRI (Figs. 26.5 and 26.6) is more sensitive for revealing the clot in the sinuses due to the combination of sequences and high sensitivity to the magnetic susceptibility of blood degradation products, notably on GRE T2-weighted images. Flow void absence or abnormal flow signal is a frequent sign of DVST in MRI, and assessment of the abnormal flow in different sequences is fundamental to confirm the presence of DVST.[33,37] Brain parenchymal lesions of DVST are also better visualized and depicted on MRI than at CT.

Zero to 5 days after the formation of a thrombus (the deoxyhemoglobin stage) the clot appears isointense on T1-weighted images and hypointense on T2-WI and FLAIR. Because this can mimic the flow void on T2-weighted imaging, MRV and CTV are necessary for diagnosis in the acute period of thrombus formation.[32,33] Using TOF-MRV in combination with nonenhanced T1- and T2-weighted imaging can minimize the risk of mistaking hyperintensity on T1-weighted images for flow on TOF.[32,33] Contrary to the acute state, the subacute state can be reliably diagnosed with T1- and T2-weighted images because of the hyperintensities present.[38] Chronic thrombus is typically isointense on T1-weighted images iso-/hyperintense on T2-weighted images. It can be reliably diagnosed with MRV with elliptic-centric ordering.[33] DVS with normal circulation have an opposite signal on FLAIR and T2-weighted images; however, when the thrombus is present, they abnormally show the same signal intensity, irrespective of the timing of the MRI exam.[39]

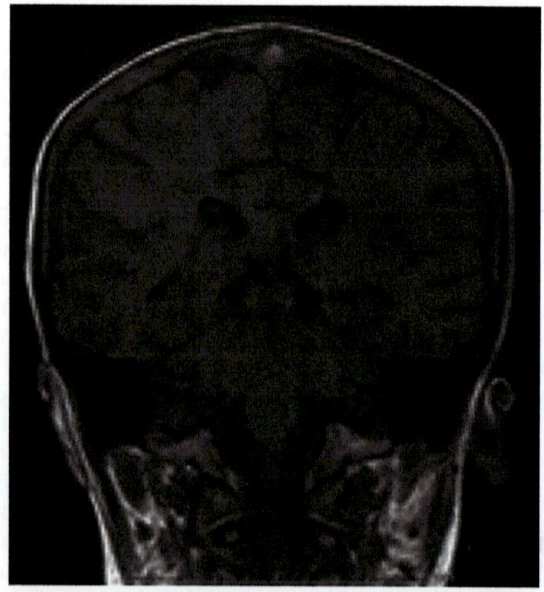

FIG. 26.5 Sagittal T1-weighted image: Nonfilling of the superior sagittal sinus, but enhancement of the sinus wall is seen in the midline superiorly.

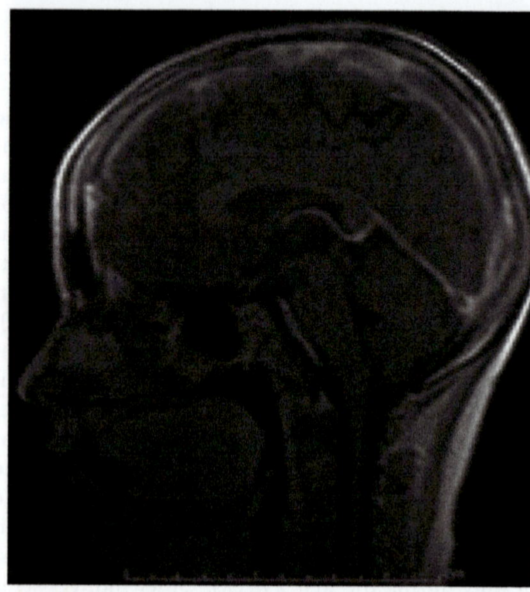

FIG. 26.6 Coronal T1-weighted image: Hyperintensity seen in superior sagittal sinus indicating thrombosis in the sinus lumen.

Magnetic Resonance Venography and Computed Tomography Venography

Both CTV and MRV are adequate vascular imaging modalities in the setting of CTV. MRV may be performed without contrast using TOF technique or PC technique or with contrast-enhanced technique. TOF-MRV is the most common nonenhanced method used for diagnosing DVST, with 2D TOF being preferred to 3D TOF. Their excellent sensitivity to slow flow and diminished sensitivity to signal loss from saturation effects make them preferred to the 3D technique.[33] The extent of the thrombosis can be measured accurately with TOF and PC MRV.[32,40] Although the sensitivity of MRI for diagnosing DVST is very high, the specificity is low and it does not replace contrast-enhanced MRV.[41] MRV sequences with injection of gadolinium are now preferred to 2D TOF sequences or MRV in-phase contrast, because of the susceptibility to flow artifacts thus resulting in too much signal loss in a small diameter venous sinus in nonenhanced sequences.[42] Another issue with TOF is that the same-plane acquisition can produce false-positive results from saturation and subsequent signal nulling, as this technique is most sensitive to orthogonal flow. Sari et al. in their comparative study reported that contrast-enhanced 3D GRE T1-weighted MRI was the most accurate imaging method for the detection of DVS and/or cortical venous thrombosis.[43] Contrast-enhanced MRV is considered the procedure of choice for the diagnosis of DVST.

CTV is reported to be superior to the unenhanced TOF-MRV for diagnosing DVST. In patients with an overlying skull fracture, CTV is the imaging modality of choice to distinguish thrombus from compression.[44] However, this technique is limited by the fact that it relies on subtracting bone, which is difficult without removing part of the sinus.[2] Further limitations of CTV are the inability to use it in pregnant patients, children, and patients with renal failure. In patients with renal failure and contrast allergies, combined noncontrast CT, T1 and T2-weight MRI, and 3D PC MRV are successful tools for diagnosing DVST.[32,45]

Digital Subtraction Angiography

DSA was previously considered the gold standard; however, the contemporary utility is often limited to cases where thrombolysis is required or for confirmation of diagnosis has been largely replaced by CTV, MRI, and MRV as the modern gold standard.[46,47]

REFERENCES

1. Casey SO, Alberico RA, Patel M, et al. Cerebral CT venography. *Radiology*. 1996;198(1):163–170. https://doi.org/10.1148/radiology.198.1.8539371.
2. Ozsvath RR, Casey SO, Lustrin ES, Alberico RA, Hassankhani A, Patel M. Cerebral venography: comparison of CT and MR projection venography. *AJR Am J Roentgenol*. 1997;169(6):1699–1707. https://doi.org/10.2214/ajr.169.6.9393193.
3. Wetzel SG, Kirsch E, Stock KW, Kolbe M, Kaim A, Radue EW. Cerebral veins: comparative study of CT venography with intraarterial digital subtraction angiography. *AJNR Am J Neuroradiol*. 1999;20(2):249–255.
4. Seo H, Choi DS, Shin HS, Cho JM, Koh EH, Son S. Bone subtraction 3D CT venography for the evaluation of cerebral veins and venous sinuses: imaging techniques, normal variations, and pathologic findings. *AJR Am J Roentgenol*. 2014;202(2):W169–W175. https://doi.org/10.2214/AJR.13.10985.
5. Gratama van Andel HA, van Boven LJ, van Walderveen MA, et al. Interobserver variability in the detection of cerebral venous thrombosis using CT venography with matched mask bone elimination. *Clin Neurol Neurosurg*. 2009;111(9):717–723. https://doi.org/10.1016/j.clineuro.2009.05.013.
6. Morhard D, Fink C, Graser A, Reiser MF, Becker C, Johnson TR. Cervical and cranial computed tomographic angiography with automated bone removal: dual energy computed tomography versus standard computed tomography. *Invest Radiol*. 2009;44(5):293–297. https://doi.org/10.1097/RLI.0b013e31819b6fba.
7. Gratama van Andel HA, Venema HW, Streekstra GJ, et al. Removal of bone in CT angiography by multiscale matched mask bone elimination. *Med Phys*. 2007;34(10):3711–3723. https://doi.org/10.1118/1.2767931.
8. Majoie CB, van Straten M, Venema HW, den Heeten GJ. Multisection CT venography of the dural sinuses and cerebral veins by using matched mask bone elimination. *AJNR Am J Neuroradiol*. 2004;25(5):787–791.
9. Mattle HP, Wentz KU, Edelman RR, et al. Cerebral venography with MR. *Radiology*. 1991;178(2):453–458. https://doi.org/10.1148/radiology.178.2.1987608.
10. Agid R, Shelef I, Scott JN, Farb RI. Imaging of the intracranial venous system. *Neurol*. 2008;14(1):12–22. https://doi.org/10.1097/NRL.0b013e318157f791.
11. Farb RI, Scott JN, Willinsky RA, Montanera WJ, Wright GA, terBrugge KG. Intracranial venous system: gadolinium-enhanced three-dimensional MR venography with auto-triggered elliptic centric-ordered sequence--initial experience. *Radiology*. 2003;226(1):203–209. https://doi.org/10.1148/radiol.2261020670.
12. Fu JH, Lai PH, Hsiao CC, et al. Comparison of real-time three-dimensional gadolinium-enhanced elliptic centric-ordered MR venography and two-dimensional time-of-flight MR venography of the intracranial venous system. *J Chin Med Assoc*. 2010;73(3):131–138. https://doi.org/10.1016/S1726-4901(10)70027-7.
13. Du YP, Parker DL, Davis WL, Cao G, Buswell HR, Goodrich KC. Experimental and theoretical studies of vessel contrast-to-noise ratio in intracranial time-of-flight MR angiography. *J Magn Reson Imaging*. 1996;6(1):99–108.
14. Boddu SR, Gobin P, Oliveira C, Dinkin M, Patsalides A. Anatomic measurements of cerebral venous sinuses in idiopathic intracranial hypertension patients. *PLoS One*. 2018;13(6):e0196275. https://doi.org/10.1371/journal.pone.0196275.
15. Srinivasan VM, Chintalapani G, Duckworth EAM, Kan P. Advanced cone-beam CT venous angiographic imaging. *J Neurosurg*. 2018;129(1):114–120. https://doi.org/10.3171/2017.2.JNS162997.
16. Lowe LH, Bailey Z. State-of-the-art cranial sonography: Part 1, modern techniques and image interpretation. *AJR*

Am J Roentgenol. 2011;196(5):1028–1033. https://doi.org/10.2214/AJR.10.6160.

17. Karl K, Heling KS, Chaoui R. Ultrasound of the fetal veins Part 3: the fetal intracerebral venous system. *Ultraschall der Med.* 2016;37(1):6–26. https://doi.org/10.1055/s-0035-1553284.
18. Lin L, Lin JH, Guan J, Zhang XL, Chu JP, Yang ZY. Falcine sinus: incidence and imaging characteristics of three-dimensional contrast-enhanced thin-section magnetic resonance imaging. *Korean J Radiol.* 2018;19(3):463–469. https://doi.org/10.3348/kjr.2018.19.3.463.
19. Chaoui R, Heling KS, Karl K. Ultrasound of the fetal veins part 1: the intrahepatic venous system. *Ultraschall der Med.* 2014;35(3):208–228. https://doi.org/10.1055/s-0034-1366316.
20. Chaoui R, Heling KS, Karl K. Ultrasound of the fetal veins part 2: veins at the cardiac level. *Ultraschall der Med.* 2014;35(4):302–318. https://doi.org/10.1055/s-0034-1366848. quiz 319–321.
21. Yang MS, Chen CC, Cheng YY, Yeh DM, Lee SK, Tyan YS. Unilateral subcortical calcification: a manifestation of dural arteriovenous fistula. *AJNR Am J Neuroradiol.* 2005;26(5):1149–1151.
22. Takahasi S. *Neurovascular Imaging: MRI and Microangiography.* London: Springer; 2010.
23. De Marco JK, Dillon WP, Halback VV, Tsuruda JS. Dural arteriovenous fistulas: evaluation with MR imaging. *Radiology.* 1990;175(1):193–199. https://doi.org/10.1148/radiology.175.1.2315480.
24. Noguchi K, Kubo M, Kuwayama N, et al. Intracranial dural arteriovenous fistulas with retrograde cortical venous drainage: assessment with cerebral blood volume by dynamic susceptibility contrast magnetic resonance imaging. *AJNR Am J Neuroradiol.* 2006;27(6):1252–1256.
25. Hirai T, Korogi Y, Ikushima I, Shigematsu Y, Morishita S, Yamashita Y. Usefulness of source images from three-dimensional time-of-flight MR angiography after treatment of cavernous dural arteriovenous fistulas. *Radiat Med.* 2003;21(5):205–209.
26. Azuma M, Hirai T, Shigematsu Y, et al. Evaluation of intracranial dural arteriovenous fistulas: comparison of unenhanced 3T 3D time-of-flight MR angiography with digital subtraction angiography. *Magn Reson Med Sci.* 2015;14(4):285–293. https://doi.org/10.2463/mrms.2014-0120.
27. Uetani H, Akter M, Hirai T, et al. Can 3T MR angiography replace DSA for the identification of arteries feeding intracranial meningiomas? *AJNR Am J Neuroradiol.* 2013;34(4):765–772. https://doi.org/10.3174/ajnr.A3284.
28. Kadooka K, Tanaka M, Sakata Y, Ideguchi M, Inaba M, Hadeishi H. Efficacy of cone beam computed tomography in treating cavernous sinus dural arteriovenous fistula. *World Neurosurg.* 2018;109:328–332. https://doi.org/10.1016/j.wneu.2017.10.026.
29. Darji PJ, Gandhi VS, Banker H, Chaudhari H. Antenatal diagnosis of aneurysmal malformation of the vein of Galen. *BMJ Case Rep.* 2015. https://doi.org/10.1136/bcr-2015-213785.
30. Gun I, Mungen E, Kurdoglu M, Babacan A, Muhcu M, Atay V. Is prenatal volumetric evaluation of aneurysm of the vein of Galen important in the prediction of adverse fetal outcome? *J Clin Ultrasound.* 2010;38(8):443–445. https://doi.org/10.1002/jcu.20672.
31. Kassem MW, Choi PJ, Iwanaga J, Mortazavi MM, Tubbs RS. Imaging characteristics of dural arteriovenous fistulas involving the vein of galen: a comprehensive review. *Cureus.* 2018;10(2):e2180. https://doi.org/10.7759/cureus.2180.
32. Haaga JR, Boll D. *CT and MRI of the Whole Body.* Mosby/Elsevier; 2016.
33. Leach JL, Fortuna RB, Jones BV, Gaskill-Shipley MF. Imaging of cerebral venous thrombosis: current techniques, spectrum of findings, and diagnostic pitfalls. *Radiographics.* 2006;26(Suppl 1):S19–S41. https://doi.org/10.1148/rg.26si055174. discussion S42-13.
34. Linn J, Ertl-Wagner B, Seelos KC, et al. Diagnostic value of multidetector-row CT angiography in the evaluation of thrombosis of the cerebral venous sinuses. *AJNR Am J Neuroradiol.* 2007;28(5):946–952.
35. Avsenik J, Oblak JP, Popovic KS. Non-contrast computed tomography in the diagnosis of cerebral venous sinus thrombosis. *Radiol Oncol.* 2016;50(3):263–268. https://doi.org/10.1515/raon-2016-0026.
36. Virapongse C, Cazenave C, Quisling R, Sarwar M, Hunter S. The empty delta sign: frequency and significance in 76 cases of dural sinus thrombosis. *Radiology.* 1987;162(3):779–785. https://doi.org/10.1148/radiology.162.3.3809494.
37. Poon CS, Chang JK, Swarnkar A, Johnson MH, Wasenko J. Radiologic diagnosis of cerebral venous thrombosis: pictorial review. *AJR Am J Roentgenol.* 2007;189(suppl 6):S64–S75. https://doi.org/10.2214/AJR.07.7015.
38. Bergui M, Bradac GB. Clinical picture of patients with cerebral venous thrombosis and patterns of dural sinus involvement. *Cerebrovasc Dis.* 2003;16(3):211–216. https://doi.org/10.1159/000071118.
39. Bonneville F. Imaging of cerebral venous thrombosis. *Diagn Interv Imag.* 2014;95(12):1145–1150. https://doi.org/10.1016/j.diii.2014.10.006.
40. Ayanzen RH, Bird CR, Keller PJ, McCully FJ, Theobald MR, Heiserman JE. Cerebral MR venography: normal anatomy and potential diagnostic pitfalls. *AJNR Am J Neuroradiol.* 2000;21(1):74–78.
41. Sadigh G, Mullins ME, Saindane AM. Diagnostic performance of MRI sequences for evaluation of dural venous sinus thrombosis. *AJR Am J Roentgenol.* 2016;206(6):1298–1306. https://doi.org/10.2214/AJR.15.15719.
42. Dmytriw AA, Song JSA, Yu E, Poon CS. Cerebral venous thrombosis: state of the art diagnosis and management. *Neuroradiology.* 2018. https://doi.org/10.1007/s00234-018-2032-2.
43. Sari S, Verim S, Hamcan S, et al. MRI diagnosis of dural sinus - cortical venous thrombosis: immediate post-contrast

3D GRE T1-weighted imaging versus unenhanced MR venography and conventional MR sequences. *Clin Neurol Neurosurg*. 2015;134:44–54. https://doi.org/10.1016/j.clineuro.2015.04.013.
44. Rischall MA, Boegel KH, Palmer CS, Knoll B, McKinney AM. MDCT venographic patterns of dural venous sinus compromise after acute skull fracture. *AJR Am J Roentgenol*. 2016:1–7. https://doi.org/10.2214/AJR.15.15972.
45. Ozturk K, Soylu E, Parlak M. Dural venous sinus thrombosis: the combination of noncontrast CT, MRI and PC-MR venography to enhance accuracy. *Neuroradiol J*. 2018. https://doi.org/10.1177/1971400918781969. 1971400918781969.
46. Janjua N. Cerebral angiography and venography for evaluation of cerebral venous thrombosis. *J Pakistan Med Assoc*. 2006;56(11):527–530.
47. Saposnik G, Barinagarrementeria F, Brown Jr RD, et al. Diagnosis and management of cerebral venous thrombosis: a statement for healthcare professionals from the American Heart Association/American Stroke Association. *Stroke*. 2011;42(4):1158–1192. https://doi.org/10.1161/STR.0b013e31820a8364.

CHAPTER 27

Surgical Nuances in Management of Intracranial Venous Sinus Injuries

MARTIN M. MORTAZAVI • SAJID S. SURIYA • FARZAD HAMI ADL • MOHSEN SADATI • GHAZALEH AHMADI JAZI • R. SHANE TUBBS

OVERVIEW

The intracranial venous sinuses are blood channels between the endosteal and meningeal layers of the dura. They provide the major drainage of cerebral blood flow. Besides venous blood drainage, the superior sagittal sinus (SSS) also serves as a main location for cerebrospinal fluid reabsorption. The incidence of intracranial venous sinus injuries due to traumatic head injury ranges from 1% to 4% in civilian life and from 4% to 12% during wartime.[1–3] Traumatic injuries to venous sinuses can be caused by direct impact of the fractured bone, or extension of the fracture line over the sinus area or suture diastase, or impact from a foreign body. Other causes are neoplastic invasion of a major venous sinus and iatrogenic injury during neurosurgical procedures (Table 27.1).

The major concerns with intracranial venous sinus injuries are massive intraoperative blood loss and/or thrombosis causing disrupted cerebral venous drainage leading to brain edema and risk of venous infarction, and air embolism. In a retrospective analysis of 39 patients with traumatic intracranial venous sinus injury, Meir et al. reported a 20% intraoperative mortality. This mortality was defined as the number of deaths during the surgical procedure.[4] In view of the high rate of intraoperative mortality, repair of injuries to intracranial venous sinuses to restore the cerebral venous drainage is always a rewarding challenge for the neurosurgeon.

LOCATION OF INJURY AND ITS EPIDEMIOLOGIC SIGNIFICANCE

The location of the injury along the venous sinus pathways, starting at the anterior SSS toward the torcular, into the transverse and sigmoid sinuses (SS) and ending in the internal jugular veins, has a major effect on clinical presentation and outcome. The most critical area is the mid and posterior third of the SSS and the torcular.

Another crucial factor for duplicated sinuses such as the transverse and SS is whether they are codominant and whether there are alternative venous pathways such as an enlarged occipital sinus draining an aberrantly degenerate transverse sinus.

Superior Sagittal Sinus Injuries

The SSS is the most common site of venous sinus injury. Injuries to it can be further divided into the anterior, middle, and posterior thirds. Multiple studies show that 66%–80% of all venous sinus injuries

TABLE 27.1
Mode of Sinus Injury and Its Mechanism

Mode of Injury	Mechanism of Injury
Direct indigenous impact	Intracranial venous sinus can be injured by direct impact of a fractured bone segment or can be caused by tearing due to extension of a fracture line.
Foreign body impact	Impact of a foreign body such as a bullet fragment in gunshot injuries to the skull.
Suture diastasis	This often occurs after trauma and usually affects newborns and infants in whom the suture lines are not yet closed.
Neoplastic invasion	Invasion of venous sinus by a tumor such as a meningioma.
Iatrogenic	Injury during resection of a tumor-invaded venous sinus. Injury to the transverse and sigmoid sinus during retrosigmoid craniotomy. Injury to the superior sagittal sinus during bicoronal craniotomy.

Anatomy, Imaging and Surgery of the Intracranial Dural Venous Sinuses. https://doi.org/10.1016/B978-0-323-65377-0.00027-1

TABLE 27.2
Incidence and Mortality Rates of Traumatic Injury to Segments of the Superior Sagittal Sinus Reported in the Literature

	MEIR et al.[4]		KIM et al.[1]	
Superior Sagittal Sinus Segment	**Incidence (%)**	**Mortality (%)**	**Incidence (%)**	**Mortality (%)**
Anterior 1/3	41.3%	17%	46.7%	0%
Middle 1/3	48.3%	50%	53.3%	25%
Posterior 1/3	10.4%	100%	0%	Not applicable

occur in the anterior and middle-third portions of the SSS.[2–4] Meier et al. reported 17% mortality from injuries to the anterior one-third, 50% mortality from injuries to the middle-third, and 100% mortality from injuries to the posterior one-third of the SSS[4] (Table 27.2). In 2015, Kim et al. reported 0% mortality from injuries involving the anterior one-third and 25% mortality due to injuries to the middle one-third of the SSS. None of their patients had injuries to the posterior one-third[1] (Table 27.2).

Meningiomas are usually benign, slow-growing tumors occasionally invading the major venous sinuses. Such invasions can be categorized on the basis of the degree of invasion. Type I is attached to the lateral wall of the venous sinus; type II invades the lateral recess of the venous sinus; type III invades the lateral wall; type IV invades the lateral wall and the roof; type V invades with total occlusion of the venous sinus; and type VI causes total venous sinus occlusion and invasion of contralateral sinus wall.

Han et al. reported that 107 of 912 cases (11.7%) with intracranial meningioma had involvement of major venous sinuses. Of the 107 cases (86%), 92 were located in the parasagittal area. Of these 92 parasagittal meningiomass, 32 (34.8%) were in the anterior one-third, 46 (50.0%) in the middle third, and 14 (15.2%) in the posterior third.[6] In a retrospective review of 36 patients, Sekhar found 26 cases with meningioma involving the SSS.[7] In a large prospective study of 100 patients, Sindou et al. found 92 patients with meningiomas involving the SSS.[5]

Torcular Injuries

The torcular Heterophili is also known as confluence of sinuses and is located at the occipital pole of the skull. It is formed by the merger of the SSS and the straight sinus draining most of the cerebral venous blood flow into the bilateral transverse sinuses. Although there is some parallel venous outflow through minor collateral sinuses, such as the petrosal sinuses, the torcular being the focal point of most of the cerebral venous outflow maintains dominance in the cerebral blood flow drainage. Isolated injury to the torcular is extremely rare, and only a few cases have been reported in the literature. These presented with the injury to the torcular, but only one case has been reported in which the patient suffered an isolated penetrating trauma to the torcular with a retained bullet fragment; this was successfully repaired.[8] Peritorcular meningiomas can involve the torcular, and their removal can cause iatrogenic injury to the torcular Heterophili. In studies of meningiomas involving venous sinuses, the torcular has been shown to be involved in as many as 19% of cases.[7]

Transverse Sinus Injuries

The transverse sinus is the second most common location of traumatic injury and accounts for 18%–24% of all venous sinus injuries. It is also a common location of neoplastic invasion most commonly caused by tentorial meningiomas. Meier et al. reported 29% mortality due to injury involving the transverse sinus.[4] Injury to the transverse sinus is often combined with the SS or at the transverse sigmoid sinus junction (TSSJ) as discussed in the following section.

Sigmoid Sinus Injuries

Traumatic injuries to the SS are rare, and few cases of combined injuries to the transverse and SS have been reported in the literature.

Iatrogenic injury to the transverse and SS or the TSSJ can occur in some approaches to the posterior fossa. Retrosigmoid craniotomy is the most commonly used approach for cerebellopontine angle (CPA) lesions. Because the transverse and SS are the natural boundaries of the retrosigmoid approach, it is crucial to place the burr hole strategically to avoid sinus injury and obtain optimal exposure of the CPA region.[9] In addition, the durotomy technique needs to be performed in such a way that the dura is based toward the transverse sinus superiorly and the SS anteriorly.

In some studies, the asterion, being the junction of the lambdoid, parietomastoid, and occipitomastoid sutures, has been used as a landmark in lateral approaches to the posterior cranial fossa; other studies have proved this anatomic landmark to be less accurate.[10] In a cadaveric study, Ucerler et al. found the asterion to be located superficial to the transverse-sigmoid junction in 87% of samples, inferior to it in 11% and superior to it in 2%.[11]

In another cadaveric study, Day et al. reported that the asterion was found over the TSSJ in 61% and 66% of right and left sides, respectively.[12] The recent use of neuronavigation for surgical planning in retrosigmoid craniotomy prevents unnecessary sinus exposure and precludes injury to the TSSJ.

Mastoid Emissary Vein Injury

A practical surgical consideration in retrosigmoid craniectomy is the significance of the mastoid emissary vein. This is a valveless vein that passes through the mastoid foramen and drains venous blood into the SS. If the bony decompression around the vein is not performed properly during retrosigmoid craniectomy, its point of drainage to the SS can be injured, leaving a hole in the SS wall. In addition, improper drilling along its course toward the SS needs to leave a sufficient extent of the vein proximal to the SS, skeletonized before bipolar cauterization. Otherwise, retraction of the vein on bipolar cauterization would risk causing retraction of the vein and a hole in the SS wall.

TECHNICAL NUANCES FOR SURGICAL REPAIR

Numerous operative techniques have been introduced to control massive bleeding from the injured venous sinus. The location and size of sinus injury are two important factors to consider for venous sinus reconstruction. Repairing an SSS injury anterior to the coronal suture or nondominant transverse sinus with ligation is well tolerated because there is adequate collateral venous drainage.[3]

An exception to this is in patients where the bridging veins have an obtuse and prolonged course, draining the eloquent posterior frontal and parietal cortices into the anterior third of the SSS.

There are various techniques for managing sinus injury.

Indirect Repair

The easiest but potentially most dangerous technique is indirect repair by putting hemostatic agents on the bleeding sinus. Artificial hemostatic agents can be administered to small injuries along with elevation of the head. A good autologous agent is macerated muscle, which is rich in tissue factor and is a strong hemostatic agent, should artificial agents fail to work.

Although application of hemostatic agents to the bleeding sinus is an easy way to manage smaller injuries, it can be dangerous for large ones, risking coagulation of the entire sinus. Bipolar cauterization of venous sinuses is dangerous as it can make the sinus wall retract, so it is not recommended.

Direct Repair

Direct repair is the technique of choice for mid-size injuries only if there are relaxed and sufficient edges at both sides of the venous sinus. Thin non-resorbable sutures such a 6.0 or 7.0 prolene can be used under a microscope to direct the suturing. The head of the bed should be elevated only as much as required to sustain light venous bleeding to avoid air embolism. The assistant needs to apply suction to both sides of the injury while the main surgeon repairs the defect.

Direct suture with patching

For larger defects or when there is a large defect in the venous sinus after tumor resection, patching is recommended. In addition, in situations where the defect is small but one or both sides of the defect are tense and traction would risk enlarging the defect, a patch is preferred. In situations where the wall width is appropriate but the dura is thin or tense, further skeletonization of the sinuses such as the SS is recommended to have enough relaxed wall for the venous sinus to be at minimal risk of tearing during suturing. The patient's head is elevated so that mild venous bleeding continues and air embolism is avoided. A dural graft is preferred, although thicker pericranium and fascia can be used.

The two poles of the graft are sutured to the two ends of the defect. A running suture with a 6.0 or 7.0 prolene or any similar nonresorbable suture is used to suture the entire graft to the sinus.

The distal and proximal flow in the sinus is confirmed with intraoperative micro-Doppler. Larger venous sinus injuries need special attention to avoid the risk of venous embolism.

In the management of brain tumors invading the major intracranial venous sinuses, some authors have suggested administration of intravenous heparin to prevent thrombosis.[7,13] This remains controversial in traumatic venous sinus injury.

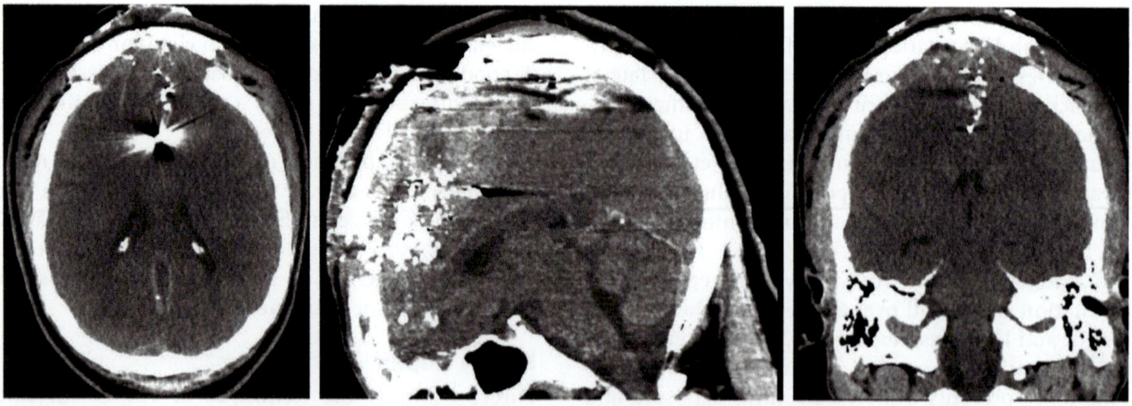

FIG. 27.1 Preoperative CT head without contrast.

Intentional venous sinus occlusion

Important bridging veins and the dominant transverse sinus must not be occluded suddenly. If it is decided to occlude owing to uncontrollable bleeding not amenable to indirect or direct repair, the occlusion should be performed stepwise and as slowly as possible so the brain has time to adapt its venous drainage. The anterior third of the SSS and a nondominant transverse and SS are the least dangerous sinuses to be closed. If a closure is planned during a surgical procedure for an interhemispheric approach or for tumor resection, the sinus can be clamped with a jeweler's forceps or bipolar while MEP and SSEP are monitored; if no major change is observed in MEP and SSEP, permanent occlusion can be performed. Attention needs to be given to the collateral venous sinuses. The important supratentorial collaterals are the superficial anastomosing veins of Trolard, Rolandic, and Labbé. In the posterior cranial fossa, the occipital sinus is sometimes engorged and works as a major drainage where tumors, over time, have occluded one side's transverse-SS and the venous blood is drained through the contralateral transverse-sigmoid route and an engorged compensating occipital sinus.

Short-term heparinization followed by 3 months of aspirin can be given if there is concern about the postoperative patency of a reconstructed sinus.

ILLUSTRATIVE CASES

Case 1

A 33-year-old right-handed male presented with a self-inflicted gunshot wound in the forehead. His neurologic exam on admission revealed withdrawal on the right side, posturing on the left side, bilateral reactive pupils, and intact cough, and gag reflexes.

CT head without contrast showed bilateral open comminuted frontal fractures extending up toward the vertex, large anterior superior frontal epidural and subdural hematomas extending 8 cm in length, multiple bone segments in the frontal lobes, a bullet piece in the right superior motor cortex, and another large bullet segment in the interface between the anterior and midportions of the SSS, causing extensive epidural and subdural hematomas. It also showed fractures of both the anterior and posterior tables of the frontal sinuses (Fig. 27.1). Because the patient was young and eloquent brain areas, including the motor cortex, thalami, basal ganglia and brainstem, appeared normal, and because he had a reactive brainstem and pupillary reflexes, and was withdrawing on neurologic exam, neurosurgical intervention was offered. He underwent bifrontal decompressive craniectomy with evacuation of the acute bifrontal epidural and subdural hematomas, removal of the bullet from the SSS and reconstruction of the injured wall of the anterior mid-third of the SSS, closure of the clotted anterior third of the SSS, and bilateral anterior frontal lobectomy of the contused frontal brain. The SSS wall was repaired directly with a nonresorbable suture, and good flow was confirmed by micro-Doppler in the sinus distal to the suture and the bridging veins draining into the sinus (Fig. 27.2).

After an extended hospital course, the patient underwent a ventriculoperitoneal shunt and improved to become alert but underwent tracheotomy. He followed commands on the right side but remained plegic on the left.

Case 2

A 69-year-old right-handed Caucasian man presented with increasing right-sided weakness and severe expressive dysphasia. Pre-operative imaging

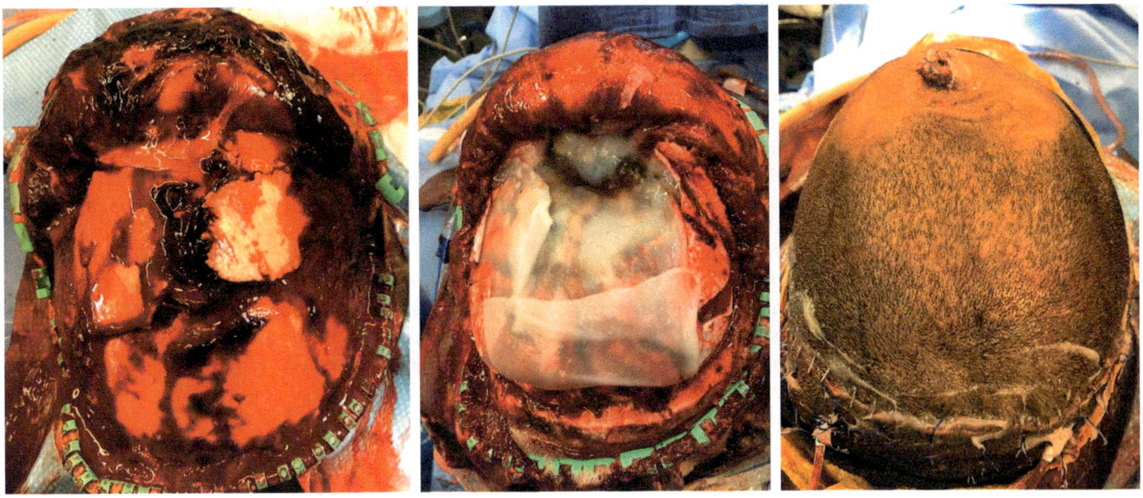

FIG. 27.2 Intraoperative images.

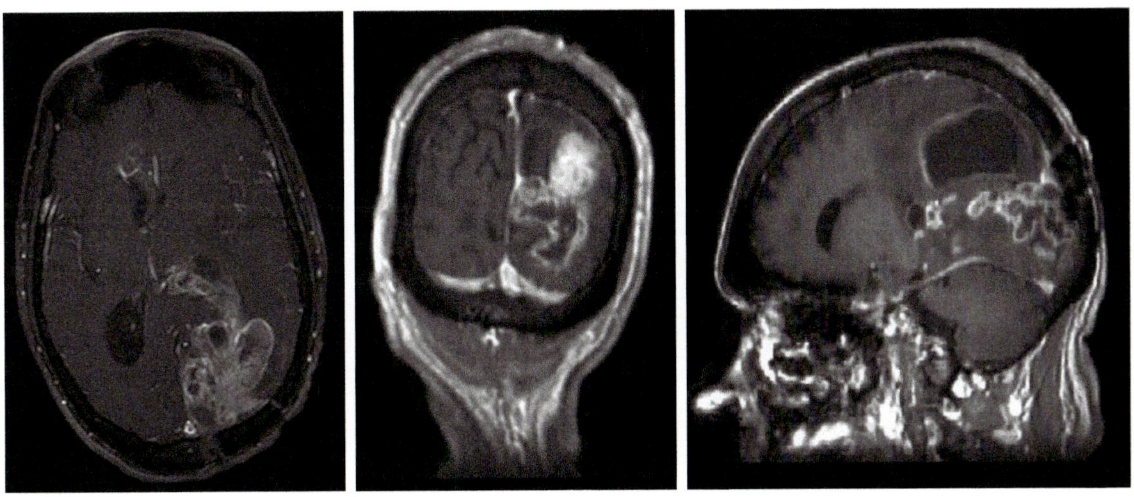

FIG. 27.3 Preoperative magnetic resonance imaging (MRI) brain.

revealed a large recurrent left paramedian parieto-occipital glioblastoma multiforme (GBM) with possible invasion of the SSS superior to the torcular. The patient underwent left occipital craniotomy for resection of the tumor. Intraoperatively, the tumor appeared to be invading the left wall of the posterior SSS approximately 5 cm superior to the torcular (Fig. 27.3). Gross total resection of the tumor was performed along with the part of the tumor invading the SSS. The invaded part of the SSS was reconstructed by direct suturing. Intraoperative Doppler confirmed good blood flow both proximal and distal to the reconstructed part.

REFERENCES

1. Kim Y-S, et al. Traumatic dural venous sinus injury. *Korean J Neurotrauma*. 2015;11(2):118–123.
2. Kapp JP, Gielchinsky I. Management of combat wounds of the dural venous sinuses. *Surgery*. 1972;71:913–917.
3. Kapp JP, Gielchinsky I, Deardourff SL. Operative techniques for management of lesions involving the dural venous sinuses. *Surg Neurol*. 1977;7:339–342.
4. Meier U, et al. The traumatic dural sinus injury—a clinical study. *Acta Neurochir*. 1992;119(1–4):91–93.
5. Sindou MP, Alvernia JE. Results of attempted radical tumor removal and venous repair in 100 consecutive meningiomas involving the major dural sinuses. *J Neurosurg*. 2006;105(4):514–525.

6. Han M-S, et al. Lessons from surgical outcome for intracranial meningioma involving major venous sinus. *Medicine*. 2016;95(35).
7. Mantovani A, et al. Management of meningiomas invading the major dural venous sinuses: operative technique, results, and potential benefit for higher grade tumors. *World Neurosurg*. 2014;82(3):455–467.
8. Pricola KL, Zou H, Chang SD. Successful repair of a gunshot wound to the head with retained bullet in the torcular herophili. *World Neurosurg*. 2011;76(3):362.e1.
9. Tubbs RS, Loukas M, Shoja MM, Bellew MP, Cohen-Gadol AA. Surface landmarks for the junction between the transverse and sigmoid sinuses: application of the "strategic" burr hole for suboccipital craniotomy. *Neurosurgery*. 2009;65(suppl 6):37–41; discussion 41. Silva, Erasmo Barros, André Giacomelli Leal, and Ricardo Ramina. "Image-Guided Surgical Planning in Retrosigmoid Approach." Skull Base 19.01 (2009): A122.
10. Ucerler H, Govsa F. Asterion as a surgical landmark for lateral cranial base approaches. *J Cranio Maxillofacial Surg*. 2006;34(7):415–420.
11. Day JD, et al. Surface and superficial surgical anatomy of the posterolateral cranial base: significance for surgical planning and approach. *Neurosurgery*. 1996;38(6):1079–1084.
12. Natarajan S, Sekhar LN. Venous reconstruction in the management of intracranial meningioma. In: Lj H, ed. *Meningioma*. Vol. 1. Springer-Velaj; 2008:603–618.
13. Sindou M, Auque J. The intracranial venous system as a neurosurgeon's perspective. *Adv Tech Stand Neurosurg*. 2000;26:131–216.

Index

Note: Page numbers followed by "f" indicate figures and "t" indicate tables.